# Quality Management in Intensive Care

## A Practical Guide

# Quality Management in Intensive Care

A Practical Guide

Edited by

**Bertrand Guidet**

Professor of Medicine and Head, Medical Intensive Care Unit, Saint Antoine Hospital, Paris, France; past president, French Intensive Care Society (SRLF)

**Andreas Valentin**

Professor, Medical University of Vienna; Head of Internal Medicine, Kardinal Schwarzenberg Hospital, Schwarzach, Austria; Chair, ESICM Working Group on Quality Improvement; founding president, Federation of Austrian Societies of Intensive Care Medicine

**Hans Flaatten**

Professor and Senior Consultant, Intensive Care Unit, Haukeland University Hospital, Bergen, Norway; Chair, ESICM Outcomes Section

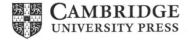

CAMBRIDGE UNIVERSITY PRESS

# CAMBRIDGE
## UNIVERSITY PRESS

University Printing House, Cambridge CB2 8BS, United Kingdom

One Liberty Plaza, 20th Floor, New York, NY 10006, USA

477 Williamstown Road, Port Melbourne, VIC 3207, Australia

314-321, 3rd Floor, Plot 3, Splendor Forum, Jasola District Centre, New Delhi - 110025, India

79 Anson Road, #06-04/06, Singapore 079906

Cambridge University Press is part of the University of Cambridge.

It furthers the University's mission by disseminating knowledge in the pursuit of
education, learning and research at the highest international levels of excellence.

www.cambridge.org
Information on this title: www.cambridge.org/9781107503861

© Cambridge University Press 2016

First published 2016

*A catalogue record for this publication is available from the British Library*

*Library of Congress Cataloging in Publication data*
Quality management in intensive care / edited by Bertrand Guidet, Andreas Valentin, Hans Flaatten.
  p. ; cm.
Includes bibliographical references and index.
ISBN 978-1-107-50386-1 (paperback)
I. Guidet, B. (Bertrand), editor.   II. Valentin, Andreas, MD, editor.   III. Flaatten, Hans, editor.
[DNLM: 1.  Intensive Care—methods.   2.  Quality Control.   3.  Intensive Care Units—organization &
administration.   4.  Quality Assurance, Health Care—methods.  WX 218]
RC86.7
616.02´8—dc23

2015032932

ISBN  978-1-107-50386-1  Paperback

....................................................................................................

# Contents

## Section 3 – Quality management on the national (and international) level

# Contributors

**Anders Aneman MD**
Assistant Professor and Senior Staff Specialist, Intensive Care, Liverpool Hospital, South Western Sydney Clinical School, University of New South Wales, Sydney, NSW, Australia

**Elie Azoulay MD**
Medical Intensive Care Unit, Saint Louis Hospital, Assistance Publique – Hôpitaux de Paris, and Faculté de Médecine Paris-Diderot, Sorbonne Paris-Cité, Paris, France

**Felix Balzer MD**
Department of Anesthesiology and Intensive Care Medicine, Campus Charité Mitte and Campus Virchow-Klinikum, Charité – Universitätsmedizin Berlin, Berlin, Germany

**Paul R. Barach BSc MD MPH**
Clinical Professor, Wayne State University School of Medicine

**Davide Bastoni MD**
Adult Critical Care, St George's University Hospitals NHS Foundation Trust, London, UK

**Ronaldo A. Sevilla Berrios**
Department of Anesthesiology, Mayo Clinic, Rochester, MN, USA

**Casper W. Bollen MD PhD**
Pediatric Intensive Care Unit, University Medical Center Utrecht, Utrecht, the Netherlands

**Rob Boots MBBS PhD MMedSci MHAIT FRACP FCICM**
Deputy Director, Department of Intensive Care Medicine, Royal Brisbane & Women's Hospital, and Associate Professor, Burns Trauma and Critical Care Research Centre, University of Queensland, Brisbane, QLD, Australia

**Maurizio Cecconi MD**
Adult Critical Care, St George's University Hospitals NHS Foundation Trust, London, UK

**Olaf L. Cremer MD PhD**
Department of Intensive Care Medicine, University Medical Center Utrecht, Utrecht, the Netherlands

**Ruth Endacott**
Professor of Critical Care Nursing, Royal Devon & Exeter Hospital/Plymouth University Clinical School, Plymouth University, UK, and School of Nursing & Midwifery, Monash University, Melbourne, Australia

**Christophe Faisy MD PhD**
Professor, Service de Réanimation Médicale, Hôpital Européen Georges Pompidou, Assistance Publique – Hôpitaux de Paris, Université Paris Descartes, Sorbonne Paris-Cité, Paris, France

**Hans Flaatten MD PhD**
Professor and Senior Consultant, Intensive Care Unit, Haukeland University Hospital, Bergen, Norway, and Chair, ESICM outcomes section

**Claire Fossard RN**
Medical Intensive Care Unit, Albert Michallon Teaching Hospital, Grenoble Alpes University, Grenoble, France

**Charles D. Gomersall MD**
Department of Anaesthesia and Intensive Care, Prince of Wales Hospital, the Chinese University of Hong Kong, Shatin, Hong Kong, China

**Pascale Gruber MBBS MRCP FRCA FICM EDIC**
The Royal Marsden Hospital NHS Foundation Trust, London, UK

**Bertrand Guidet MD**
Professor of Medicine and Head, Medical Intensive Care Unit, Saint Antoine Hospital, Paris, France, and past president, French Intensive Care Society (SRLF)

**Matthias Haenggi MD**
Department of Intensive Care Medicine, Bern University Hospital (Inselspital) and University of Bern, Bern, Switzerland

**Ken Hillman MBBS MD FRCA(Eng) FCICM**
Professor of Intensive Care, Liverpool Hospital, South Western Sydney Clinical School, and Director of the Simpson Centre for Health Services Research, University of New South Wales, Sydney, NSW, Australia

**Gaetano Iapichino MD**
Dipartimento di Fisiopatologia Medico-Chirurgica e dei Trapianti, Università degli Studi di Milano, Unità Operativa di Anestesia e Rianimazione, Azienda Ospedaliera San Paolo–Polo Universitario, Milano, Italy

**Gavin M. Joynt MBBCh FCICM FRCP(Edin)**
Department of Anaesthesia and Intensive Care, Prince of Wales Hospital, the Chinese University of Hong Kong, Shatin, Hong Kong, China

**Göran Karlström MD**
Executive Director, Swedish Intensive Care Registry, Sweden

**Oliver Kumpf MD**
Department of Anesthesiology and Intensive Care Medicine, Campus Charité Mitte and Campus Virchow-Klinikum, Charité – Universitätsmedizin Berlin, Berlin, Germany

**Caroline Landelle PharmD PhD**
Infection Control Program, University of Geneva Hospitals and Faculty of Medicine, Geneva, Switzerland

**Asad Latif MD MPH**
Assistant Professor, Department of Anesthesiology and Critical Care Medicine, Johns Hopkins University School of Medicine, and Johns Hopkins Medicine Armstrong Institute for Quality and Patient Safety, Baltimore, MD, USA

**Czarina C.H. Leung**
Department of Anaesthesia and Intensive Care, Prince of Wales Hospital, the Chinese University of Hong Kong, Shatin, Hong Kong, China

**Jeffrey Lipman MBBCh MD FFA(SA) FFA(Critical Care-SA) FCICM**
Director, Department of Intensive Care Medicine, Royal Brisbane & Women's Hospital, and Professor, Burns Trauma and Critical Care Research Centre, University of Queensland, Brisbane, QLD, Australia

**Tanja Manser MD**
Director, Institute for Patient Safety, University Hospital Bonn, Bonn, Germany

**Joana Manuel MD**
Unidade de Cuidados Intensivos Polivalente, Hospital Garcia de Orta, Almada, Portugal

**Clémence Minet MD**
Medical Intensive Care Unit, Albert Michallon Teaching Hospital, Grenoble Alpes University, Grenoble, France

**Rui P. Moreno MD PhD**
Unidade de Cuidados Intensivos Neurocríticos (UCINC), Hospital de São José, Centro Hospitalar de Lisboa Central, E.P.E., and Professor, Nova Medical School (Faculdade de Ciências Médicas da Universidade Nova de Lisboa), Lisbon, Portugal

**Yên-Lan Nguyen MD MPH**
Anesthesiology and Critical Care Medicine
Department, Cochin Academic Hospital,
Assistance Publique – Hôpitaux de Paris;
Institut Pierre Louis d'Epidémiologie et de
Santé Publique, Paris Descartes University,
Sorbonne Universities; INSERM U707,
Pierre and Marie Curie University,
Paris, France

**John C. O'Horo**
Department of Anesthesiology, Mayo
Clinic, Rochester, MN, USA

**Lotti Orvelius MD**
Department of Intensive Care, Linköping
University Hospital, Department of
Medical and Health Sciences, Linköping
University, Linköping, Sweden

**Michael Parr MD**
Assistant Professor and Director of
Intensive Care, Liverpool Hospital, South
Western Sydney Clinical School, University
of New South Wales, Sydney, NSW,
Australia

**Iris Pélieu MD**
Senior Registrar, Service de Médecine
Intensive Adulte, Centre Hospitalier
Universitaire Vaudois, Lausanne,
Switzerland

**Brian W. Pickering MB BAO BCh
FFARCSI MSc**
Department of Anesthesiology, Mayo
Clinic, Rochester, MN, USA

**Didier Pittet MD MS**
Director, Infection Control Programme
and WHO Collaborating Centre on
Patient Safety, University of Geneva
Hospitals and Faculty of Medicine, Geneva,
Switzerland

**Peter J. Pronovost MD PhD**
Johns Hopkins University School of
Medicine, Johns Hopkins Medicine
Armstrong Institute for Quality and Patient
Safety, Baltimore, MD, USA

**Dinis dos Reis Miranda MD PhD FCCM**
Professor Emeritus of Critical Care
Medicine, University Medical Centre
Groningen, Groningen, the Netherlands

**Andrew Rhodes MD**
Adult Critical Care, St George's University
Hospitals NHS Foundation Trust,
London, UK

**Mark Romig MD**
Johns Hopkins University School of
Medicine, Johns Hopkins Medicine
Armstrong Institute for Quality and Patient
Safety, Baltimore, MD, USA

**Hans U. Rothen MD PhD**
Department of Intensive Care Medicine,
Bern University Hospital (Inselspital) and
University of Bern, Bern, Switzerland

**Francesca Rubulotta MD PhD FRCA FFICM**
Centre for Perioperative Medicine
and Critical Care Research, Charing
Cross Hospital and St Mary's Hospital,
and Anaesthesia and Intensive Care
Medicine, Imperial College NHS Trust,
London, UK

**Katerina Rusinova MD**
Department of Anaesthesia and Intensive
Care, Institute for Medical Humanities,
First Medical Faculty, Charles University,
General University Hospital, Prague,
Czech Republic

**Damon C. Scales MD PhD**
Department of Critical Care Medicine,
Sunnybrook Health Sciences Centre
and Sunnybrook Research Institute, and
Interdepartmental Division of Critical Care
Medicine, University of Toronto, Toronto,
ON, Canada

**Carole Schwebel MD PhD**
Medical Intensive Care Unit, Albert
Michallon Teaching Hospital, Grenoble
Alpes University, Grenoble, and INSERM
U1039, Grenoble Alpes University, La
Tronche, France

**Jeffrey M. Singh MD MSc**
Toronto Western Hospital, University
Health Network, and Interdepartmental
Division of Critical Care Medicine,
University of Toronto, Toronto, ON, Canada

**Folke Sjöberg MD PhD**
Director, Burn Center, Department of
Clinical and Experimental Medicine,
Linköping University, Linköping, Sweden

**Rebecca-Lea Smith MBChB FRCA**
The Royal Marsden Hospital NHS
Foundation Trust, London, UK

**Claudia Spies MD**
Department of Anesthesiology and Intensive
Care Medicine, Campus Charité Mitte and
Campus Virchow-Klinikum, Charité –
Universitätsmedizin Berlin, Berlin, Germany

**Andreas Valentin MD MBA**
Head of Internal Medicine, Kardinal
Schwarzenberg Hospital, Schwarzach,
Austria; Chair, ESICM working group on
quality improvement; founding president,
Federation of Austrian Societies of
Intensive Care Medicine

**Peter van der Voort MD**
Professor of Health Care, Tilburg
University School for Business and Society,
Utrecht, the Netherlands

**Nelleke van Sluisveld MSc**
Scientific Institute for Quality of Healthcare
(IQ Healthcare), Radboud University
Medical Center, Nijmegen, the Netherlands

**Sten M. Walther MD**
Department of Cardiothoracic Anesthesia and
Intensive Care, Linköping University Hospital
and Division of Cardiovascular Medicine,
Department of Medical and Health Sciences,
Linköping University, Linköping, Sweden

**Neil Widdicombe MBBS FRCA FCICM**
Senior Staff Specialist, Department
of Intensive Care Medicine, Royal
Brisbane & Women's Hospital, and Burns
Trauma and Critical Care Research
Centre, University of Queensland,
Brisbane, QLD, Australia

**Hub Wollersheim MD**
Scientific Institute for Quality of
Healthcare (IQ Healthcare), Radboud
University Medical Center, Nijmegen,
the Netherlands

**Adrian Wong BSc MBBS MRCP FRCA
FFICM EDIC**
Clinical Fellow, Department of Critical
Care, John Radcliffe Hospital, Oxford, UK

**Wai-Tat Wong MBBS EDIC FRCP(Edin)**
Department of Anaesthesia and Intensive
Care, Prince of Wales Hospital, the Chinese
University of Hong Kong, Shatin, Hong
Kong, China

**Marieke Zegers MSc PhD**
Scientific Institute for Quality of
Healthcare (IQ Healthcare), Radboud
University Medical Center, Nijmegen, the
Netherlands

# Introduction

## Hans Flaatten, Bertrand Guidet, and Andreas Valentin

The world is rapidly changing, with demographic, ecologic, and financial constraints. Societal expectations are also rapidly changing with easy access to information (websites, smart phones, etc.): reduced delays, requests for rapid decisions, a need for understanding, being part of the decision (shared-decision model). These changes have translated into the hospital, including our critical care services.

The population expects high-quality care given in a timely fashion. They expect this to be without adverse events and side-effects from the treatment in the short and long term. Since very few (if any) of our intensive care units (ICUs) are in this position, most of us have to improve performance on various levels. This means we must improve the quality of care, and as a consequence, we must work together on quality management.

This book addresses several aspects of quality and safety in critical care. Although the main focus is the ICU, several concepts can be generalized to many other settings within the hospital, or even in other institutions.

Today the ICU plays a fundamental role in all modern hospitals worldwide. The ICU provides coverage 24/7, all year round, and is expected to perform equally well, at the same capacity, in the middle of the night and during weekends as within ordinary daytime working hours. Increasingly the ICU team is solicited for patients that are not admitted to the ICU ("ICU without walls"). This may be prior to admission through medical emergency teams (MET) or to address the goal/level of care after an ICU discharge.

During the ICU admission, several interactions with colleagues with different specialties occur. Hence, in term of management we cannot focus only on the ICU, but we must consider the ICU in its environment. As a consequence, frequently ICU physicians are involved in local committees, regional or national professional groups.

We have been educated as medical students using the diagnosis and treatment approach. It means that for the diagnosis we need tools to assess management skills – indicators of quality. Regarding treatment, we need to implement individualized medicine and not simply apply guidelines regardless of patients' specificities. We need also to build a team with common goals.

We need to work as a team, to share the same goals and values, to work on a safety climate, and to build a common culture. We need leaders to inspire such an approach but still maintain a flat hierarchy. We need an atmosphere to enhance information exchange, allowing for different points of view to be expressed. We need to think together in order to implement corrective actions and to adjust behavior according to expectations and results. A good example is the way serious adverse events are handled in the ICU: declaration, mitigation, analysis, proposals for improvement, and follow-up. If people are not confident, or fear being stigmatized or punished, adverse events are not declared and there is no room for improvement.

---

*Quality Management in Intensive Care*, ed. Bertrand Guidet, Andreas Valentin and Hans Flaatten. Published by Cambridge University Press. © Cambridge University Press 2016.

The paradox of modern medicine is that we should endorse individualized treatment adapted to a number of personal factors at the same time as we promote the use of bundles and guidelines in order to reduce the heterogeneity of practice. This means we need initial and continuous training aiming at reaching high competency, but also to diffuse and use protocols locally. This new approach requires active participation of all actors: both new and experienced doctors, in addition to nurses and allied health personnel. Protocols cannot be applied passively; they need to be adapted, tailored according to each unit's culture, case-mix, and environment.

A great step forwards will be to work on communication skills. Important information may be lost on the way from hospital admission to discharge; interpersonal conflicts might arise if people belonging to the same team do not share information. This is true between physicians and between nurses, but also between physicians and nurses. This implies that handover procedures must be formalized and all documentation must be available and shared by the team (medical files and nurses' reports). The electronic ICU management system contributes to easing this sharing approach.

How to improve quality and safety? Several chapters of this book open new horizons and can hopefully be of value to the individual ICUs and ICU clusters at regional and national levels. The number of quality improvement tools we can use has increased substantially in the last decades, and many of these are covered in this book. We do not expect you to use all of them, but hope you will find one or more of the chapters interesting enough to decide to test it out in your ICU.

The development of new ways and methods to improve quality will certainly continue, and with time our "toolbox" will grow. It is hence the hope that some of you will be inspired to find your own way to improve quality and safety of care toward critically ill patients. If you do, share your results and let us all know. In that way we can continue building even better intensive care in the future.

Chapter

# Use of checklists

Mark Romig, Asad Latif, and Peter J. Pronovost

## Introduction

The complexity of medicine in the modern era is increasing on an almost daily basis. Nowhere is this more obvious than in the intensive care unit (ICU), where a vast array of cutting-edge practices, potent medications, and advanced technologies are brought to bear in support of failing organs and critical illness. The care of ICU patients is also time-sensitive. The typical ICU patient requires an average of 178 activities per day [1]. The care of one patient can easily require dozens of healthcare providers to carry out thousands of activities properly, at the right time, and in the correct order. This choreography can be challenging under normal circumstances, given the natural limitations of human memory and attention. In the stressful, high-stakes environment of the ICU, it can be nearly impossible.

The high levels of stress and fatigue that caregivers experience can compromise their cognitive function [2] and lead to decreased compliance with proper protocols, increased error rates, and reduced efficiency [3,4]. Using checklists to standardize processes ensures that all steps and activities are addressed, thereby reducing the risk of costly oversights or mistakes and improving overall outcomes. Checklists are typically an organized list of essential elements or steps that need to be considered or performed for a given task. They differ from other tools in that they lie somewhere between an informal cognitive aid and a protocol. They provide guidance to users and serve as verification after task completion, without leading to a predetermined conclusion [5]. Checklists can function in several ways, including as memory aids, evaluation frameworks, diagnostic tools, and tools to standardize and regulate processes or methodologies. Ultimately, checklists need to highlight the critical issues: facilitating care delivery, decreasing variability, and improving performance.

Most literature regarding checklist use in the workplace comes from outside medicine. Industries that require precise execution for quality and safety, such as aviation and product manufacturing, depend on checklists as simple aids to achieve consistent quality and minimize error. In aviation, checklists are now a mandatory part of routine operations and are highly regulated. They are used both in the course of normal practice and during emergency situations, providing a systematic approach to situation recovery. Today, many aircraft manufacturers have transitioned from paper to electronic checklist systems. In product manufacturing, the smallest error during development can affect the quality of the final product, increase costs, and potentially harm the consumer. Checklists play a central role in ensuring

*Quality Management in Intensive Care*, ed. Bertrand Guidet, Andreas Valentin and Hans Flaatten. Published by Cambridge University Press. © Cambridge University Press 2016.

that proper operating procedures are followed and quality standards are maintained. Quality assurance personnel use them routinely at multiple stages of the production process to evaluate whether required regulatory standards are being met. Checklists are frequently the most important component of standard operating procedures for manufacturing and distribution processes because they help to maintain product quality standards.

Healthcare has begun to follow the example of other industries in adopting the use of checklists in select high-intensity fields like trauma, anesthesiology, and critical care [6–8]. However, they have not yet fully permeated the healthcare industry. The reasons for their lack of use are both operational and sociocultural. Operationally, it can be challenging to standardize processes for the wide variability that exists between and even within patients. Physiologic differences, the nuances of patient comorbidities, the occurrence of unforeseen events, and other unpredictable dynamics all influence the approach to diagnosis, treatment, and even recovery, making the design and implementation of a standardized approach very difficult. Socioculturally, healthcare providers, especially physicians, are often resistant to standardization tools, viewing them as a limitation on their autonomy and even infantilizing. As memory aids, checklists can be perceived to undermine a physician's claim to expertise, and their use tantamount to an admission of weakness.

## Types of checklists

Checklists can be divided into four basic types: static parallel, static sequential with verification, static sequential with verification and confirmation, and dynamic [9]. The main differences between these types are the number of people involved and the degree to which required elements or actions are substantiated.

Static parallel checklists require only one person and consist of a series of read-and-do tasks. An example is the machine checklist used by anesthesiologists on a daily basis.

The static sequential with verification checklist requires two people, usually performing a challenge and response. The first person reads off a series of items (challenge) that the second person confirms as having been addressed (response). An example is the central line insertion checklist, in which the nurse challenges the completion of each task or behavior while the proceduralist confirms whether it has been addressed.

The static sequential with verification and confirmation checklist is usually used in group settings, and the tasks or action items are completed by a variety of team members. A person is selected to state each item (challenge), after which the responsible team member(s) confirms the completion of that particular task (response). An example of this type is the surgical safety checklist performed in the operating room for patients undergoing surgery [10]. Before making an incision, the surgeon calls a "time out" and states the patient's identifying information, specific procedure type, side, and site. He/she then asks about the presence of necessary equipment, which is confirmed by the circulating nurse, and about the patient's medical condition and availability of blood products, which is confirmed by the anesthesiologist.

Dynamic checklists utilize tools like flowcharts to facilitate complex decision-making. They usually have an algorithmic progression with multiple possible options; healthcare providers must choose options sequentially to determine the optimal pathway. An example is the difficult airway algorithm developed by the American Society of Anesthesiologists [11]. In difficult airway scenarios, the team leader uses it to provide guidance on securing the airway and to communicate the plan and required roles to other team members based on progression along the predetermined algorithm.

Checklists can also be further categorized according to the context of their use: normal or non-normal. Normal checklists are used in the course of routine day-to-day operations, such as preflight checks in aviation or instructions on preoperative preparation for patients in healthcare. Non-normal, or emergency, checklists are used to troubleshoot errors or mitigate harm when individual or system failures occur. Completion of the checklist provides a systematic approach to situational recovery that facilitates reliable communication, enables consistent operations, and prevents further errors.

# Development and implementation of checklists

Recent reviews have started addressing the current gap in robust strategies and standardized methodologies for the development of medical checklists [9,12]. When checklists are well thought through, they can standardize the how, why, where, what, and by whom regarding performance of tasks. This standardization can improve quality by reducing variability and error in both routine and emergent situations. Checklists democratize knowledge, allowing healthcare providers to support each other by verifying work performance. Appropriate development of novel and effective checklists is complex. Necessary steps include assembling a multidisciplinary team to guide development, reviewing the existing literature for evidence-based best practices, understanding the local context and environment, and using an iterative approach to test and validate the tool [9].

It is essential to have a definitive objective in mind before creating a checklist. One way to set an appropriate goal is to use the S.M.A.R.T. criteria [13]. A multidisciplinary team should be assembled to provide diverse perspectives in a collaborative development process. The team should review and incorporate empiric and implicit evidence from the evidence-based literature and their own experience before deciding on the content of the checklist. The Translating Evidence into Practice (TRiP) model is a framework that helps frontline healthcare providers summarize the evidence-based recommendations and determine how to effectively evaluate the focus of their improvement effort, e.g., the checklist [14] (Figure 1.1). The first step is to summarize the evidence. Recommendations should be made on the basis of established evidence-based interventions as found in the literature (explicit knowledge). Some elements will be known to improve patient outcomes (e.g., using aseptic technique for central-line insertion). However, when elements lack empiric evidence, teams can tap into the "wisdom of crowds" to obtain diverse input on potential checklist items [15]. Once an exhaustive list of prospective interventions is compiled, the multidisciplinary team should decide which components can be expected to have the strongest impact in practice.

The next step is to identify local barriers to implementation. Frontline staff often have implicit knowledge of existing barriers and how they might hamper delivery of the proposed checklist components. Engaging these providers in a non-judgmental manner can uncover these barriers. One potential barrier to implementation occurs when providers are unware of or disagree with recommendations or the evidence behind them. Alternatively, providers may not be properly supported in efforts to deliver the prescribed practices. Most commonly, failure to use evidence-based practices results when caregivers forget to perform a process or the process is at odds with the care delivery environment, making it difficult to do the right thing each time for every patient.

A checklist of tasks and action items must remain manageable in size and scope. Attention must be paid to the number of items, their arrangement, and operator workflow. Formative work in cognitive psychology recognizes that most people can remember only 7–9 items with relative accuracy [16]. As the complexity of the task, provider stress, or fatigue levels increase, the memory becomes increasingly unreliable [17]. If a process necessitates that the checklist contains more items, it is better to separate out the components into sections or subsets organized as their own individual checklists. Such organization needs to be cognitively and operatively

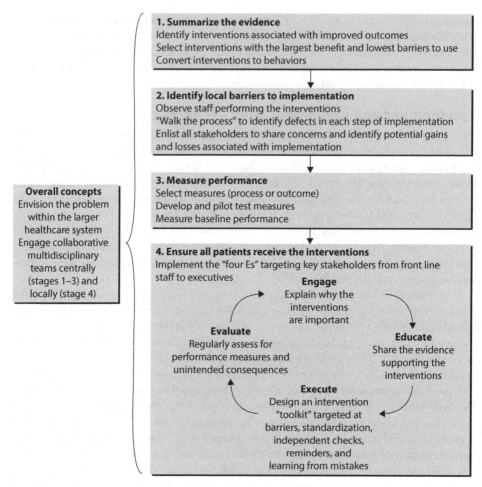

**Figure 1.1** Strategy for translating evidence into practice.

From: Pronovost PJ, Berenholtz SM, Needham DM. Translating evidence into practice: a model for large scale knowledge translation. *BMJ* 2008 6;337:a1714.

functional. For example, our Daily Goals checklist is organized by organ/disease system into 7–9 sections with no more than 7–9 items under each system [18]. Expanding beyond these limits can result in the creation of an unmanageable tool that is neither useful nor used.

Once consensus has been achieved on the checklist components, appropriate measures need to be developed to monitor the practical performance. Such measures are used to evaluate how consistently individual components are performed (process measures) or how outcomes of interest are affected (outcome measures). The accuracy and validity of the selected measures must be tested and verified. Feedback on results must be given to frontline providers in a manner that ensures transparency and accountability.

The last step of the TRiP model provides a framework for implementation of the developed checklist. The model engages and educates frontline staff about the necessity of the checklist, executes the checklist, evaluates its effect on performance, and monitors for any unintended consequences. The checklist is developed in collaboration with frontline operators, who are also encouraged to be educated to support its use. This education includes evidence specific to the checklist being developed as well as general principles related to the science of safety and safe design, and the utility of cognitive tools in improving quality and safety. Engagement with frontline healthcare providers should focus on identifying barriers to implementation and defining solutions to overcome them. The opinions of all providers who will potentially use the checklist are valuable, as even "dissenters" provide valuable insights that may lead to a more successful implementation. Evaluation and data collection are also important components of engagement. The data should be shared with healthcare providers, operators, and other stakeholders as they are collected so that users can gauge whether the intervention is working and track progress over time. The ultimate goal is to make the process an iterative one that incorporates new evidence, provides continuous education, and ensures engagement and automatic evaluation.

## Changing the story

The reductions in mortality and costs associated with central line-associated bloodstream infections (CLABSI) seen in the Michigan Keystone project [8,19] led to other health systems and nations attempting to replicate the results [20–22]. Media accounts of the program have provided a one-dimensional narrative about the miraculous results achieved through the implementation of a technologically simple tool – a checklist. This narrative is an oversimplification. While checklists were an important tool in generating long-term sustainable outcomes, the narrative ignores the complex social interactions that were necessary to create a cultural change to eliminate CLABSI [23].

For an outsider, the checklist is often seen as the entire intervention, instead of one facet of a larger and more holistic quality improvement effort, which can involve changing an entire system of care and/or its delivery. Failure to address this system as a whole leaves the bedside healthcare provider as the singular "hero" who must prevent harm despite the odds. When engaging or emulating other successful systems, healthcare providers must recognize all aspects that were required for the successful implementation of a quality improvement initiative, and not just focus on the use of a checklist.

The narrative surrounding preventable harm in healthcare is often more important than the use of any individual tool aimed at eliminating harm. In the past, CLABSI was considered inevitable – central lines are necessary for the care of critically ill patients, and infection is an unfortunate but inevitable consequence of their use. With the persistence of such a narrative, it can be difficult to engage bedside providers in quality improvement efforts to prevent harm, as they may view these efforts as a waste of time and resources. Likewise, a checklist should be considered only one component of a broader quality improvement perspective. These initiatives must start with the belief that the efforts put forth will result in real gains. Without these overarching themes, the checklist is doomed to fail and may even have a negative impact on future quality improvement efforts involving them.

## Beyond checklists: engineering toward zero harm

Although checklist use has improved patient safety, it is not a panacea for eliminating all preventable harm that patients may experience. Checklists are being used increasingly in safety efforts in part because of their success as a component of efforts to eliminate CLABSI. The resulting expansion of checklist use has led to the checklist itself sometimes being perceived as a burden and detraction from patient care. The risk of "checklist fatigue" threatens to undo the initial benefits gained from their development and implementation.

In the field of patient safety and quality improvement, we must look beyond the checklist itself and instead understand its ultimate goal – ensuring adequate delivery of evidence-based therapies to eliminate a specific harm. Though an individual checklist may serve this function at the time of its use, it is a static tool that may become irrelevant over the dynamic course of a patient's care. Likewise, a checklist targeting one harm may sometimes overlap or even contradict with another checklist targeting a different harm. Our siloed approach of targeting harms individually belies a lack of understanding regarding when and where these synergies and discordances may be occurring, leading to unintended, and sometimes harmful, consequences.

If we are to continue to build upon our past successes in eliminating preventable harm, we must learn from other high-reliability industries such as aviation, nuclear power, and product manufacturing. In these industries, harm is not perceived as inevitable, but rather as a problem that can be overcome through a systems engineering approach. Such an approach is not merely theoretical. An active prototype (Project Emerge) is being developed at the Johns Hopkins Medical System and the University of California San Francisco.

Project Emerge simultaneously addresses seven common harms in ICU patients: venous thromboembolic events, CLABSI, delirium, ICU-acquired weakness, ventilator-associated events, care inconsistent with patient goals, and loss of respect and dignity. The first step in creating this prototype was to catalog all the stakeholders, resources, and workflows associated with the evidence-based practices that contribute to prevention of each harm (Figure 1.2) This detailed assessment was used to gain an understanding of the interdependencies within the existing system. The knowledge was coalesced into a generalizable, scalable framework that explicitly details the steps necessary for harm reduction. These steps broadly consist of proactively identifying each of the harms for which a patient is at risk, which of the predetermined strategies is needed to eliminate the specific harm, who is responsible for performing the tasks aimed at harm elimination, when these tasks should be performed, and how to ensure that all tasks have been performed as prescribed.

The adoption of methodologies used by other industries, specifically checklists, has revolutionized modern healthcare by targeting adequate delivery of practices proven to improve care quality and reduce patient harm. However, the current permutation of checklists tends to focus on some harms at the expense of others. Likewise, the ubiquitous use of checklists is becoming increasingly time- and labor-intensive at the cost of efficiency. Future improvements in healthcare quality and patient safety will need to depend on a more integrated approach that uses technology to improve delivery of healthcare processes through automated process monitoring, thus removing this unsustainable burden from the individual healthcare provider.

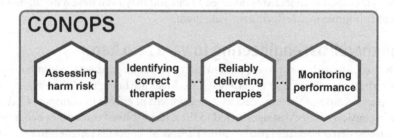

**Figure 1.2** The ConOps for Emerge has four components that can be generalized for any harm.

## Conclusion

Harm has long been understood to be either an inevitable part of healthcare, or worse, a failure of provider vigilance. This view is antiquated and ignores the nature of systems as applied to harm. That is, every system is perfectly designed to achieve the results it achieves [24]. True harm elimination requires not just the adoption of checklists, but also the understanding that harm is a preventable part of a system, and that we must design systems with the end goal of harm elimination in mind.

New technologies, such as device integration and sensor technologies, provide us with the opportunity to remove the bedside clinician from the burdens of process assurance. Leveraging these new technologies will also give us the ability to scale our harm elimination efforts and to address multiple potential harms simultaneously. Only through this broad systems approach can we realistically hope to eliminate the burden of preventable harm in our healthcare system.

## References

1. Donchin Y., Gopher D., Olin M., et al. A look into the nature and causes of human errors in the intensive care unit. Crit Care Med 1995;23(2):294–300.

2. Bourne L.E., Yaroush R.A. Stress and cognition: a cognitive psychological perspective. Technical report NAG2-1561, 2003.

3. Sexton J.B., Thomas E.J., Helmreich R.L. Error, stress, and teamwork in medicine and aviation: cross sectional surveys. BMJ 2000;320(7237):745–749.

4. Hockey G.R., Sauer J. Cognitive fatigue and complex decision making under prolonged isolation and confinement. Adv Space Biol Med 1996;5:309–330.

5. Hales B.M., Pronovost P.J. The checklist: a tool for error management and performance improvement. J Crit Care 2006;21(3):231–235.

6. Harrahill M., Bartkus E. Preparing the trauma patient for transfer. J Emerg Nurs 1990;16(1):25–28.

7. Hart E.M., Owen H. Errors and omissions in anesthesia: a pilot study using a pilot's checklist. Anesth Analg 2005;101(1): 246–250.

8. Pronovost P., Needham D., Berenholtz S., et al. An intervention to decrease catheter-related bloodstream infections in the ICU. N Engl J Med 2006;355(26):2725–2732.

9. Winters B.D., Gurses A.P., Lehmann H., Sexton J.B., Rampersad C.J., Pronovost P.J. Clinical review: checklists – translating evidence into practice. Crit Care 2009;13(6):210.

10. WHO Safe Surgery. 2015; Available at: www.who.int/patientsafety/safesurgery/en/.

11. Apfelbaum J.L., Hagberg C.A., Caplan R.A., et al. Practice guidelines for management of the difficult airway: an updated report by the American Society of Anesthesiologists Task Force on Management of the Difficult Airway. Anesthesiology 2013;118(2):251–270.

12. Hales B., Terblanche M., Fowler R., Sibbald W. Development of medical checklists for improved quality of patient care. Int J Qual Health Care 2008;20(1):22–30.

13. Doran G.T. There's a SMART way to write management's goals and objectives. Manage Rev 1981;70(11):35–36.

14. Pronovost P.J., Berenholtz S.M., Needham D.M. Translating evidence into practice: a model for large scale knowledge translation. BMJ 2008;337:a1714.

15. Surowiecki J. The Wisdom of Crowds: Why the Many are Smarter than the Few and How Collective Wisdom Shapes Business, Economies, Societies and Nations, New York: Doubleday, 2004.

16. Schwarb H., Nail J., Schumacher E.H. Working memory training improves visual short-term memory capacity. Psychol Res 2015, Epub.

17. Lorist M.M., Boksem M.A., Ridderinkhof K.R. Impaired cognitive control and reduced cingulate activity during mental fatigue. Brain Res Cogn Brain Res 2005;24(2):199–205.

18. Schwartz J.M., Nelson K.L., Saliski M., Hunt E.A., Pronovost P.J. The daily goals communication sheet: a simple and novel tool for improved communication and care. *Jt Comm J Qual Patient Saf* 2008;34(10):608–613.

19. Pronovost P.J., Watson S.R., Goeschel C.A., Hyzy R.C., Berenholtz S.M. Sustaining reductions in central line-associated bloodstream infections in Michigan intensive care units: a 10-year analysis. *Am J Med Qual* 2015, Epub.

20. Bion J., Richardson A., Hibbert P., *et al.* "Matching Michigan": a 2-year stepped interventional programme to minimise central venous catheter-blood stream infections in intensive care units in England. *BMJ Qual Saf* 2013;22(2):110–123.

21. Palomar M., Alvarez-Lerma F., Riera A., *et al.* Impact of a national multimodal intervention to prevent catheter-related bloodstream infection in the ICU: the Spanish experience. *Crit Care Med* 2013;41(10):2364–2372.

22. Latif A., Kelly B., Edrees H., *et al.* Implementing a multifaceted intervention to decrease central line-associated bloodstream infections in SEHA (Abu Dhabi Health Services Company) intensive care units: the Abu Dhabi experience. *Infect Control Hosp Epidemiol* 2015, in press.

23. Dixon-Woods M., Bosk C.L., Aveling E.L., Goeschel C.A., Pronovost P.J. Explaining Michigan: developing an ex post theory of a quality improvement program. *Milbank Q* 2011;89(2):167–205.

24. Berwick D.M. A primer on leading the improvement of systems. *BMJ* 1996;312(7031):619–622.

# Daily goal discussions

Hans U. Rothen and Matthias Haenggi

## Introduction

Caring for the critically ill patient is the main mission of an ICU. To ensure optimal patient care, a complex interaction between a wide range of medical specialties and between professionals of diverse occupational groups is essential. In addition, delivery of care is complex, dynamic, and often highly fragmented, with many shared or overlapping tasks. Thus, integration of the caring teams' individual actions into one single network of patient-centered activities is a challenge.

Effective communication is a key element in teamwork and one of the main prerequisites of well-functioning patient care [1]. Failures in communication account for the majority of critical incidents and adverse events in an ICU. Furthermore, poor communication is considered an important cause of nurse–physician conflicts in the ICU [2]. To change workflow and to enhance patient safety, improving communication and changing the culture of teamwork is therefore critical. Besides staff communication and collaboration, several other issues need to be taken into account when addressing problems related to patient care. In the setting of hospital care, they include staffing levels and team composition, standardization of the process of care, early recognition and treatment of the deteriorating patient, and, finally, the local safety climate [1].

Transfer of information relevant to patient care is practiced almost continuously. In addition, medical responsibility is transferred several times per day from one caregiver to another. These processes of handover are complex, and up to now they have been only poorly analyzed and understood. To ensure quality of care, a well-designed handover with clearly defined aims and tasks of the various participants is needed. As outlined in the following paragraphs, using systematic, standardized daily goal discussions has the potential to improve the process of care in respect of several of the problems outlined above.

## Daily goal discussions as a key element in care of the critically ill patient

The daily goals concept as a tool to improve communication in the ICU was presented for the first time in 2003 by Peter Pronovost and his team [3]. The concept aims at improving communication within the caring team during patient rounds while encouraging the use of

*Quality Management in Intensive Care*, ed. Bertrand Guidet, Andreas Valentin and Hans Flaatten. Published by Cambridge University Press. © Cambridge University Press 2016.

**Table 2.1** General aspects of a daily care plan in critically ill patients

- List of the patient's clinical problems.
- Interpretation of lab results, cultures, imaging procedures, and other investigations.
- Defining physiological targets and aims.
- Management plan.
- Effective and efficient handover.
- Issues for discharge planning.

(Modified from [9])

all possible information resources to prevent errors and increase efficiency [4]. It does so by facilitating a systematic, standardized, and well-structured approach, while simultaneously allowing for multidisciplinary input. This concept is founded on theories of crew resource management [5]. A key element is a shared understanding of goals and, based on this, a well-coordinated and organized process of patient care. This can be further supported by clearly assigning clinical and educational responsibilities [6].

Ultimately, the daily care plan (a brief outline is presented in Table 2.1) should be based on a shared understanding of patients' problems, underlying diseases, and measures to ensure optimal outcome. In the ICU, the ultimate result will either be an improved or restored quality of life, or compassionate and supportive palliative or end-of-life care. Using the daily goals concept aims at enhancing the understanding and implementation of all these activities.

In general, patient care rounds are used as a key mechanism to ensure and coordinate communication within the team responsible for patient care, to serve as a platform for effective exchange of information relevant to patient care, to ensure shared perception of a patient's situation, to support decision-making, and to agree on patient management and on each participant's role and tasks [7,8]. Virtually the same aims are also relevant for the process of handover. A well-designed daily goals tool (e.g., a checklist or specifically designed form) will not only support patient care rounds, but may also be used as the basis for handover. It will contribute to a safe, effective, efficient, timely, and patient-centered process of care. Eventually, it will be one of the key elements ensuring optimal patient outcome.

## Daily goal discussions: beneficial effects and challenges

As shown by Pronovost *et al.* [3], a daily goals checklist for morning rounds in the ICU improves interprofessional communication and increases nurses' and residents' understanding of the goals of care for the day in the ICU. In addition, these authors observed that patients' length of stay in their ICU was reduced after the introduction of this concept.

A number of beneficial effects of the daily goals concept were confirmed in subsequent research, but due to limited space only a few examples can be mentioned here. These studies vary in design and setting, and they were all performed as single-center studies. Karalapillai *et al.* [9] found distinct improvements of ICU nurses' self-reported understanding of the medical plan, including, among other elements, the patient's clinical problems, the management plan, and issues for discharge. Similar findings were reported for a pediatric ICU by Agarwal *et al.* [10]. As described by Rehder *et al.* [11], using a bedside whiteboard for documentation can support shared agreement of patients' daily goals. Siegele [12] proposed that a daily goals tool may also have a positive effect on the communication between the caring team and the patients' families. Based on their mixed-methods study, Centofanti *et al.* [13] note that a daily goals checklist may have a direct impact on patient care by fostering a systematic approach, by encouraging participation from all team members, and by minimizing errors of omission and commission. Interestingly, as noted by Seigel *et al.* [14], the implementation of a multidisciplinary standardized rounding structure including a daily goals form may result in a decrease in the overall length of daily rounds. Last but not least, a daily goals checklist may also prompt teaching opportunities [6,13].

Mnemonics such as SBAR (situation, background, assessment, and recommendation) or FAST-HUG (feeding, analgesia, sedation, thromboembolic prophylaxis, head-of-bed elevation, stress ulcer prevention, and glucose control) typically support the structured approach to some aspects of patient care. Similarly, care bundles (sepsis, mechanical ventilation, etc.) encompass a specific subset of patient care. However, neither mnemonics nor care bundles are a substitute for the systematic review of all relevant aspects of clinical care as covered by the daily goals concept.

Introducing a daily goals concept to ensure or improve quality of care can be challenging. In general, implementing a change in clinical practice should be based on multifaceted interventions [15]. Even though there is face-validity that interventions aiming at improved interprofessional rounds will improve the process of patient care, until now there has been rather limited scientific evidence, supporting this assumption [16]. As a consequence, it is difficult to draw any firm, generalizable conclusions on the effect of such interventions on the process of care or on patients' outcomes. A daily goals form or checklist may be viewed by some as repetitive or a duplication of information [13]. Furthermore, there is a risk that during very busy times, completion of a daily goals form may be superficial, imprecise, or incomplete (see also Chapter 1). Indeed, orally stated goals are at times not reliably documented in the written health record [17], and such problems most probably will also be observed while using a daily goals form. Finally, filling out a daily goals form or checklist never should be considered as a substitute for verbal communication [13].

## Implementing the daily goals concept

Implementing the daily goals concept includes more than the mere creation of a checklist. However, it is important to remember some prerequisites. Such a form or checklist should be simple but well structured, and must be developed with the active involvement of those who will use them [14,15]. Adapting the tool to local needs most likely improves acceptance and compliance in its use. Table 2.2 suggests some elements that might be included in a daily goal form or checklist.

As a general approach, a daily goals form might be introduced using the plan–do–check–act (PDCA) model. This iterative four-step management method is used for continuous improvement of processes and products, and it is also known as the Deming circle (but referred to by Deming as the "Shewhart cycle"). A similar but slightly expanded model has recently been proposed with the "5E" approach (Evaluate – engage – educate – execute – estimate impact) [15].

The PDCA model is probably the most often cited tool in quality management. It relies on repeated, often short, sequences of learning by "trial and error" [14,18]. This methodology was also used by Pronovost when introducing the first daily goals form [3]. In many cases, the PDCA model seems the appropriate approach to a daily goals form as opposed to a large-scale change, based on endless discussions and workshops, and never-ending trials to reach a common consensus on what is accepted as the best solution. The PDCA cycle is certainly also to be preferred to a "quick and dirty" action that aims at a change in workflow without assessment of its results.

Implementing the daily goals concept demands commitment of the caring team while establishing common grounds. In fact, using an interdisciplinary communication tool *per se* may be more important than the specific statements on that form [3]. It should also be

**Table 2.2** Elements of a daily goals checklist

Communication and code status

- Communication with primary service updated?
- Family communication up-to-date, any need for a family conference or spiritual care?
- Code status addressed? Re-addressed?

Safety and patient transfer

- What is this patient's greatest safety risk? How to reduce that risk?
- Any events that need to be reported (e.g., as a note in CIRS)?
- Is this patient receiving deep venous thrombosis and peptic ulcer disease prophylaxis?
- What needs to be done for the patient to be discharged from the ICU?

Neurological and pain management

- Neurological status, delirium, and pain assessed?
- Is there any change in neuro status?
- Is the cervical spine cleared?
- Are pain, sedation, and delirium protocols used appropriately?

Hemodynamics and volume status

- Hemodynamic system assessed?
- Volume status (including urinary output) assessed?
- Adequate organ perfusion confirmed?

Pulmonary and respiratory support

- Patient's status in terms of the weaning protocol?
- Readiness to be extubated assessed?
- Ventilator bundle checked (safe limits of tidal volume and plateau pressure, elevate head of bed)?

Gastro-intestinal, nutrition, and renal

- Bowel sounds checked? Abdomen distended?
- Parenteral and/or enteral feeding checked?
- Tube feeding operational? Residuals?
- Glucose control assured?

Infectious disease

- Febrile? Any other signs of infectious disease?
- Results of cultures?
- Resistant germs? Screening for MRSA needed/performed?
- Sepsis bundle operational?

Skin, wounds, and mobilization

- Skin integrity and dressings checked?
- Pressure reduction mattress and skin bundle used?
- Early mobilization assured?
- Eye protection adequate?

Medication

- Drug levels adequate?
- Can any medication be discontinued?

Instrumentation: Catheters, tubes, drains, and other devices

- Sites of insertion checked?
- Can catheters or tubes be removed?

**Table 2.2** (cont.)

Tests, procedures, and consultations

- Review scheduled labs, chest radiograph, and any other imaging procedure.
- New tests and imaging procedures to be ordered?
- Need of any procedures?
- Consultations needed?

This table is not meant to be exhaustive. It has to be adapted according to local needs, patient mix and diagnostic or therapeutic procedures used in a specific ICU.

ICU: intensive care unit; CIRS: critical incidence reporting system; MRSA: methicillin resistant *S. aureus*.

Modified from [3,9,12,14,20,21].

remembered that strategies using only one single intervention, or that are based solely on didactic education and passive dissemination, most probably will be less effective [19]. In addition, implementation is impeded if the concept is too difficult to understand, if there is lack of support from peers or local opinion leaders, or if there are restrictions in time or shortage of staff [15,19]. Finally, implementation of the daily goals concept is enhanced if it is supported by a user-friendly, easily adaptable documentation system.

# Conclusions

In the future, focusing on workflow and teamwork will be an integral part of ICU management. Most healthcare professionals are hard workers. What matters, however, is not how many patients a nurse cares for or how many procedures a physician performs, but rather the result of the team's activities. Workflow has to be re-organized by eliminating unnecessary variation in practice as well as failures in communication. The daily goals concept is a tool with the potential to support this process. It is not unlikely that more lives can be saved by appropriate use of already existing knowledge and by optimizing patient care with tools such as the daily goals concept, rather than by generating new knowledge or by developing new drugs.

# References

1. Pannick S., Beveridge I., Wachter R.M., Sevdalis N. Improving the quality and safety of care on the medical ward: a review and synthesis of the evidence base. *Eur J Intern Med.* 2014;25:874–887.

2. Hartog C.S., Benbenishty J. Understanding nurse–physician conflicts in the ICU. *Intensive Care Med.* 2015;41:331–333.

3. Pronovost P., Berenholtz S., Dorman T., Lipsett P.A., Simmonds T., Haraden C. Improving communication in the ICU using daily goals. *J Crit Care.* 2003;18:71–75.

4. Rawat N., Berenholtz S. Daily goals: not just another piece of paper. *Crit Care Med.* 2014;42:1940–1941.

5. Kosnik L.K. The new paradigm of crew resource management: just what is needed to re-engage the stalled collaborative movement? *Jt Comm J Qual Improv.* 2002;28:235–241.

6. Dodek P.M.,Raboud J. Explicit approach to rounds in an ICU improves communication and satisfaction of providers. *Intensive Care Med.* 2003;29:1584–1588.

7. Manser T. Teamwork and patient safety in dynamic domains of healthcare: a review of the literature. *Acta Anaesthesiol Scand.* 2009;53:143–151.

8. Lane D., Ferri M., Lemaire J., McLaughlin K., Stelfox H.T. A systematic review of evidence-informed practices for patient

care rounds in the ICU. *Crit Care Med.* 2013; 41:2015–2029.

9. Karalapillai D., Baldwin I., Dunnachie G., *et al.* Improving communication of the daily care plan in a teaching hospital intensive care unit. *Crit Care Resusc.* 2013;15:97–102.

10. Agarwal S., Frankel L., Tourner S., McMillan A., Sharek P.J. Improving communication in a pediatric intensive care unit using daily patient goal sheets. *J Crit Care.* 2008;23:227–235.

11. Rehder K.J., Uhl T.L., Meliones J.N., Turner D.A., Smith P.B., Mistry K.P. Targeted interventions improve shared agreement of daily goals in the pediatric intensive care unit. *Pediatr Crit Care Med.* 2012;13:6–10.

12. Siegele P. Enhancing outcomes in a surgical intensive care unit by implementing daily goals tools. *Crit Care Nurse.* 2009;29:58–69.

13. Centofanti J.E., Duan E.H., Hoad N.C., *et al.* Use of a daily goals checklist for morning ICU rounds: a mixed-methods study. *Crit Care Med.* 2014;42:1797–1803.

14. Seigel J., Whalen L., Burgess E., *et al.* Successful implementation of standardized multidisciplinary bedside rounds, including daily goals, in a pediatric ICU. *Jt Comm J Qual Patient Saf.* 2014;40:83–90.

15. Bion J.F., Abrusci T., Hibbert P. Human factors in the management of the critically ill patient. *Br J Anaesth.* 2010;105:26–33.

16. Zwarenstein M., Goldman J., Reeves S. Interprofessional collaboration: effects of practice-based interventions on professional practice and healthcare outcomes. *Cochrane Database Syst Rev.* 2009:CD000072.

17. Collins S.A., Bakken S., Vawdrey D.K., Coiera E., Currie L.M. Agreement between common goals discussed and documented in the ICU. *J Am Med Inform Assoc.* 2011;18:45–50.

18. Berwick D.M. Developing and testing changes in delivery of care. *Ann Intern Med.* 1998;128:651–656.

19. Francke A.L., Smit M.C., de Veer A.J., Mistiaen P. Factors influencing the implementation of clinical guidelines for health care professionals: a systematic meta-review. *BMC Med Inform Decis Mak.* 2008;8:38.

20. Khorfan F. Daily goals checklist: a goal-directed method to eliminate nosocomial infection in the intensive care unit. *J Healthc Qual.* 2008;30:13–17.

21. Braun J.P., Kumpf O., Deja M., *et al.* The German quality indicators in intensive care medicine 2013: second edition. *Ger Med Sci.* 2013; 11: Doc09.

# Common ICU procedures

## Central venous catheters insertion and management

**Davide Bastoni, Maurizio Cecconi, and Andrew Rhodes**

## Introduction

Treatment of critically ill patients in the intensive care unit (ICU) requires the deployment of multiple routine and on-demand procedures to deliver the highest level of care. Many of these procedures have specific benefits that enable and facilitate treatment and monitoring to be delivered, but also can have adverse consequences. Robust quality improvement programmes (including audit) are therefore necessary to ensure quality and to prevent harm occurring [1]

Every quality-procedure improvement should follow the RUMBA rule [1,2]:

- *Relevant*: important to the patient care improvement.
- *Understandable*: critical care staff must be able to understand it.
- *Measurable*: it must be able to be measured, quantified, and, hence, assessed.
- *Behaviourable*: it must bring changes in routine staff actions.
- *Achievable*: the aim of it must be possible to attain.

In this chapter we will explore the 'state of art' of central venous catheter (CVC) insertion, care, and infection control; we will review the catheter-related bloodstream infection (CR-BSI) guidelines; and we will shortly discuss new approaches to prevent CVC colonization and CR-BSI.

## Practicalities for CVC insertion, management, and removal

Central venous catheters are important devices to deliver intravenous fluids, blood components, drugs, parenteral nutrition, and chemotherapy in a large set of patients [3].

They are percutaneously inserted intravascular tubes which have their tip in a central vein (jugular, subclavian, or femoral). Different sizes and lengths of devices are available.

There are several kinds of CVC:

- *Peripherally inserted central catheters (PICCs)*. Using an ultrasound-guided technique, these catheters are inserted from a peripheral vein, such as the basilica, cephalic, or brachial vein, and have 1–4 lumens. They are, on average, 20 cm long and usually a first choice for relatively long-term parenteral nutrition or fluid support, lasting in place for a maximum of one year. In comparison to short-term CVCs, PICCs are less prone to infection; however, they frequently become dysfunctioning due to thrombi formation in the lumen. Patients

*Quality Management in Intensive Care*, ed. Bertrand Guidet, Andreas Valentin and Hans Flaatten. Published by Cambridge University Press. © Cambridge University Press 2016.

with compulsory arm position, spasticity, and un-intact skin are not eligible for PICC insertion because of higher risk of thrombus formation and catheter-related infections.

- *Tunnelled catheters.* These are defined as CVCs with a particular skin-to-vein entry site, such as a cuff, which reduces the risk of CR-BSI. Usually inserted for long-term IV therapy, they are longer than non-tunnelled catheters, being at least 8 cm long, depending on patient size. Internal jugular access has been shown to be safer, with less thrombotic complications, than the subclavian vein [4].
- *Implanted port catheter systems.* These CVCs have a subcutaneous tunnel (port) which remains in place beneath the skin and permits IV access through a needle. This is the favourite choice for oncologic patients needing chemotherapy for a long period of time. They have no need for CVC care, but the removal requires a surgical approach.
- *Short-term CVCs* with single, double, triple, or quadruple lumen. The most common type of CVCs, they have a length of 8–24 cm. The length choice depends upon the insertion site: the right internal jugular access usually requires the shortest length, while the femoral one the longest. They also account for the majority of CR-BSI. A specific type is the 'vasc-cath', a triple-wide lumen CVC used for veno-venous renal replacement therapy.

## The *decision* to insert a CVC can be taken on an urgent or elective basis

In the emergency setting, the most available site and type of CVC is inserted. On the contrary, if the insertion is planned, CVC duration, location of insertion and patient's preferences should be considered and reviewed daily [5].

Reasons for CVC:

1. *Need for multiple lumen IV access to infuse different kind of fluids and drugs simultaneously.* Also, some medications, such as chemotherapy, can only be given via a central line due to the irritating and damaging effect they would trigger on peripheral veins and soft tissues.
2. *Central venous pressure monitoring* for hemodynamic purposes and as part of the evaluation for fluid responsiveness.
3. *Difficulty finding peripheral venous access.*
4. *Need for a dedicated central line for parenteral nutrition.*

## Some situations can increase the procedural risk related to CVC insertion

Several characteristics of the patient can increase the insertion difficulty: neck shortness for jugular approach; obesity, agitation, haemodynamic instability, scars, and bullous emphysema for all approaches.

The only relative contraindication to CVC insertion is a coagulopathy that augments the bleeding risk during the procedure. In those cases, CVC must be inserted only if strictly necessary and the operator must be expert in the procedure, even though the incidence of peri-procedural bleeding has been reported as 0.5–1.6% and it is usually controlled with the application of mechanical pressure to the source of bleeding. In the rare reports of fatal outcome, human errors during the procedures were the cause rather than bleeding diathesis.

Before inserting a CVC, it is recommended to have a clotting test and a full blood count available in order to assess the bleeding risk. In a patient receiving anti-platelet drugs or oral anticoagulation, the risk of bleeding must be considered and related to the risk of thrombo-embolism if the therapy was stopped. In a patient with a coagulopathy, the choice of subclavian access is less advisable, as it is more difficult to compress a source of bleeding.

A platelet count of $50 \times 10^9$ / L is considered the cut-off under which the risk of bleeding increases.

Moderately prolonged activated partial thromboplastin time (aPTT) levels (up to 1.3 times the upper reference interval) do not increase the risk of bleeding or haematoma formation in the absence of other coagulation disorders.

Levels of prothrombin time-international normalized ratio (PT-INR) at or below 1.8 are also considered safe to proceed with CVC insertion. In selected patients (and in haemophiliac patients) in which bleeding can be disastrous, correction of clotting test abnormalities or low platelet counts can be considered [6] before starting the procedure.

## Insertion of central venous catheters

*Ultrasound-guided CVC insertion* is recommended to reduce the risk of immediate complications, thrombosis, and the duration of insertion [5,7]. In the UK, the National Institute for Health and Care Excellence (NICE) advises the use of two-dimensional ultrasound for CVC insertion in the internal jugular vein [8] for both adults and children. This guidance method is associated with reduced failed catheter insertion attempts (86% reduction in relative risk in comparison to the landmark traditional method). Secondary to the reduced time of insertion, ultrasound guidance diminishes also the time from CVC insertion to the start of IV therapy. The ultrasound guidance is particularly important when the physician is not experienced with the procedure (<50 successful insertions) because in that case the reduction of immediate complications is more important. The probe used is the linear one or that with the highest frequency, in order to have the best resolution for small depths. Use of audio-Doppler to differentiate between vein and artery is not recommended [8]. The differentiation can be on anatomic (depth and location) and physiological basis (pulsatile vs non-pulsatile, compressible vs non-compressible). Two kinds of images can be screened: the longitudinal axis and the transverse axis. The former allows for the appreciation of the vein in its full length and to follow the needle in the moment of the insertion in the vein. The latter allows seeing both the vein and the artery, but the needle will be visualized as a spot and no insertion point will be appreciated. The needle insertion on the longitudinal axis is called *in-plane needle approach*, whereas that on the transverse axis is called *out-of-plane needle approach*. Whatever approach is chosen, the probe and the needle must be as aligned as possible to avoid partial images; of course, on transverse approach only the tip of the needle will be displayed.

New two-dimensional ultrasound probes have been developed. One new approach, called the AxoTrack® system (from Soma Access Systems), includes an ultrasound probe with a needle guide that extends through the body of the ultrasound probe, making the path of the needle coincident and coplanar within the ultrasound beam. This device has been shown to be safe and has the advantage of giving the operator real-time knowledge of the probe's exact position [9].

Recently, three-dimensional ultrasound probes have been released [10]. These combine the images of both the transverse and longitudinal view simultaneously on the screen. The three-dimensional probes can be either a mechanically steered array or matrix array. The mechanically steered array probes provide three different real-time images on the screen, permitting the operator to visualize the longitudinal, transversal, and coronal plane. The drawbacks of these probes are their dimensions – they are bigger than the standard two-dimensional probes, which increases the difficulty of the insertion.

The matrix array probe is smaller and lighter than the mechanically steered array probe; it allows three-dimensional views of the site and also volumetric post-insertion reconstruction to show the correct position of the needle in the vein. These two new probes still need to be trialled on a large scale, but it is expected they will help in reducing the number of attempts and procedural errors during CVC insertion.

## The antiseptic non-touch technique (ANTT)

The antiseptic non-touch technique (ANTT) for CVC insertion is composed of a number of fundamental elements including reducing environmental risks, hand cleansing and protection of 'key parts' to minimize the risk of microbial colonization and infection of the catheter.

The key parts include:

- sterile equipment that will be used invasively;
- the surface of the sterile dressing that will be in direct contact with the exit site;
- surfaces of intravenous connectors;
- skin after it has been disinfected;
- open wounds and invasive device sites;
- the ultrasound probe used for echo-guided CVC insertion, after it has been wrapped in a sterile dressing;
- the transparent dressing – this will be replaced 24 hours post-insertion.

All the steps of CVC insertion must be performed in an aseptic way. A completed checklist must always accompany the insertion. In particular, the hotspots during the procedure are [11]:

- *Skin antisepsis.* The aim is to minimize the resident microbial count on the skin before the CVC insertion. On the basis of recent evidence, the common and most used means to maximize microbial kill involves applying 2% chlorhexidine in 70% alcohol with friction and allowing the solution to air-dry before the procedure.
- *Avoid contamination during the insertion.* Drapes and sterile cloth to border and limit the access skin area must be put in place. Minimize gloves-to–skin contact using an ultrasound guided approach that reduces the clinician's palpation manoeuvres.
- *Sterile field.* Creating a sterile field and adhering to maximal barrier precautions by the clinician and assisting staff is thought to be among the key elements in preventing CR-BSIs. These involve sterile apron and gloves, the use of mask and hat; removing all sorts of tools and objects that can be in contact to sterile things. It is important to emphasize that meticulous attention should be paid to the set up of the equipment required for the CVC insertion. Sterile sets should only be opened immediately prior to use. Personnel not involved in the procedure and staff movement should be reduced to a minimum within the procedural space.

After the insertion, the daily CVC lines and dressing care is equally important. Every contact with lines, taps, bungs, and the insertion site must be undertaken with gloves and disinfection. One of the most sensitive moments in the post-insertion CVC care is the dressing change (not intact or not sterile) and caps and taps replacement [12]. The interval between scheduled changes can be safely increased to seven days in the ICU, provided soiled and loosened dressings are changed immediately. In particular patients, such as burn patients, recent findings suggest CVC change after 72 hours from insertion [13].

## The *insertion* of a CVC is correlated to some complications

Immediate complications occur during or soon after the procedure; these are:

- arterial puncture and arterial incannulation;
- artero-venous fistula;
- nerve damage;

- haemorrhage, especially in patients with coagulopathies;
- pneumothorax and haemothorax, mainly for subclavian approach;
- tracheal tear;
- air embolism;
- arrhythmias, due to mechanical stimulation of CVC tip in the right atrium or ventricle.

Late complications occur in the days after the insertion and depend on the quality of care and the duration of CVC; these are:

- catheter occlusion and thrombosis;
- infection and CR-BSI;
- catheter dysfunction.

## With expert personnel, subclavian CVC is the best choice because it has the lowest risk of infection

The *location* of the CVC insertion is still a matter of debate. Although guidelines have been recommending for years to prefer jugular or subclavian access over femoral [5], some recent literature reviews and meta-analyses have suggested no difference in the rate of CR-BSI between the three sites [14,15]. More clear evidence from large-scale meta-analysis with enough power and the data quality is needed to analyse the factors that can potentially affect the site selection (physician skills and experience, BMI, patient risk of injury or thrombotic complications, duration of catheterization and bundle implementation). Until universal agreement on this issue is reached, it is still reasonable to avoid femoral site insertion in non-emergency situations when other locations are available, in accordance with HICPAC 2011 Guidelines [5].

## CVC tubes are long and hence not suitable for resuscitation purposes as the resistance to fluid infusion is higher

The *length of CVC*, the number of lumens, and the deep tip position are proportionally related to an increased risk of thrombosis. Hence, CVC type choice should be carefully evaluated, balancing the benefits–risks ratio, and the number of lumens must be kept to a minimum [5,16].

The optimal position for the catheter tip is still a matter of debate. For jugular or subclavian catheters the tip has been suggested to be positioned within the inferior part of the superior caval vein or within the right atrium. In the last situation, the risk of thrombosis can be augmented, in particular if the CVC is due to stay in place for a longer time. For femoral catheters, the tip is considered to be safe above the inferior caval entry points for renal veins.

In all cases, an X-ray after insertion is recommended to evaluate the correct position of the CVC. Indirect assessment of CVC position can also be made by connecting the central venous pressure transducer and measuring the central venous pressure, which should be between 0 and 20 mmHg. Also, a blood sample from the CVC, processed for a blood gas analysis, can help differentiate between arterial and venous blood.

## New materials and prevention procedures are being evaluated [17]

- *Antiseptic-impregnated dressings.* Chlorhexidine-impregnated dressings prevent microorganism re-growth in the epidermis and their main side-effect is a local dermatitis with no systemic involvement. Another option, in particular for neonates, is silver-alginate-coated dressings, which have been shown to reduce PICC-associated BSI in neonates. Still, a clear benefit–cost ratio must be assessed for both in large-scale trials.

- *Antithrombotic prophylaxis*. The formation of thrombi in CVC lines is a major risk factor for bacteria colonization and CR-BSI. Use of heparin or fibrinolytic drugs in CVC lines has been tested and a decrease in CR-BSI is suggested. As the risk of thrombi formation is proportional to the time the CVC remains in place, these agents are so far considered just for longstanding CVCs. We do not know yet the exact rate of thrombocytopenia or bleeding risks correlated to their use.
- *Antimicrobial-coated catheter and antibiotic lock solutions*. These CVCs are added with chlorhexidine and silver sulfadiazine on the outer surface. Some studies suggest the reduction of bacteria colonization and CR-BSI for short-term CVCs (CVC in place fewer than eight days) owing to the withering of the impregnation. New extra and intraluminally coated CVC types with minocycline and rifampicin are being tested and to date no clear benefits in comparison to the chlorhexidine and silver sulfadiazine ones have been shown. Concerns for both types regarding the development of resistance in bacterial strains are still present.

Antibiotic lock solutions refer to intraluminal application of an antimicrobial drug solution in catheters that are used only intermittently as the CVCs for dialysis. In this setting, they have been shown to reduce CR-BSI.

Recently, specific criteria have been developed for the application of antibiotic-impregnated catheters [18]. At least two of the following three criteria must be met:

1. CVC need estimated to be more than seven days;
2. total parenteral nutrition;
3. CR-BSI in the same admission.

Until new materials and guidelines become available, following the quality improvement effort and the CR-BSI reduction goal is of greatest importance to provide the best care possible to patients.

# CR-BSI

CR-BSI is a well-known source of morbidity and mortality in critically ill patients. The incidence of CVC-related infections has been estimated to be as high as 2.7 per 1000 catheter-days using classical non-cuffed CVCs that are introduced primarily for short-term use [3].

The CDC defines a catheter-*associated* BSI (CA-BSI) as a BSI caused by an organism not related to another infection when a central line has been in place at some time during the 48 hours prior to the collection of the blood culture. In contrast, a catheter-*related* BSI (CR-BSI) is defined as a BSI with either a positive catheter tip culture or a positive blood culture drawn from the CVC consistent with a culture drawn simultaneously from a peripheral site (see Table 3.1). The difference between the two definitions is relevant: CA-BSIs are a clinical entity derived from a suspected and an exclusion source of infection process; CR-BSI is based on a microbiological diagnosis and is more specific [19]. Actually, several pathogens identified as CA-BSI responsible, have been shown not to cause catheter-related infections. Hence, CR-BSI definition is more accurate to catheter-specific interventions designed to reduce rates of BSI in the ICU [19].

Most infections are caused by skin flora colonization of the catheter external side. Bacteria can also be transferred from health carers' hands. Coagulase-negative staphylococci (such as *Staphylococcus epidermidis*) and enterobacteria are the most common species. Also, *Pseudomonas aeruginosa* and *S. aureus* can cause catheter-related infections and, in these

**Table 3.1** US Centers for Disease Control and Prevention Definitions of Catheter-Associated (CA) and Catheter-Related (CR) Blood Stream Infection (BSI)

| CA-BSI | Positive blood culture |
|---|---|
| | Catheter in place |
| | No other site with the same bacteria as blood culture isolate |
| | Catheter is *assumed* to be the cause of the BSI |
| | |
| | Criterion 1: patient has a recognized pathogen cultured from one or more blood cultures and organism cultured from blood is not related to an infection at another site. |
| | Criterion 2: patient has at least one of the following signs or symptoms: fever (>38 °C), chills, or hypotension with signs and symptoms and positive laboratory results are not related to an infection at another site, and at least one of the following: common skin contaminant (e.g., diphtheroids, *Bacillus* spp., *Propionibacterium* spp., coagulase-negative staphylococci, or micrococci) is cultured from two or more blood samples drawn on separate occasions; common skin contaminant is cultured from at least one blood culture from a patient with an intravascular catheter; and the physician institutes appropriate antimicrobial therapy |
| CR-BSI | Positive blood culture |
| | Catheter in place |
| | Positive culture of catheter tip (confirming colonization) with the same bacteria in blood culture |
| | Catheter is *confirmed* to be the cause of the BSI |
| | |
| | Attributed to patients who have a CVC and who have been in the ICU for at least 48 hours |
| | Patients with a CVC who develop a bloodstream infection within 48 hours of ICU discharge are also defined as having a CA-BSI or CR-BSI. |
| | If a patient has more than one CVC, counts only as one catheter–day. |
| | Catheter colonization is defined as significant growth of a microorganism (>15 colony-forming units) from the catheter tip, subcutaneous segment of the catheter, or catheter hub. |

latter cases, the virulence and antimicrobial resistance is higher. Coagulase-negative and gram-negative bacteria other than *P. Aeruginosa* usually have a weak virulence, and infections usually respond well to antibiotic therapy [16,20].

One of the main risk factors for CR-BSI is the intrinsic catheter structure. In fact, the irregular microscopial surface and the fibrin sheath that develops after insertion are both stimuli for bacterial colonization and growth, which can be extraluminal and intraluminal, in particular in long-term CVC.

Clinical presentation involves local swelling, erythema, oozing, CVC dysfunction, pain, and sore skin. In CVC infection-related sepsis, systemic symptoms such as fever can be present as well as increased inflammatory markers. The sensitivity of clinical symptoms in predicting BSI is low [21]. In critically ill patients suspicion of CR-BSI must be confirmed by blood cultures from the CVC and peripheral vein. If the CVC is no longer strictly necessary, the following step is the immediate removal; if it is still necessary and there are signs of sepsis, the CVC must be replaced, the tip sent for culture, and empiric antibiotic therapy started.

Figure 3.1 shows a flow chart to assist in the decision-making process when CVC infection is suspected.

## The Keystone-ICU project in Michigan hospitals: USA [22]

In the USA, there are up to 80,000 CR-BSI cases, which result in 28,000 deaths per year in intensive care patients. These infections cost up to $2.3 billion annually and the median rate of CR-BSI is reckoned to be in the range between 1.8 to 5.2/1000 catheter-days [23].

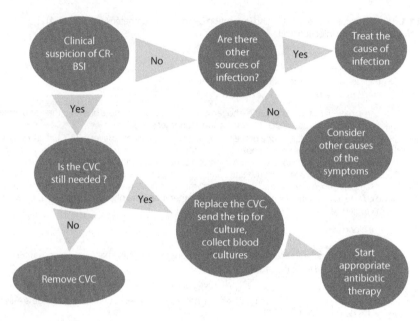

**Figure 3.1** Suspected CVC infection decision-making flow chart.

To tackle this phenomenon, in 2003 all Michigan hospitals with ICUs for adults were invited to participate in the Keystone-ICU project. The interventions were as follows:

- Implementation of five evidence-based procedures recommended by the CDC and identified as having the greatest effect on the rate of CR-BSI:
  1. hand washing;
  2. using full-barrier precautions during the insertion of CVC;
  3. cleaning the skin with chlorhexidine;
  4. avoiding the femoral site, if possible;
  5. removing unnecessary catheters.
- Checklist form to ensure the application of the above procedures.
- Educational training on safety and infection control procedures for all the ICU staff.
- Implementation of staff communication, daily sheet, and checklist regarding CVC management.
- Designation of doctor and nurse leaders for CVC management.

The period given to complete the staff training and procedures deployment was three months.

At the baseline, and then each month, data from each ICU were collected and aggregated into three-month periods for a total of six three-month periods. Procedure compliance and CR-BSI rate were calculated.

This study, even with some limitations (study design not capable of making a causal connection between the intervention and reduced rates of CR-BSI; the possibility of under-reporting of CR-BSI; no collection of organisms responsible for CR-BSI) showed that decreasing CR-BSI with a focused pack of interventions, even on a large scale such as in a whole state, is possible (from 7.7 to 1.4 CR-BSIs per 1000 CVC-patient days). This would bring morbidity and mortality reduction and also huge cost savings for hospitals. Of great interest, the three-year follow-up period reported sustained improvement when the interventions were continuously applied.

## The "Matching Michigan" English project [24]

Following an increasing awareness on quality improvement in English ICUs and an effort to reduce CR-BSI, in 2009 a two-year programme, known as 'Matching Michigan', was started (see Table 3.2).

As you can see from the table, the debate around hospital-acquired infections, infection control, and CR-BSI had been growing since the early years of the new century. In those years, the necessity of a national reporting system concerning CR-BSI was stated. In this context, the 'Matching Michigan' study aimed to examine the impact of a series of focused quality interventions and best-practice guidance on minimizing CVC BSIs in English ICUs. For the study, 139 English hospitals with ICUs agreed to participate. Of these, 79% were general adult ICUs, 9% were paediatric ICUs, and 11.5% were subspecialties. Interventions were technical (procedural) and non-technical.

*Technical interventions* were: hand cleansing and use of 2% chlorhexidine for skin antisepsis, full barrier operator–patient protection (hat, mask, sterile scrubs and gloves, CVC insertion checklist, CVC insertion packs).

*Non-technical* interventions were: teaching and training sessions, safety and incident reviews, teamwork, and communication.

The programme demonstrated a 60% reduction in reported CVC BSIs in adult ICUs in England; for paediatric ICUs the 48% reduction did not achieve statistical significance. Mean adult ICU CR-BSIs diminished from 3.7 CR-BSIs/1000 CVC-patient days to 1.48. The important and significant reduction was due to the training and procedural guidance

**Table 3.2** History of infection control efforts relevant to central venous catheters

2001 Mandatory reporting to the Health Protection Agency (HPA) of MRSA bacteraemia.

2003 Report of the Chief Medical Officer: *Winning ways: guidance to reduce healthcare associated infection in England*.

2004 Mandatory reporting of *Clostridium difficile* infection (HPA website).

2004 Hospital in Europe Link for Infection Control through Surveillance of Nosocomial Infections in ICUs protocol: http://helics.univ-lyon1.fr/helicshome.htm

2005 DoH Saving Lives programme: NHS High Impact Interventions (NHS-HII), modelled on Institute for Healthcare Improvement bundles.

2006 Health Act 2006: Department of Health Code of Practice gives new powers of inspection to the Healthcare Commission. Superseded by the Health & Social Care Act 2008.

2008 Health and Social Care Act 2008: required registration with the Care Quality Commission: duty to protect patients against HCAIs. New code of practice: www.dh.gov.uk/en/Publicationsandstatistics/Publications/PublicationsPolicyAndGuidance/DH_081927

2008 Patient Safety First sponsored by National Patient Safety Agency (NPSA), NHS HII, and Health Foundation, includes interventions to reduce CVC BSIs: www.patientsafetyfirst.nhs.uk/content.aspx?path

2009 Some NHS trusts participated in CQUIN (Commissioning for Quality and Innovation) schemes that made a percentage of their incomes dependent on demonstrating compliance.

2011 Mandatory reporting of MRSA and *Escherichia coli* bacteraemia.

for CVC insertion and management brought about by this study, as well as by the concurrent and preceding improvement efforts and consciousness-raising effect of a nationwide programme already in place before the 'Matching Michigan' study.

The key point to highlight is that a common nationwide programme aiming to reduce rates of infection could deliver health gains for patients and benefits for health systems.

Later, in 2011, another independent quality improvement report showed that the goal of the elimination of CR-BSI is reachable [25]. In the ICU of Stirling Royal Infirmary (a general hospital in Forth Valley, Scotland), the authors conducted a multiple-step study on daily CVC insertion and management practices. During the first year (2006), they focused on infection surveillance, establishing that full aseptic technique and prevention of CR-BSI procedures were not always performed. In the following year (2007) they implemented a fully protocolized approach to CVC insertion and maintenance. This protocol comprised two bundled packages of care:

1. The *insertion bundle*: procedural steps to follow, such as hand cleaning, antiseptic technique, full barrier precautions, avoidance of the femoral site, and CVC insertion checklist.
2. The *maintenance bundle*: removal of CVC as soon as possible, cleaning of ports with alcohol before use, parenteral nutrition dedicated line, no blood sampling from CVC if possible.

The implementation of the bundles programme was supported by educational and training sessions, measurement of outcomes, and reviewing the unit organization.

The study carried on till 2009 and, after 2007, an impressive reduction of CR-BSI was noted, from 3.38/1000 device-days at the start of the study to 0 when the adherence to the bundle was higher than 80%, demonstrating the importance of having common and shared rules and behaviours for CVC insertion and management.

## The upcoming frontier against CR-BSI: nanotechnologies application

Modern catheter materials are silicone-, polyurethane-, or propylene-based, and are highly bio-compatible. They are also resistant to some chemicals, drugs, and clotting formation. Nevertheless, the formation of a biofilm on the outer and inner surface of CVCs represents a serious problem, being the origin of CR-BSIs.

Several approaches have recently been developed to improve the antimicrobial quality of CVC materials.

- *Silver nanoparticle connectors.* These are valved connectors with a silicone membrane embedded with silver nanoparticles in the polycarbonate matrix and also on the external casing. The coat releases minute quantities of bactericidal ionic silver from the surface into the fluid path, thus preventing contamination and biofilm formation on the internal surface of the CVC. They have been studied only on models; trials on humans are still to be carried out.
- *Liposomes* (artificially prepared vesicles made of a lipid bio-layer that can carry an antimicrobial drug). These substances could be administered like lock solutions into the CVC lumen, permitting their contact with the biofilm and thus resulting in a bactericide action. Trials on humans will have to analyse the benefit–cost ratio, safety, and efficacy.
- *Polymer-associated drug nanocarriers* are polymer compounds mixed with drugs that could carry antimicrobial agents directly to the site of colonization, passing through the biological membranes. These polymers could be connected and deployed as part of the CVC structure.

- *Bacteriophages.* Use of phages that attack and kill selectively and locally the bacterial biofilm is another promising possibility. Also, the advantage would be that phages replicate in-situ, increasing the efficacy against the biofilm formation. Still, some queries are unsolved, such as the development of bacterial resistance against the phages, virulence genes in phages that can be incorporated in the bacteria genetic code, immune system phage inactivation, and the presence of endotoxins in the phage preparation.
- *Bioelectric effect* is an approach that uses tiny-voltage electrical current to prevent biofilm formation and to enhance the activity of antimicrobials against established biofilms.

All the above approaches are still under investigation in terms of large-scale efficacy, human safety, benefit–cost ratio, and applicability in different clinical settings [26].

# References

1. Martin J., Braun J.P. Quality management in intensive care medicine. *Anaesthesist.* 2014;108:521–529.

2. Valentin A., Ferdinande P. Recommendations on basic requirements for intensive care units: structural and organizational aspects. *Intensive Care Med.* 2011. DOI: 10.1007/s00134-011-2300-7

3. Linnemann, Birgit. Management of complications related to central venous catheters in cancer patients: an update. *Semin Thromb Hemost.* 2014;40: 382–394.

4. Trerotola S.O., Kuhn-Fulton J., Johnson M.S., Shah H., Ambrosius W.T., Kneebone P. Tunneled infusion catheters: increased incidence of symptomatic venous thrombosis after subclavian versus internal jugular venous access. *Radiology.* 2000;217:89–93.

5. O'Grady N.P., Alexander M., Burns L.A., et al. Guidelines for the prevention of intravascular catheter-related infections. *Clin Infect Dis.* 2011;52:e162–193.

6. Frykholm P., Pikwer A., Hammarskjöld F., et al. Clinical guidelines on central venous catheterisation: Swedish Society of Anaesthesiology and Intensive Care Medicine. *Acta Anaesthesiol Scand.* 2014;58:508–524.

7. Peris A., Zagli G., Bonizzoli M., et al. Implantation of 3951 long-term central venous catheters: performances, risk analysis, and patient comfort after ultrasound-guidance introduction. *Anesth Analg.* 2010;111:194–201.

8. NICE. Guidance on the use of ultrasound locating devices for placing central venous catheters. www.nice.org.uk/guidance/ta49.

9. Ferre R.O., Mercier M. Novel ultrasound guidance system for real-time central venous cannulation: safety and efficacy. *West J Emerg Med.* 2014;15:536–540.

10. French J.L., Raine-Fenning N.J., Hardman J.G., Bedforth N.M. Pitfalls of ultrasound guided vascular access: the use of three/four-dimensional ultrasound. *Anaesthesia.* 2008;63:806–813.

11. Yacopetti N., Davidson P., Blacka J., Spencer T. Preventing contamination at the time of central venous catheter insertion: a literature review and recommendations for clinical practice. *J Clin Nurse.* 2013;22:611–620.

12. Shapey I.M., Foster M.A., Whitehouse T., Jumaa P., Bion J.F. Central venous catheter-related bloodstream infections: improving post-insertion catheter care. *J Hosp Infect.* 2009;71:117–122.

13. Kagan R.J., Neely A.N., Rieman M.T., et al. A performance improvement initiative to determine the impact of increasing the time interval between changing centrally placed intravascular catheters. *J Burn Care Res.* 2014;35:143–147.

14. Marik P.E., Flemmer M., Harrison W. The risk of catheter-related bloodstream infection with femoral venous catheters as compared to subclavian and internal jugular venous catheters: a systematic review of the literature and meta-analysis. *Crit Care Med.* 2012;40:2479–2485.

15. Timsit J.F., Bouadma L., Mimoz O., *et al.* Jugular versus femoral short-term catheterization and risk of infection in intensive care unit patients: causal analysis of two randomized trials. *Am J Respir Crit Care Med.* 2013;15:1232–1239.

16. Schiffer C.A., Mangu P.B., Wade J.C., *et al.* Central venous catheter care for the patient with cancer: American Society of Clinical Oncology clinical practice guideline. *J Clin Oncol.* 2013;31:1357–1370.

17. Timsit J.F., Dubois Y., Minet C., *et al.* New materials and devices for preventing catheter-related infections. *Ann Intensive Care.* 2011;18:34.

18. Gozu A., Clay C., Younus F. Hospital-wide reduction in central line-associated bloodstream infections: a tale of two small community hospitals. *Infect Control Hosp Epidemiol.* 2011;32:619–622.

19. Sihler K.C., Chenoweth C., Zalewski C., Wahl W., Hyzy R., Napolitano L.M. Catheter-related vs. catheter-associated blood stream infections in the intensive care unit: incidence, microbiology, and implications. *Surg Infect (Larchmt).* 2010;11:529–534.

20. Lorente L., Martín M.M., Vidal P., Rebollo S., Ostabal M.I., Solé-Violán J. Should central venous catheter be systematically removed in patients with suspected catheter related infection? *Crit Care.* 2014;18:564.

21. Borchardt R.A., Raad I. Bloodstream infections: the risks and benefits of intravascular catheters. *JAAPA.* 2012;25: 21–22.

22. Pronovost P., Needham D., Berenholtz S., *et al.* An intervention to decrease catheter-related bloodstream infections in the ICU. *N Eng J Med.* 2006;355:2725–2732.

23. Surveillance, National Nosocomial Infections. National Nosocomial Infections Surveillance (NNIS) report data summary from January 1992 through June 2004. *Am J Infect Control,* 2004;32:470–485.

24. Bion J., Richardson A., Hibbert P., *et al.* 'Matching Michigan': a 2-year stepped interventional programme to minimise central venous catheter-blood stream infections in intensive care units in England. *BMJ Qual Saf.* 2013;22: 110–123.

25. Longmate A.G., Ellis K.S., Boyle L., *et al.* Elimination of central-venous-catheter-related bloodstream infections from the intensive care unit. *BMJ Qual Saf.* 2011;20;174–180.

26. Zhang L., Keogh S., Rickard C.M. Reducing the risk of infection associated with vascular access devices through nanotechnology: a perspective. *Int J Nanomedicine.* 2013;8:4453–4466.

# Use of guidelines and bundles

Oliver Kumpf, Felix Balzer, and Claudia Spies

## Introduction

Guidelines aim to facilitate medical decision-making incorporating the most recent evidence on particular topics into daily clinical routine. Especially in intensive care medicine – with its complex nature – evidence-based approaches are needed to avoid unnecessary variations in care that negatively influence clinical outcome.

In contrast to simple therapy standards, guidelines exceed a summary of textbook evidence regarding a certain topic. They should be thought of as tools that use the most recently published evidence to provide the best solution for a common clinical problem.

A search of internet databases like PubMed for clinical guidelines in the context of intensive care medicine reveals more than 250 guidelines involving aspects of critical care. There are different sources of guidelines that can be found online – for example, on the sites of the Agency for Healthcare Research Quality (AHRQ), the Guideline International Network (GIN), and the Arbeitsgemeinschaft der Wissenschaftlichen Medizinischen Fachgesellschaften (AWMF), among others [1–3]. However, not all those guidelines exclusively cover aspects of critical care medicine. In this chapter we provide an overview of aspects of development, current use, and implementation of guidelines.

## Level of evidence and grade of recommendation

As mentioned above, there is a difference between recommendations included in clinical guidelines and simple therapy standards. Clinical guidelines are developed with the clear aim to include robust evidence that has been evaluated by a group of experts in a predefined process. Usually, to fulfil adequate quality criteria a certain level of evidence (LoE) is determined. Second, the grade of recommendation (GoR) is agreed according to the underlying LoE following discussion within and vote by the group.

The assessment of the LoE is usually achieved by systematic literature research regarding a topic, and afterwards a systematic evaluation of this literature. The LoE can be assessed either regarding an outcome of interest across several studies (e.g. GRADE-system) [4] or by evaluating individual studies (e.g. Oxford classification, SIGN classification) [5]. The question of whether the LoE should be outcome-based or study-based is a matter of current discussion among guideline developers. The outcome-based LoE assessment has the advantage that the

*Quality Management in Intensive Care*, ed. Bertrand Guidet, Andreas Valentin and Hans Flaatten. Published by Cambridge University Press. © Cambridge University Press 2016.

'body of evidence' – which is all the evidence available regarding a topic – is evaluated for a very specific question. This allows assessment of negative effects ('harms') of a certain intervention and weighing them against benefits. Nevertheless, the outcome-based LoE evaluation needs key questions (so-called PICO questions (Patient–Intervention–Control–Outcome)) to be addressed and requires several studies with a comparable method and a robust outcome measurement, which are often not available. In addition, PICO questions might not be suitable for all relevant aspects of clinical practice. In this context, the study-based assessment of LoE allows a more general view, with the disadvantage of less precision and a possible over- or underestimation of evidence.

The GoR of a guideline statement can be either determined solely by the LoE (solely evidence-based guideline), a consensus conference where members of the guideline committee vote on the GoR with respect to the LoE and consideration of, for example, clinical factors (evidence- and consensus-based guidelines) or solely relying on expert opinions (solely consensus-based guideline). This depends on the methodological concept of the guideline.

LoR and GoR are not identical because evidence of the current literature does not necessarily reflect practical recommendations. In addition, there are important – e.g. ethical – exceptions: if we consider a widely used example of the necessity for sedation in patients treated with neuro-muscular blocking agents (NMBAs), we will find no randomised controlled trial that ever compared non-sedation vs sedation in patients treated with NMBAs. This example stresses the utmost relevance of clinicians in clinical guideline development to evaluate the LoE and the statement in a meaningful way.

## Appraisal of guidelines

Instruments for guideline appraisal are necessary to ensure a standardised quality assessment of the guideline before it is implemented into practice, because the term 'guideline' is not protected, and the quality of guidelines is heterogeneous. A prominent example for an appraisal tool for guidelines is the Appraisal of Guidelines for Research and Evaluation Instrument (AGREE) – first published in 2003, in 2010 it was revised and renamed AGREE II [6,7]. AGREE II consists of 23 items for guideline evaluation, arranged in six domains: (1) scope and purpose; (2) stakeholder involvement; (3) rigour of development; (4) clarity of presentation; (5) applicability; and (6) editorial independence. The domains reflect that a critical appraisal exceeds evaluation of the methodological rigour of development and the way an LoE has been evaluated, but also covers aspects like applicability and the possibilities of translation into clinical practice. As medical decisions in critically ill patients have an immediate effect on outcome, a guideline appraisal is mandatory before considering implementation of a guideline.

Stakeholder involvement should be mentioned separately as this is a critical point in guideline appraisal: panels should thus consist of experts on all areas of interest, including nurses, patient representatives, and physicians from different subspecialties. Since the opinions and demands of various stakeholders may differ considerably, they should be considered to find a consensus that is approved by all participating stakeholders in a guideline-development process. This plays an important role in intensive care medicine as *not* all guidelines that cover aspects of intensive care medicine do cover it exclusively (e.g. guidelines on chronic-obstructive pulmonary disease or guidelines on prevention and management of pressure ulcers).

Another key element is the update process of a guideline as the body of evidence grows: a guideline undergoes continuous development to take the most recent evidence into consideration to ensure best clinical practice. Besides the provision of knowledge, a guideline can also address a research demand, which should be re-evaluated regularly.

## ICU bundles

One option to increase applicability of guidelines is that recommendations are translated into a 'set of treatment goals (usually three to seven) that when grouped and achieved together over a finite time span are believed to promote optimum outcomes' [8].

In essence, a bundle aims at performing a treatment process in an optimal, most reliable way. The most important characteristic of a treatment bundle is to make adherence to the process elements mandatory. So a bundle differs substantially from a checklist, although checklists may be used to perform a bundle. Because all elements of a bundle consist of high levels of evidence, it is believed that complete adherence has the most positive influence on outcome. Therefore an (ICU) bundle is not only closely related to a guideline (it is the upstream link to evidence), but it is also to the treatment standard (the downstream link to practice). The package of interventions has to be followed by caregivers for every patient every single time. The accountability of the providers of a bundle has to be checked every single day since it has to be performed as a set, with no exceptions.

The development of bundles has to take into account that it should be unsusceptible to local specifics and can be performed collectively and reliably. The bundle approach is widely considered as a practical and feasible way to implement the parts of a guideline with the strongest effect on outcome [9].

## Considerations before implementation

Despite the quality of a guideline, guideline statements are *per definition* not mandatory or enforced by law. In contrast, there are cases where clinicians should deviate from recommendations, because limitations are inherent to guidelines [10]. Obviously, guideline recommendations can never account for all problems in the context of a specific patient. When healthcare professionals neglect the clinical situation of a patient in its complexity, guidelines may sometimes harm rather than benefit. Especially physicians with limited experience may be led to initiate therapeutic steps that could be clinically inappropriate, futile, or potentially harmful if a guideline is applied too rigorously. In summary, guidelines in intensive care medicine provide a framework of aggregated evidence and expertise, but they do not substitute individual decisions. They limit an arbitrary variability of treatment but they do not limit the possibility of a reasonable variability.

## Practical approaches for the implementation of a clinical practice guideline (CPG)

Implementation of evidence-based medicine in daily practice is difficult [11]. There are four steps that are needed to implement new treatment guidelines. When initiating a change in treatment strategies, first, *adoption* of a change in practice has to take place, meaning the care team has to commit to a change. *Diffusion* of the necessary knowledge is the next step, making the new practice recommendations available for all members of the team. With *dissemination*, this diffusion is actively pursued in the team based on the recommendations to improve knowledge and skills. *Implementation*, then, is dissemination with an additional focus to deal also with obstacles to a practice change.

These obstacles are referred to as barriers of implementation. Cabana *et al.* found a variety of those barriers [12]. In their article they included 120 different surveys investigating

293 potential barriers to physician guideline adherence. In general, lack of awareness ($n = 46$), familiarity ($n = 31$), agreement ($n = 33$), self-efficacy ($n = 19$), and outcome expectancy ($n = 8$) were prominent among the surveyed. Also, the inability to overcome the inertia of previous practice ($n = 14$) and the presence of external barriers to performing recommendations ($n = 34$) were found, representing institutional obstacles. There are in principle two ways to overcome these barriers. They are either focused on the personal behaviour or on the structural circumstances, and in most instances they influence each other. In the following paragraph we describe a potential strategy for CPG implementation.

For all clinical practice guidelines there is a need for personnel, time, and motivation. When deciding to include a new CPG into the treatment standards of an ICU before such an intervention, the current standard of practice should be evaluated. This evaluation has to include all groups taking part in a process. Ideally, in this step potential barriers of implementation are also identified that can be approached directly during the implementation process.

How can the implementation of a guideline be achieved – for example, a sedation guideline? There are two clinical practice guidelines on practice in analgesia, sedation, and delirium (PASD) available. Both guidelines offer some recommendations for implementation and evaluation. One of these guidelines also includes a bundle approach to support implementation and both state that educational measures are important but no specific interventions are proposed [13,14].

After evaluating local treatment habits, the first step is to develop a local treatment protocol that defines sedation goals, gives specific timeframes for measurement of sedation scores and other refined excerpts from the guideline. This protocol needs to be developed by all stakeholders involved in the process. The goal of the protocol is maximal adherence. A documentation tool for the protocol has to be included, providing a measurement of adherence to it. In a next step, ICU staff as a whole have to become familiar with the new CPG. Accompanying education efforts are critical to bringing about *diffusion* of knowledge. The next step is often the first problem in a real-life change process. Regular measurement of adherence to the protocol by using a reporting system developed for that purpose is a cornerstone of sustainable guideline implementation. However, measurement is time consuming and potentially needs additional personnel. The use of electronic patient records might help with measurements via predefined queries. The data gathered with these queries should be processed and ideally a regular report should be produced. Making this report available to the care team is one of the most important aspects in CPG implementation. Furthermore, only a form of feedback enables action by the leadership of an ICU. Those reports can be used to investigate non-adherence to the protocol, and also for benchmarking with other collaborating ICUs. However, feedback doesn't increase adherence to treatment guidelines automatically; audits or peer review might help to elucidate factors leading to non-adherence. Figure 4.1 gives an overview of elements involved in implementation of clinical guidelines.

In general, the use of quality improvement techniques will help in these circumstances, like the Plan–Do–Check–Act (PDCA) cycle. To facilitate guideline implementation, *care bundles* can be integrated in these situations. Regarding, for example, PASD care, the American Critical Care Society provides a specific care bundle to facilitate introduction of the guideline. This bundle is designed to integrate the core elements of a guideline into practice. But also checklists might help as they additionally provide reminders on certain practices. Quality management techniques should be used to help evaluate effects for all

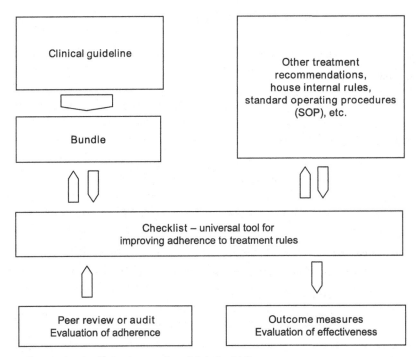

**Figure 4.1** Elements involved in implementation of clinical guidelines.

implementation strategies of a CPG or care bundles [15]. We recommend a tailored approach to local circumstances using protocolised bundles or checklists flanked by PDCA cycles to continuously measure adherence to CPG, ideally with reporting of key performance indicators to staff. Table 4.1 summarises theories and models that are important in implementing change and offers general approaches to practical change management. Overall it can be stated that for implementation of a CPG it is helpful to adopt common quality improvement techniques [15].

## How do guidelines and bundles affect patient outcome?

There is increasing evidence that the incorporation of guidelines and bundles into clinical practice improves treatment quality measurably. Both have been shown to positively influence patient outcome [16]. The evaluation and report of (positive) effects of guidelines on treatment is of key importance for further large-scale implementation and also for future guideline development. An example for guideline effects is the presently available CPG for treatment of sepsis [17]. The guideline includes a sepsis bundle that has been evaluated very recently. It is shown that implementation of guidelines including bundles is improving treatment quality in sepsis patients [18]. For PASD we have shown in a large observational study that oversedation due to non-adherence to an institutional sedation bundle resulted in a more than two-fold increase in hospital mortality that persisted up to two years in follow-up [19]. The overall effect of guidelines in ICU treatment was recently evaluated in a systematic review by Sinuff *et al.* in which they concluded that 'knowledge transfer interventions' such as protocols and education are effective in changing processes [20]. They also stated that the benefit of these interventions

**Table 4.1** Theories/models relating to implementing change to improve practice in analgesia, sedation, and delirium (PASD)

| Theories/models | Important factors | Lessons for improving care |
|---|---|---|
| **Relating to individual professionals** | | |
| Cognitive | Mechanisms of thinking and deciding; balancing benefits and risks | Provide convincing information on, for example, analgesia, sedation, and delirium evidence |
| Educational | Individual learning needs and styles | Involve professionals in improving care; define improvement plan |
| Attitudinal | Attitudes, perceived behavioural control, self-efficacy, social norms | Convince key professionals of importance; show that they can do it and that others will follow |
| Motivational | Different motivational stages with different factors/barriers | Tailor interventions to different target groups (doctors, nurses) within sedation practice |
| **Relating to social context** | | |
| Social learning | Incentives, feedback, reinforcement, observed behaviour of role models | Model best practices of care; give feedback on progress |
| Social network and influence | Existing values and culture of network, opinion of key people | Use opinion leaders in network to improve routines |
| Patient influence | Perceived patient expectations and behaviour | Involve patients actively in improving their care; stimulate self-management |
| Leadership | Leadership style, type of power, commitment of leader | Obtain commitment of management to improving care |
| **Relating to organisational and economic context** | | |
| Innovativeness of organisation | Extent of specialisation, decentralisation, professionalisation, functional differentiation | Take into account type of organisation; encourage teams to develop their own plans for change |
| Quality management | Culture, leadership, organisation of processes, customer focus | Reorganise processes; develop systems for continuous improvement |
| Complexity | Interactions between parts of a complex system, behavioural patterns | Focus on system as a whole; find main 'attractors' for improving care |
| Organisational learning | Capacity and arrangements for continuous learning in organisation | Encourage continuous exchange of expertise at all levels of the organisation |
| Economic | Reimbursement arrangements, rewards, incentives | Reward achievement of treatment targets |

Adapted from [21].

on clinical outcome was sparse. This was mostly due to the methodology of studies, of which 94% were observational with small populations causing large effects. In general it appears that conducting large studies on practice change is difficult. Moreover, as was shown for sepsis mortality over time, there was an actual effect following the first development of guidelines [18] – however, it was never proven that this was due to the new guidelines. It seems safe to assume that certain effects of knowledge transfer via other channels have led to increased awareness of sepsis, and therefore might also have improved outcome.

## Conclusion

Guidelines and derived bundles are helpful tools that are intended to aid knowledge transfer into clinical practice to reduce the well-known gap between evidence-based therapy principles and daily clinical routine. They provide clinicians with up-to-date surrogate knowledge on frequently encountered clinical problems. However, there are barriers to implementation of guidelines and bundles. To overcome these barriers, methods of quality management are needed for sustainable effects of full guideline and bundle implementation. Most guidelines do not provide sufficient support on how they should be implemented in practice. Research of recent years has shown that the use of guidelines and bundles can improve treatment quality. Yet it has to be noted that high-quality research on this topic is still lacking because large trials are extraordinarily complicated to perform and suitable outcome measures are difficult to define.

## References

1. Guidelines International Network. *International Guideline Library*. 2014. www.g-i-n.net/library/international-guidelines-library (accessed 18 November 2014).

2. Agency for Healthcare Research and Quality (AHRQ). *National Guideline Clearinghouse*. 2014. www.guideline.gov/search/advanced-search.aspx (accessed 18 November 2014).

3. AWMF online. *Das Portal der wissenschaftlichen Medizin. Leitliniensuche*. 2014. www.awmf.org/leitlinien/aktuelle-leitlinien.html (accessed 18 November 2014).

4. Atkins D, Eccles M, Flottorp S, *et al.* Systems for grading the quality of evidence and the strength of recommendations I: critical appraisal of existing approaches. The GRADE Working Group. *BMC Health Serv Res.* 2004;4(1):38.

5. Petrie JC, Grimshaw JM, Bryson A. The Scottish Intercollegiate Guidelines Network Initiative: getting validated guidelines into local practice. *Health Bulletin.* 1995;53(6):345–348.

6. Brouwers MC, Kho ME, Browman GP, *et al.* Development of the AGREE II, part 1: performance, usefulness and areas for improvement. *CMAJ.* 2010;182(10):1045–1052.

7. Brouwers MC, Kho ME, Browman GP, *et al.* Development of the AGREE II, part 2: assessment of validity of items and tools to support application. *CMAJ.* 2010;182(10):E472–478.

8. Dellinger RP, Townsend SR. Point: are the best patient outcomes achieved when ICU bundles are rigorously adhered to? Yes. *Chest.* 2013;144(2):372–374.

9. Institute for Healthcare Improvement (IHI). What is a bundle? 2014. www.ihi.org/resources/Pages/ImprovementStories/WhatIsaBundle.aspx (accessed 18 November 2014).

10. Wollersheim H, Burgers J, Grol R. Clinical guidelines to improve patient care. *Neth J Med.* 2005;63(6):188–192.

11. Grol R, Grimshaw J. From best evidence to best practice: effective implementation of change in patients' care. *Lancet.* 2003;362(9391):1225–1230.

12. Cabana MD, Rand CS, Powe NR, *et al.* Why don't physicians follow clinical practice guidelines? A framework for improvement. *JAMA.* 1999;282(15):1458–1465.

13. Martin J, Heymann A, Basell K, *et al.* Evidence and consensus-based German guidelines for the management of analgesia, sedation and delirium in intensive care: short version. *Ger Med Sci.* 2010;8:Doc02.

14. Barr J, Fraser GL, Puntillo K, *et al.* Clinical practice guidelines for the management of pain, agitation, and delirium in adult patients in the intensive care unit. *Crit Care Med.* 2013;41(1):263–306.

15. Curtis JR, Cook DJ, Wall RJ, *et al.* Intensive care unit quality improvement: a 'how-to' guide for the interdisciplinary team. *Crit Care Med.* 2006;34(1):211–218.

16. Resar R, Pronovost P, Haraden C, *et al.* Using a bundle approach to improve ventilator care processes and reduce ventilator-associated pneumonia. *Jt Com J Qual Patient Saf.* 2005;31(5):243–248.

17. Dellinger RP, Levy MM, Carlet JM, *et al.* Surviving Sepsis Campaign: international guidelines for management of severe sepsis and septic shock: 2008. *Crit Care Med.* 2008;36(1):296–327.

18. van Zanten AR, Brinkman S, Arbous MS, *et al.* Guideline bundles adherence and mortality in severe sepsis and septic shock. *Crit Care Med.* 2014;42(8):1890–1898.

19. Balzer F, Weiss B, Kumpf O, *et al.* Early deep sedation is associated with decreased in-hospital and two-year follow-up survival. *Crit Care.* 2015;19(1):197.

20. Sinuff T, Muscedere J, Adhikari NK, *et al.* Knowledge translation interventions for critically ill patients: a systematic review. *Crit Care Med.* 2013;41(11): 2627–2640.

21. Grol R, Wensing M. What drives change? Barriers to and incentives for achieving evidence-based practice. *Med J Aust.* 2004;180(6 Suppl):S57–60.

# Nosocomial/healthcare-associated infections

Caroline Landelle and Didier Pittet

## Introduction

Nosocomial infection – today most appropriately termed healthcare-associated infection (HAI) – is one of the most common medical complications affecting patients in intensive care units (ICUs). In developed countries, HAI affects about 30% of patients admitted to ICUs [1]. The burden of HAI is even higher in developing countries [2]. Although ICU beds account for only 5% of all hospital beds and care for less than 10% of patients admitted, ICU-acquired HAI (ICU-HAI) account for more than 20% of all HAI. An assessment of mortality attributable to HAI in the ICU setting is difficult as it shares common risk factors with both the underlying disease and acuity of illness. Crude mortality rates vary from 12% to 80% [1] and attributable morbidity and mortality due to ICU-HAI may be in excess of corresponding rates for the infections that initially led to the patient's hospitalization. Associated costs are equally high.

## Risk factors for ICU-HAI

Patients' underlying conditions play an important role in the high rates of ICU-HAI. Natural and specific host defense mechanisms might be impaired by underlying diseases or as a result of medical (e.g., immunosuppressive medications) and surgical interventions. Another reason for the high rates of ICU-HAI is the selective pressure for resistant organisms induced by the large amount of antimicrobial use. Importantly, almost all ICU patients are equipped with at least one vascular access or device breaking the normal skin barrier, thus enabling a direct connection with the external environment. A large quantity of equipment and devices surround patients in ICU and almost every item of equipment has been shown to be a source of ICU-HAI. Furthermore, new devices are constantly introduced into ICUs, mostly increasing the workload and the opportunity for cross-transmission of bacterial pathogens.

Several studies show that overcrowding, understaffing, or an imbalance between workload and resources are important determinants of HAI and microorganism cross-transmission in ICUs. The higher the workload, the lower the compliance with preventive measures, and the higher the risk for HAI. Importantly, not only the number of staff, but also the level of staff training affect outcomes. The causal pathway between understaffing and infection is complex and several factors may contribute, including primarily lack of time to comply with infection control recommendations.

*Quality Management in Intensive Care*, ed. Bertrand Guidet, Andreas Valentin and Hans Flaatten. Published by Cambridge University Press. © Cambridge University Press 2016.

The most important vehicle of transmission remains healthcare workers' (HCWs) hands. Lack of or inadequate hand hygiene practice is the direct cause of cross-transmission in many endemic and epidemic situations.

Host colonization is a prerequisite for the subsequent development of infection, particularly in critical care. Although factors favoring the progression from colonization to infection are not completely understood, it is estimated that almost 50% of ICU-HAI are preceded by colonization with the same microorganism. Factors associated with colonization are similar to those associated with infection and include duration of hospitalization, high exposure to invasive devices, and prolonged antibiotic therapy. Studies have shown that severity of illness and ICU admission contributed to rapid colonization with Gram-negative bacteria. These are endemic in the ICU and the patient physiological flora can be substituted by the local endemic flora after some days in this setting.

## Epidemiology

HAI include infections acquired in the healthcare facility but appearing after discharge, as well as occupational infections among HCWs of the facility. The most commonly used definitions are those of the United States Centers for Disease Control and Prevention [3], although several European countries use also the definitions of the "Hospital Infection Link for Infection Control through Surveillance" (HELICS) network for ICUs [4]. Concordance between US and European definitions of pneumonia and primary bloodstream infection exists, and these infections can be compared if some issues are taken into account [5]. In particular, work is being conducted on the definition of ventilator-associated pneumonia (VAP) to decrease the complexity and subjectivity of the definition and to allow for a more reliable assessment and comparison of quality of care for ventilated patients [6].

In 1992, the European Prevalence of Infection in Intensive Care (EPIC) study [7] included data from 1417 ICUs in 17 West European countries and provided valuable information on the prevalence and epidemiology of infection in critically ill European patients. Fifteen years later, the Extended Prevalence of Infection in Intensive Care (EPIC II) study was conducted to provide a picture of the extent and patterns of infection in ICUs worldwide [8]. In 2007, 14,414 patients in 1265 ICUs from 75 countries participated in a one-day point prevalence survey. Of 13,796 patients aged >18 years, 7087 (51%) were considered to be infected. Patients who had longer ICU stays prior to the study day had higher infection rates. Infection prevalence varied markedly by geographical region, ranging from 46% to 60%.

Gram-negative organisms were more commonly isolated than Gram-positive organisms (62% vs. 47%). In patients with positive microbiologic results, the most common Gram-positive organism was *Staphylococcus aureus* (20.5%), including 10.2% of methicillin-resistant *S. aureus* (MRSA); the most common Gram-negative organisms were *Pseudomonas* spp. (19.9%), *Escherichia coli* (16.0%), and *Klebsiella* spp. (12.7%); 17.0% were *Candida* spp. There is a significant relation between the time spent in the ICU before the study day and the development of infection, particularly for infections due to MRSA, *Acinetobacter*, *Pseudomonas*, and *Candida* spp. Significant regional differences in the organisms isolated from microbiologic cultures were described, with a particularly striking variation in the prevalence of *Acinetobacter* spp. (ranging from 3.7% in North America to 19.2% in Asia).

There also was a significant relation between the percentage of infected patients and hospital mortality rate. But being hospitalized in an ICU in a region with high levels of antimicrobial resistance is not associated *per se* with a worse outcome. This likely reflects differences in critical care practices between countries and underlines the importance of controlling for case-mix when interpreting and comparing HAI rates between hospitals or countries.

The frequency of the occurrence of infection may also differ among different sites in the ICU and within a hospital, as well illustrated by the annual United States National Healthcare Safety Network (NHSN) report [9]. While urinary tract infections predominate in general wards, the most common ICU-HAI are lower respiratory tract infections. The type of ICU also plays a role. Infection rates tend to be higher in surgical than in medical ICUs, and higher in adult ICUs than in pediatric units, with the exception of neonatal ICUs. In adult ICUs, the lower respiratory tract is the most common site of infection, whereas bloodstream infections are more prominent in pediatric and neonatal ICUs. High rates of pulmonary infections are unique to adult ICUs, where patients are frequently admitted because of respiratory distress and require mechanical ventilation. Although primary bacteremia and infections due to vascular devices are less common than lower respiratory tract infections, morbidity and mortality associated with these infections are particularly high.

HAI does not only occur individually; they can develop also as outbreaks. Epidemics are associated with specific organisms sometimes introduced from outside and remaining within the ICU because of the continuous selection pressure of antibiotics. These do not necessarily need to be virulent – it is sufficient to be resistant enough in order to persist. Leading pathogens are MRSA, multiresistant non-fermentative Gram-negative rods, such as *Pseudomonas* sp., *Enterobacter* sp., *Serratia* sp., *Stenotrophomonas maltophilia*, and *Acinetobacter* sp., all of which can become longlasting problems. Pathogens producing extended-spectrum beta-lactamases (ESBL), such as *Klebsiella* sp. or *E. coli*, are equally a major concern in many countries worldwide. In some parts of the world, vancomycin-resistant enterococci (VRE) and carbapenem-resistant Enterobacteriae have recently completed this list of worrisome pathogens. Last but not least, non-bacterial pathogens can become a problem, e.g., the steady increase of HAI caused by non-albicans *Candida* sp.

# Control and prevention

Two types of measures are needed to control HAI. Engineering controls are those controls that are incorporated into the structural design of the unit or equipment and over which there is limited human control. Administrative controls are guidelines that must be learned and executed by HCWs. The latter are effective only if appropriate changes in behavior are incorporated into the routine activities of HCWs.

Although resource-demanding, correctly performed surveillance is a condition *sine qua non* for effective infection control. Surveillance may help to define and detect common or unusual sources of cross-infection or failures in care management. It summarizes rates and reports feedback for corrective actions and is best performed by dedicated, specifically trained, infection control staff in close collaboration with the ICU team. Controversy exists over whether surveillance should be continued post-discharge. It is wise to prolong it for a brief period after the patient has left the ICU because ICU-HAI may become evident only in the following days while the patient stays in the general ward. Of note, this approach is labor-intensive and may not always be justified, as few HAI may be detected after discharge. Target-oriented, post-discharge surveillance could be a rational alternative.

Surveillance has a major impact on the incidence of infections. However, to understand the meaning of infection rates implies comparisons. On a micro-epidemiological level, this implies comparison of endemic rates over time within the same population, before and after an intervention or system change, or outbreak detection. Inter-institutional comparison, termed "benchmarking," is increasingly common, with the aim of improving the effectiveness of healthcare and promoting patient safety. Similar comparisons might soon be made between different healthcare settings. Benchmarking among healthcare structures requires meticulous adjustment for case-mix, and failure to adjust adequately for infection-associated factors will erroneously punish commitment to more challenging medical tasks and hinder quality improvement [10]. Standardization of the surveillance method is a second challenge that has to be addressed to make comparisons possible [11]. This obviously clashes with the will to improve and adapt definitions to medical progress and local specificities. Adjustment should be implemented according to variations in the use of microbiological investigation within the different healthcare settings and type of diagnostic techniques applied. Diagnostic power and accuracy largely impact on infection rates. Voluntary participation in a surveillance network, confidentiality, and adequate feedback of results are the prerequisites for healthcare settings' adherence to the method and dedication to data quality. Caution must be used regarding data obtained by mandatory public reporting.

Prevention must be guided by the measurement of indicators that identify gaps and point to the most appropriate solutions. These indicators are composed of HAI rates, structure indicators (e.g., alcohol-based handrub available at the point of care), process indicators (e.g., hand hygiene compliance rates), and audits using checklists to assess whether correct procedures and equipment are in place. This is known as the "recognize–explain–intervene" concept, which was validated for the first time on a large scale by the Study on the Efficacy of Nosocomial Infection Control (SENIC) project carried out in US hospitals in the 1980s [12]. While demonstrating that 35–50% of HAI are preventable by a few fundamental practices (e.g., correct use of urinary catheters and vascular access lines, therapy and support of pulmonary functions, surveillance of surgical procedures, timely hand hygiene, and application of isolation precautions), the SENIC project identified key elements for the success of an infection control program: one infection control nurse per 200–250 beds; one epidemiologist per hospital (1000 beds); organized surveillance for HAI; and systematic feedback of HAI rates to administrators and HCWs. Facing today's challenge in healthcare in general and in ICUs in particular, the respective needs are one infection control nurse per 100–150 acute care hospital beds and one per ~25–35 ICU beds.

HCWs' hands are the principal instruments in the course of complete nursing and highly invasive care in the ICU. Although hand hygiene is the single most important measure to prevent cross-transmission and to reduce the rate of nosocomial colonization and infection, compliance among HCWs is unacceptably low worldwide, usually 30–50%. Explanations for such a low compliance include insufficient time due to high workload, inconvenient access to hand cleansing facilities, inferior priority compared with other patient needs, emergency nature of care, lack of institutional priority for hand hygiene, lack of institutional safety climate, lack of leadership of senior medical and nursing staff, allergy or intolerance to hand hygiene agents, and lack of awareness of recommendations or skepticism regarding their effect on HAI. Not surprisingly, high workload is correlated with an increasing number of hand hygiene opportunities per hour of patient care. To overcome the time constraint factor, hand hygiene indications have been condensed into five moments when action is required during healthcare [13,14] (Figure 5.1). During the past decade the strength of evidence favoring the use of alcohol-based handrubbing, unless hands are visibly soiled, has become simply overwhelming. If actively promoted, the preferential recourse to alcohol-based handrubbing improves compliance with hand hygiene recommendations and reduces HAI and transmission rates [15]. In high-demand settings such as ICUs, handrubbing appears to be the only method that might allow reasonable compliance [16]. Handrubs can be made available at the point of care, for immediate accessibility to reduce time to action as much as possible and to make it realistic to ICU care practices. In addition, alcohol-based handrubs in the form of gels, rinses, or foams containing emollients

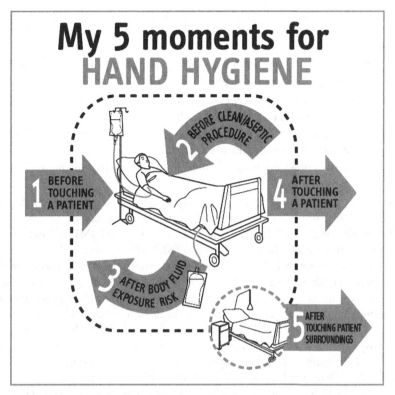

**Figure 5.1** The "my 5 moments for hand hygiene" concept.

Adapted with permission from [13].

are less harmful to the skin than regular handwashing with soap and water. Finally, there is no bacterial resistance to alcohol.

Other selected measures of prime importance in the ICU are standard precautions (the principles are the same throughout the hospital).

Scrutiny by government agencies, competition among hospitals for reputation, and increased awareness by patients and families have all contributed to efforts by hospitals to improve issues like hand hygiene, environmental cleaning, and standardization of practice.

However, it is unclear what proportion of HAI is potentially preventable under routine working conditions. Several reports suggest that great potential exists to decrease HAI rates, from a minimum reduction effect of 10% to a maximum effect of 70%, depending on the setting, study design, baseline infection rates, and type of infection. The most important reduction effect was identified for catheter-related bacteremia, whereas a smaller, but still substantial, potential for prevention seems to exist for other types of HAI.

Although the optimal approach to reducing HAI in critically ill patients is unclear, education-based programs with multiple interventions can decrease infection rates in different ICUs and settings.

The bundle concept was first implemented for the prevention of HAI via improved compliance with hand hygiene [15]. In 2001, the US Institute for Healthcare Improvement (IHI) defined the bundle concept as: "a small set of evidence-based interventions for a defined patient segment/population and care setting that, when implemented together, will result in significantly better outcomes than when implemented individually" [17]. Bundle design guidelines for IHI, are:

- The bundle has three to five interventions (elements), with strong clinician agreement.
- Each bundle element is relatively independent.
- The bundle is used with a defined patient population in one location.
- The multidisciplinary care team develops the bundle.
- Bundle elements should be descriptive rather than prescriptive, to allow for local customization and appropriate clinical judgment.
- Compliance with bundles is measured using all-or-none measurement, with a goal of 95% or greater.

The Ventilator Bundle and the Central Line Bundle were the first bundles developed by IHI (Table 5.1). The Ventilator Bundle was used subsequently in IHI's critical care initiative in the IMPACT network starting in July 2002. Data from 35 ICUs in the IMPACT network showed that, with high Ventilator Bundle compliance (>95%), VAP rates were reduced by 44.5% [18]. In analyzing these improved outcomes, the authors determined that it was more than just measuring these care elements as a bundle that led to success. The changes made to how work was done and how the team interacted contributed to the high levels of performance (>95% compliance with the bundle). Examples of such changes included use of checklists, revising the structure and process of daily multidisciplinary rounds, and use of daily goal sheets.

Many hospitals have continued to use these two bundles in ICU patients and reported on their improved outcomes, which have repeatedly been linked to sustained compliance with the bundle. Others have made local modifications to this bundle and reported on their success as well. For example, a French multifaceted prevention program with eight targeted VAP preventive measures implemented during a 30-month intervention period resulted in a 43% decrease in VAP rates among ICU patients who received mechanical ventilation [19]. But no large randomized study has demonstrated that reducing VAP using any VAP prevention strategy, including those in the IHI bundle, is associated with improvements in clinical outcomes such as mortality. Furthermore, it remains difficult to assess the significance and effect of each individual measure on VAP prevention.

Similar decreasing trends have been published regarding the Central Line Bundle. The Keystone ICU project has demonstrated that a multifactorial approach, including adherence

**Table 5.1** Institute for Heathcare Improvement IHI Infection Prevention Bundles for ICU settings

**IHI Ventilator Bundle**

1. Elevation of the head of the bed to between 30 and 45 degrees.
2. Daily "sedation vacations" and assessment of readiness to extubate.
3. Peptic ulcer disease prophylaxis.
4. Deep venous thrombosis prophylaxis.

**IHI Central Line Bundle**

(A fifth bundle element, "Daily oral care with chlorhexidine," was added in 2010.)

1. Hand hygiene.
2. Maximal barrier precautions.
3. Chlorhexidine skin antisepsis.
4. Optimal catheter site selection, with avoidance of using the femoral vein for central venous access in adult patients.
5. Daily review of line necessity, with prompt removal of unnecessary lines.

to the five evidence-based procedures in the Central Line Bundle, when combined with a daily goals sheet, team training and communication, a unit-based program to improve the safety culture, and other factors, can lead to a sustained reduction, up to 66%, in catheter-related bloodstream infections rates [20]. It is of note that other intervention studies, using multifaceted, multimodal approaches to reduce vascular-catheter infections rates, had shown similar or higher impact in single- or multisite settings, without using the term "bundle" in the methodology applied.

The bundle concept has also been applied in other clinical areas, including sepsis, which also has led to improvements in outcomes.

The use of a bundle appears attractive in many ways, although the choice of practices incorporated in the bundle needs critical evaluation. Consequently, physicians should first consider preventive measures with a demonstrated impact on patient outcomes, such as optimal infection control practices (particularly hand hygiene). Various strategies exist to implement bundles, including educational meetings, feedback, reminders, financial incentives, and revision of professional roles. Unfortunately, there is no superior strategy or so-called magic bullet that works for all innovations in all circumstances. The challenge lies in building a strategy on the careful assessment of barriers and facilitators, and on a coherent theoretical base. Finally, a great deal of attention must be given to factors that might improve adherence with preventive measures.

# References

1. Vincent J.L. Nosocomial infections in adult intensive-care units. *Lancet* 2003;361: 2068–2077.

2. Allegranzi B., Bagheri Nejad S., Combescure C., *et al.* Burden of endemic health-care-associated infection in developing countries: systematic review and meta-analysis. *Lancet* 2011;377:228–241.

3. Horan T.C., Andrus M., Dudeck M.A. CDC/NHSN surveillance definition of health care-associated infection and criteria for specific types of infections in the acute care setting. *Am J Infect Control* 2008;36:309–332.

4. Hospitals in Europe Link for Infection Control through Surveillance (HELICS) Surveillance of Nosocomial infections in intensive care units: master protocol. 2004. http://helics.univ-lyon1.fr/helicshome.htm (accessed 30 October 2012).

5. Hansen S., Sohr D., Geffers C., *et al.* Concordance between European and US case definitions of healthcare-associated infections. *Antimicrob Resist Infect Control* 2012;1:28.

6. Klompas M., Kleinman K., Khan Y., *et al.* Rapid and reproducible surveillance for ventilator-associated pneumonia. *Clin Infect Dis* 2012;54:370–377.

7. Vincent J.L., Bihari D.J., Suter P.M., *et al.* The prevalence of nosocomial infection in intensive care units in Europe: results of the European Prevalence of Infection in Intensive Care (EPIC) Study. EPIC International Advisory Committee. *JAMA* 1995;274:639–644.

8. Vincent J.L., Rello J., Marshall J., *et al.* International study of the prevalence and outcomes of infection in intensive care units. *JAMA* 2009;302:2323–2329.

9. Dudeck M.A., Weiner L.M., Allen-Bridson K., *et al.* National Healthcare Safety Network (NHSN) report, data summary for 2012: device-associated module. *Am J Infect Control* 2013;41:1148–1166.

10. Sax H., Pittet D. Interhospital differences in nosocomial infection rates: importance of case-mix adjustment. *Arch Intern Med* 2002;162:2437–2442.

11. Gastmeier P., Kampf G., Wischnewski N., *et al.* Importance of the surveillance method: national prevalence studies on nosocomial infections and the limits of comparison. *Infect Control Hosp Epidemiol* 1998;19:661–667.

12. Haley R.W., Morgan W.M., Culver D.H., *et al.* Update from the SENIC project: hospital infection control. Recent progress and opportunities under prospective payment. *Am J Infect Control* 1985;13:97–108.

13. Sax H., Allegranzi B., Uckay I., *et al.* 'My five moments for hand hygiene': a user-centred design approach to understand, train, monitor and report hand hygiene. *J Hosp Infect* 2007;67:9–21.

14. World Health Organization. The World Health Organization guidelines on hand hygiene in health care. 2009. http://whqlibdoc.who.int/ publications/2009/9789241597906_eng. pdf?ua=1 (accessed 30 October 2014).

15. Pittet D., Hugonnet S., Harbarth S., *et al.* Effectiveness of a hospital-wide programme to improve compliance with hand hygiene: infection control programme. *Lancet* 2000; 356:1307–1312.

16. Hugonnet S., Perneger T.V., Pittet D. Alcohol-based handrub improves compliance with hand hygiene in intensive care units. *Arch Intern Med* 2002;162:1037–1043.

17. Resar R., Griffin F.A., Haraden C., *et al.* Using care bundles to improve health care quality. IHI Innovation Series white paper. 2012. www.IHI.org (accessed 30 October 2014).

18. Resar R., Pronovost P., Haraden C., *et al.* Using a bundle approach to improve ventilator care processes and reduce ventilator-associated pneumonia. *Jt Comm J Qual Patient Saf* 2005;31:243–248.

19. Bouadma L., Deslandes E., Lolom I., *et al.* Long-term impact of a multifaceted prevention program on ventilator-associated pneumonia in a medical intensive care unit. *Clin Infect Dis* 2010;51:1115–1122.

20. Pronovost P., Needham D., Berenholtz S., *et al.* An intervention to decrease catheter-related bloodstream infections in the ICU. *N Engl J Med* 2006;355: 2725–2732.

# Optimal handover of ICU patients

Marieke Zegers, Nelleke van Sluisveld, and
Hub Wollersheim

Handover of patients is an everyday practice of intensive-care professionals, while physicians and nurses receive little formal training in this important responsibility [1]. Patients who need critical care are admitted to the ICU from the emergency room, operating theatre, or general ward, and discharged to a step-down unit, general ward, or to another intensive care unit (ICU) or hospital. Handovers also take place at change of shift, occurring two or more times daily, seven days a week [1]. The number of handovers has increased as a result of duty hours restrictions of resident physicians and part-time working doctors, resulting in increased opportunities for discontinuity of care.

## Consequences and causes of suboptimal handover

### Consequences

Patient handover is a high-risk episode in patient care. Incomplete or incorrect information transfer and communication errors between healthcare professionals lead to information breakdowns and misunderstandings. As an example, one-third of patients discharged from the ICU have one or more of their chronic medications omitted at hospital discharge. They leave the hospital without a note of their previously prescribed chronic medications [2]. Another study found that communication errors are involved in one-third of major cardio-respiratory events in the ICU, occurring more frequently during the late shift [3].

Information breakdowns may result in poor continuity of care and subsequently in adverse outcomes for patients. These adverse outcomes can be either physical and psychological complications, like feelings of fear, anxiety, and depression; or adverse (drug) events that may ultimately lead to life-threatening situations [4,5]. For example, anaesthesia care transitions are significantly associated with higher rates of in-hospital mortality and morbidity, with incidence rates of 8.8, 11.6, 14.2, 17.0, and 21.2% occurring in patients with 0, 1, 2, 3, and ≥4 transitions, respectively [6].

Other consequences of suboptimal handover procedures are greater healthcare professional and patient dissatisfaction; patients dislike having to answer the same questions over and over again. But also legal claims of malpractice and higher healthcare costs as a result of inefficiencies has been identified, such as avoidable ICU readmissions and rehospitalisations; increased length of ICU and hospital stay; delays in medical diagnoses and treatments; and

*Quality Management in Intensive Care*, ed. Bertrand Guidet, Andreas Valentin and Hans Flaatten. Published by Cambridge University Press. © Cambridge University Press 2016.

over- or underuse of diagnostics, treatments, and medications [5]. Intensive care is the most expensive service provided by hospitals; costs of ICU beds are 3–6 times higher than a ward bed [7,8]. Based on available data, a reduction of the ICU readmission rate by 1%, incorporating an overall mean ICU stay of 6.6 days, could save the US government $1.4 billion per year [7].

## Causes

Patient handover is a complex process. It consists of several tasks, involves a broad range of professionals (e.g. nurses, physicians, allied health professionals, pharmacists) from multiple specialties (e.g., surgery, internal medicine, anaesthesiology, intensive care, emergency care), and it depends on the changing condition of patients, contextual factors, and supporting facilities.

Factors adversely affecting information transfer and communication between professionals can be categorised into five groups [1,5,9]:

1. *Patient risk factors* are older age, physical condition, presence of co-morbidities, polypharmacy, and communication barriers, including consciousness, alertness, language problems, and low health literacy. Critically ill patients are particularly vulnerable to poor handovers because of their complex physiology, their acute and unstable condition, their special needs and the significant decrease in monitoring these patients undergo when transferred to a general ward. In these complex patients, more information should be transferred, resulting in a higher risk of miscommunication and errors.

2. *Individual healthcare professional factors* are lack of knowledge, experience and skills, sensory and information overload, not using protocols, lack of awareness, lack of priority – competing priorities (administrative handover work considered to be burdensome), lack of patient involvement, and conflict between patient preferences and medical needs.

3. *Interpersonal factors (team and cultural factors)* are lack of collaborative attitude, lack of shared communication language (e.g. use of abbreviations), relational problems, lack of mutual respect, inward attitude, lack of leadership support, no feedback culture, hierarchical problems, and confusion about roles and responsibilities.

4. *Organisational factors* are no standardisation, lack of guidelines, policies, protocols, or tools, premature ICU discharge, after-hours discharge (evenings and weekends), high workload, lack of skilled staff, high staff turnover, pressure on available beds, high bed occupancy, lack of training and education, lack of shared information systems, time constraints, and lack of financial resources.

5. *Environmental factors* include interruptions, distractions, chaotic work environment, multitasking, too much noise, and lack of privacy.

# Conceptual model of the handover procedure

## Definition

The term 'handover' refers to 'the process whereby professional responsibility and accountability for some or all aspects of care for a patient, or group of patients, is transferred to another person or professional group on a temporary or permanent basis' [10]. It involves communication of patient care-related information between or among members of healthcare teams during shift changes, when patients are transferred between units or facilities, and during admission, referral, and discharge (see Figure 6.1).

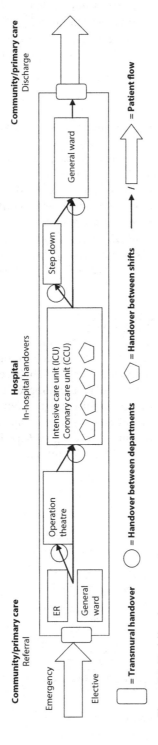

**Figure 6.1** Model handover moments.

The purpose of handover is to provide accurate information about a patient's care and treatment, their preferences, current condition, and any recent or anticipated changes [10]. Effective handovers should facilitate continuity of patient care across care settings, promote coordination of care among healthcare providers, and maintain high-quality, safe patient care [11]. Synonyms for handover are handoff, transfer, transition, sign off, and sign out.

## Settings and persons

Handovers occur in several settings and between several types of healthcare providers. Transmural handovers occur between institutions (nursing homes, hospitals, etc.) and between institution and community (home, primary care, ambulance). In-hospital handovers take place between departments (e.g. from the ER to the operating theatre and from the operating theatre to recovery, ICU, and/or ward), or shifts (between nurses, between physicians, within teams/multidisciplinary handover). The venue where handover takes place is at the patient's bedside or in a central location, e.g. in the professional's work area (staff area) in front of a computer or a whiteboard. The latter is more efficient because of easy access to patient information, and also affords greater privacy. The bedside handovers gives the ability to integrate patient input into the handover and to introduce the patient to the receiving healthcare professional [9,10].

## Components of the handover procedure

Although handover procedures vary considerably, there are commonalities in structure and purpose [9]. Essential components of the procedure of handover are information exchange (the quality of information that is exchanged between healthcare professionals), coordination of care (the quality of assessment, planning, and organisation of diagnostics, treatments, and medications prescribed and provided by different healthcare professionals), and communication (the quality of exchanging information in terms of personal and direct contact, accessibility, and timeliness) (see Figure 6.2). To ensure continuity of care, information needs to be accurate, complete, relevant, understandable/clear, on time, and available [5,12].

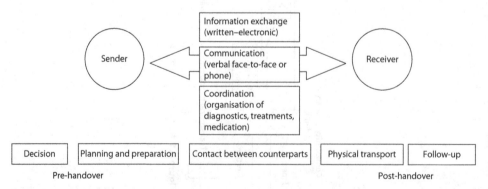

**Figure 6.2** Model handover phases and components.
Adapted from [1,8,9,15,16]

## Handover methods

Methods of handover are verbal (face-to-face or via telephone) and written (orders, documentation on paper or electronic). There have been many studies that show the inadequacies of information transfer using different handover methods. Greenberg and colleagues [13] showed that 92% of the identified information breakdowns in surgical malpractice claims were verbal and the majority occurred between a single transmitter and a single receiver (64%). Another study showed that 20–30% of the information transmitted during handovers is not documented in the medical record [14].

## Phases of the handover process at ICU admission and discharge

Five phases in time of the handover process can be distinguished (see Figure 6.2):

1. Decision (triage) to admit or discharge patients from the ICU. The decision to admit and discharge patients should involve both the patient's consultant and the consultant in critical care. Criteria are used to assess whether patients (still) need intensive care. Admission to intensive care should occur within four hours of making the decision to admit. Minimising delays to definitive treatment is associated with better outcomes [8].

2. Planning and preparation. Avoid transfers between 22:00 and 07:00, since transfers at night are associated with an increased hospital mortality rate and higher ICU readmission rates. Healthcare professionals should ensure timely preparation for the upcoming handover, including organisation and updating information (patient record, progress note, and supporting documentation, e.g. lab test results, anaesthesia chart), and organisation of follow-up services tailored to patient needs and preferences [9,15]. UK standards and guidelines state that the handover from a critical care area should include [8]:
   - a summary of critical care stay including diagnosis, treatment, and changes to chronic therapies;
   - a monitoring and investigation plan including drugs and therapies, nutrition plan, infection status, and any agreed limitations of treatment;
   - a plan for ongoing treatment;
   - physical and rehabilitation needs;
   - psychological and emotional needs;
   - specific communication needs.

3. Actual personal contact and information exchange between healthcare providers. All relevant team members of the sending and receiving team should be present during the handover. Both written information and that the person receiving information understands and accepts transfer of responsibility should be verified. If possible, staff should offer patients information about their condition and encourage them to participate in discussion of plans and goals and in decisions that relate to their recovery [1,15].

4. Physical transport of patient. Because inter- and intrahospital transport of critically ill patients is associated with an increased risk of morbidity and mortality, qualified transport personnel, appropriate transport equipment, and monitoring during transport should be arranged [17].

5. Follow-up. Post-handover time in which the receiving healthcare providers assume the responsibility for providing care and perform patient care tasks pending from the previous shift, as well as newly assigned tasks [14,16].

# Improving the safety and effectiveness of handover procedures

The literature regarding interventions to improve the effectiveness and safety of handover procedures is growing [1,5,9,15,18,19,20,21,22]. A summary of these interventions is given in Table 6.1 and includes standardisation of the handover content and procedure, enhancing verbal communication, coordination, team work, and patient involvement, using electronic tools, and improving the physical work environment.

Standardised handover forms that facilitate timely, complete, and accurate clinical information exchange between healthcare providers and settings lead to a reduction in the incidence of adverse events. Williams and colleagues showed that using a multidisciplinary form and discharge checklist, completed by nurses and the medical staff at ICU discharge, reduced the proportion of preventable adverse events significantly from 65% to 42% [23].

To structure verbal communication, mnemonics can be used. Examples of these are SBAR (situation–background–assessment–recommendation of clinical handover), ISOBAR (identity–situation–observations–background–agreed plan–read back), I PASS the BATON (introduction–patient–assessment–situation–safety concern–the background–actions–timing–ownership–next), HANDOFFS (hospital location–allergies and adverse reactions–name–do not attempt resuscitation–ongoing medical/surgical problems–facts about this hospitalisation–follow-up on–scenarios), and SIGN OUT (sick or DNR–identifying data–general hospital course–new events of the day–overall health status–upcoming possibilities with plan–tasks to complete [9,24].

The teach-back method means that the care provider asks the counterpart professional and/or patient to recall what he or she has just heard, if they understood all information needed, and whether they have any questions (cross-checking). This is an effective method to ensure that the receiving professionals and/or patients understood the information provided, to clarify issues, to improve shared understanding and to detect errors in assessments and plans [5,9].

Liaison persons and critical care outreach teams are useful tools for bridging coordination gaps between healthcare settings and to improve the communication between ICU and ward professionals. Coordination of care of critically ill patients after ICU discharge by a liaison person or critical care outreach team was associated with a reduced risk of ICU readmissions (pooled RR, 0.87 [95% CI, 0.76–0.99]). The risk of ICU readmissions did not depend on the presence of an intensivist in the critical care outreach team [18].

Medication reconciliation at ICU discharge, a standardised procedure using a checklist to identify medication discrepancies and to create an up-to-date complete medication overview, resulted in a dramatic drop in medication errors for patients discharged from an ICU [25].

The evidence of handover interventions is, however, thin and the number of interventions evaluated in the critical care setting is limited [5,9,19,21]. Research on this topic and testing handover interventions in the ICU setting is necessary. Thereafter, one should be aware that the effects of interventions in practice might differ from the research setting because of implementation problems.

# Implementation of handover improvement interventions

Adoption of improvement interventions in clinical practice has proven to be difficult. Figure 6.3 provides insight into the process of the implementation of interventions, and factors influencing this process [26]. The grey boxes reflect the temporal sequence of the implementation process from scientific evidence to improved patient outcomes: (I) scientific research results

**Table 6.1** Handover improvement interventions

### Standardisation of handover documentation and process

Standardised handover forms, templates, discharge letter, clinical decision-support to facilitate structured discharge summary generation

Standardised discharge planning (guidelines, policies, standard operating protocols (SOPs), checklists, tools)

Redesigned handover process

Medication reconciliation: standardised procedure and checklist to identify medication discrepancies and to create an up-to-date complete medication overview at patient handover

Timely communication (verbal communication and up-to-date documentation) – early discharge planning

Follow-up protocol

### Improvement of verbal (face-to-face) communication

Training and education in general communication skills (assertiveness and listening skills)

Teach-back (cross-checking): care providers check whether counterpart and/or patient received and understood all information needed

Verbal *and* visual discharge information

Mnemonics, such as SBAR technique, 5-Ps, I PASS the BATON, HANDOFF, SIGNPOUT, JUMP technique, ISOBAR

### Coordination

Multidisciplinary transition team: face-to-face or telephone meetings between providers of different disciplines

Pre-handover assessments of patient needs and organising post handover services and follow-up

Liaison person coordinating the handover process, follow-up care and communication between healthcare providers from different departments (e.g. liaison nurse, transition coach, pharmacist transition coordinator)

Post-discharge monitoring of follow-up: providing routine follow-up to patients recently discharged from ICU. Visiting patient to evaluate follow-up, giving provider additional instructions and answering questions (e.g. consulting nurse, critical care outreach team)

### Team work/culture

Team training: training in team skills and communication; address hierarchical and social issues; discuss social and cultural norms

Meetings between care providers of different departments/specialties to increase mutual understanding and respect between parties

Stimulate structural feedback (standard feedback forms along with discharge information)

### Patient-targeted interventions

Patient or caregiver education

Patient-centred discharge instructions

Use of patient-friendly, non-medical language: discharge summary in language that is understandable for patients and relatives

### Electronic tools/information technology

Shared electronic information system: multi-disciplinary electronic patient record accessible for all relevant stakeholders (healthcare providers and patients)

Electronic reminders for writing handover summaries

Mandatory administrative tasks

Electronic Patient Journey Board

Electronic tools to facilitate quick and clear handover summary generation

### Environmental strategies

Choose a quiet and dedicated location to limit interruptions and distraction

Complete urgent clinical tasks before the information transfer

Allow only patient-specific discussions during verbal handovers

Require that all relevant team members be present

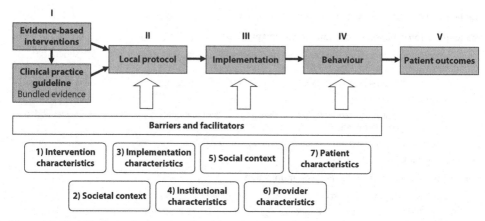

**Figure 6.3** Model for the implementation of guidelines and interventions.

in evidence about effective interventions that are recommended in clinical practice guidelines; (II) the evidence should be tailored to local circumstances in local protocols; (III) implementation efforts, such as a detailed and feasible implementation plan, and engaging stakeholders at an early stage, will improve the implementation process; leading to (IV) improved healthcare professional behaviour and adherence to the intervention; and ultimately resulting in (V) improved patient outcomes. Several factors influence the implementation process and could explain why effective and evidence-based interventions are not (fully) implemented. Barriers and facilitators to implementation can be categorised in seven main domains, represented by the white boxes in Figure 6.3. The domains are related to the (1) characteristics of the intervention, (2) societal context, (3) characteristics of the implementation efforts, (4) characteristics of the healthcare facility, (5) social context (e.g. interpersonal, interdepartmental, and interinstitutional relationships), (6) professional characteristics, and (7) patient characteristics [26].

Several guides, checklists, and toolboxes exist to guide the implementation process of handover improvement programmes and to tackle the factors that may influence this process [11,27,28]. Common mentioned strategies are:

- Education and training to creating awareness of the consequences of suboptimal handover procedures and to give insight into existing interventions to improve handovers. Training in handover should be part of the medical and nursing curriculum [1,5,22].
- Organisation-wide governance and leadership to support effective handover policy, procedures, and resources, including dedicated staff time, appropriate requirements, and training [11].
- Staff involvement in the development of the intervention programme, guidelines, protocols, tools, policies, procedures, implementation strategies, and training programmes. Commitment from and ownership by the target group is essential to successful implementation. Uptake of policies and interventions is enhanced when they are involved from the beginning of the process of improving the handover procedure [1,5].
- An ongoing evaluation of the effects of the implementation will ensure future adaption of the improvement intervention [11].

## Evaluation of the handover process and improvements

The development and effect evaluation of a strategy to improve handovers in local settings starts with measuring the quality of current handover practice. The following measures are available: scores on patient outcomes related to handover (e.g. ICU readmissions, adverse (drug) events, mortality after ICU discharge, patient satisfaction); quality gaps in the handover procedure (e.g. information gaps, amount of time for handover, number of interruptions, adherence to handover protocols and interventions); and presence of causal factors for suboptimal handover.

Several evaluation techniques are available to assess the quality of handovers using information from (video) observations of handover situations, audio recordings of handover communication, interviews with healthcare professionals and patients, surveys, and studying documents, including patient records and progress notes [11,29–31]. With a systematic insight into local problems, best practices can be selected tailored to the identified barriers for effective handover and to local needs. Given the wide variety of factors influencing the handover process, handover improvement interventions need to be multifaceted and integrated into a so-called intervention programme [5,26].

## References

1. L.A. Riesenberg, J. Leitzsch, J.M. Cunningham. Nursing handoffs: a systematic review of the literature. *Am J Nurs* 2010; 110: 24–34.

2. C.M. Bell, P. Rahimi-Darabad, A.I. Orner. Discontinuity of chronic medications in patients discharged from the intensive care unit. *J Gen Intern Med* 2006; 21: 937–941.

3. M. Williams, N. Hevelone, R.F. Alban, *et al.* Measuring communication in the surgical ICU: better communication equals better care. *J Am Coll Surg* 2010; 210: 17–22.

4. S. Bench, T. Day. The user experience of critical care discharge: a meta-synthesis of qualitative research. *Int J Nurs Stud* 2010; 47: 487–499.

5. G. Hesselink, M. Zegers, M. Vernooij-Dassen, *et al.* Improving patient discharge and reducing hospital readmissions by using Intervention Mapping. *BMC Health Serv Res* 2014; 14: 389.

6. L. Saager, B.D. Hesler, J. You, *et al.* Intraoperative transitions of anesthesia care and postoperative adverse outcomes. *Anesthesiology* 2014; 121: 695–706.

7. N.A. Halpern, S.M. Pastores. Critical care medicine in the United States 2000-2005: an analysis of bed numbers, occupancy rates, payer mix, and costs. *Crit Care Med* 2010; 38: 65–71.

8. National Institute for Health and Care Excellence. Acutely ill patients in hospital: Recognition of and response to acute illness in adults in hospitals. 2007. www.nice.org.uk/guidance/cg50/resources/guidance-acutely-ill-patients-in-hospital-pdf (accessed 23 October 2014).

9. D.S. Cheung, J.J. Kelly, C. Beach, *et al.* Improving handoffs in the emergency department. *Ann Emerg Med* 2010; 55: 171–180.

10. Australian Commission on Safety and Quality in Health Care. Safety and quality improvement guide standard 6: clinical handover. 2012. www.safetyandquality.gov.au/wp-content/uploads/2012/10/Standard6_Oct_2012_WEB.pdf (accessed 23 October 2014).

11. Australian Commission on Safety and Quality in Health Care. OSSIE guide to clinical handover improvement. 2010. www.safetyandquality.gov.au/wp-content/uploads/2012/01/ossie.pdf (accessed 23 October 2014).

12. R. Hellesø, M. Lorensen, L. Sorensen. Challenging the information gap: the patient's transfer from hospital to home health care. *Int J Med Inform* 2004; 73: 569–580.

13. C.C. Greenberg, S.E. Regenbogen, D.M. Studdert, *et al.* Patterns of communication breakdowns resulting in injury to surgical patients. *J Am Coll Surg* 2007; 204: 533–540.

14. E.S. Patterson, R.L. Wears. Patient handoffs: standardized and reliable measurement tools remain elusive. *Jt Comm J Qual Patient Saf* 2010; 36: 52–61.

15. N. Segall, A.S. Bonifacio, R.A. Schroeder, *et al.* Can we make postoperative patient handovers safer? A systematic review of the literature. *Anesth Analg* 2012; 115: 102–115.

16. J. Abraham, T.G. Kannampallil, V.L. Patel. Bridging gaps in handoffs: a continuity of care based approach. *J Biomed Inform* 2012; 45: 240–254.

17. J. Warren, R.E. Fromm, R.A. Orr, *et al.* Guidelines for the inter- and intrahospital transport of critically ill patients. *Crit Care Med* 2004; 32: 256–262.

18. D.J. Niven, J.F. Bastos, H.T. Stelfox. Critical care transition programs and the risk of readmission or death after discharge from an ICU: a systematic review and meta-analysis. *Crit Care Med* 2014; 42: 179–187.

19. M.C. Wong, K.C. Yee, P. Turner. A structured evidence-based literature review regarding the effectiveness of improvement interventions in clinical handover. 2008. eHealth Services Research Group, University of Tasmania, Australia.

20. L.O. Hanssen, R.S. Young, K. Hinami, *et al.* Interventions to reduce 30-day rehospitalisation: a systematic review. *Ann Intern Med* 2011; 155: 520–528.

21. S. Rennke, O.K. Nguyen, M.H. Shoeb, *et al.* Hospital-initiated transitional care interventions as a patient safety strategy: a systematic review. *Ann Intern Med* 2013; 158: 433–440.

22. L.A. Riesenberg, J. Leitzsch, J.L. Massucci, *et al.* Residents' and attending physicians' handoffs: a systematic review of the literature. *Acad Med* 2009; 84: 1775–1787.

23. T.A. Williams, G.D. Leslie, N. Elliott, *et al.* Introduction of discharge plan to reduce adverse events within 72 hours of discharge from the ICU. *J Nurs Care Qual* 2010; 25: 73–79.

24. L.A. Riesenberg, J. Leitzsch, B.W. Little. Systematic review of handoff mnemonics literature. *Am J Med Qual* 2009; 24: 196–204.

25. P. Pronovost, B. Weast, M. Schwarz, *et al.* Medication reconciliation: a practical tool to reduce the risk of medication errors. *J Crit Care* 2003; 18: 201–205.

26. N. van Sluisveld, M. Zegers, G. Westert, *et al.* A strategy to enhance the safety and efficacy of handovers of ICU patients: study protocol of the pICUp study. *Implement Sci* 2013; 14: 67.

27. H. Drachsler, W. Kicken, M. van der Klink, *et al.* The handover toolbox: a knowledge exchange and training platform for improving patient care. *BMJ Qual Saf* 2012; 21: i114–120.

28. New South Wales Department of Health. Implementation toolkit: standard key principles for clinical handover. 2009. www.archi.net.au/documents/resources/qs/clinical/clinical-handover/implementation-toolkit.pdf (accessed 23 October 2014).

29. T. Manser, S. Foster, S. Gisin, *et al.* Assessing the quality of patient handoffs at care transitions. *Qual Saf Health Care* 2010; 19: e44.

30. B.W. Pickering, K. Hurley, B. Marsh. Identification of patient information corruption in the intensive care unit: using a scoring tool to direct quality improvements in handover. *Crit Care Med* 2009; 37: 2905–2912.

31. J. Apker, L.A. Mallak, E.B. Applegate III, *et al.* Exploring emergency physician–hospitalist handoff interactions: development of the Handoff Communication Assessment. *Ann Emerg Med* 2010; 55: 161–170.

# Diagnostic pathways

### Hans Flaatten

To achieve the correct diagnosis is frequently a challenge in the ICU setting. Naturally, a correct diagnosis is essential for the appropriate treatment, and is hence often included in therapeutic bundles, such as the Surviving Sepsis campaign [1]. The challenge in critically ill patients is that we often have limited time to achieve a certain diagnosis, and very often have to start treatment of a suspected diagnosis immediately. The ultimate example is, of course, cardiac arrest, where appropriate CPR has to be started immediately, most often with little or no knowledge of the cause of cardiac arrest.

Another problem is that intensivists in the first phase of intensive care are more occupied with the immediate consequence of disease or trauma than the initiating underlying causes. The immediate consequences are most often described as acute organ dysfunction(s) and also have to be given first priority in the initial phase.

On the other hand, it is obviously vital for patient recovery that the intensivists at an early stage also start to look for the cause or causes of the acute organ dysfunction(s). In that respect it may be of importance to have clear steps for further diagnosis, or the diagnostic pathways. Figure 7.1 highlights these three parallel processes run during the first 'golden' hours in the ICU.

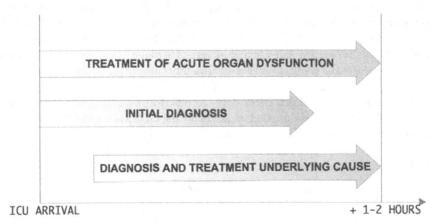

TREATMENT OF ACUTE ORGAN DYSFUNCTION

INITIAL DIAGNOSIS

DIAGNOSIS AND TREATMENT UNDERLYING CAUSE

ICU ARRIVAL                                    + 1-2 HOURS

**Figure 7.1** Initial priority in the first 1–2 hours after admission. Showing how treatment and diagnosis of acute organ dysfunction have initial priority, but increasingly important are diagnosis (and hence treatment) of the underlying processes.

*Quality Management in Intensive Care*, ed. Bertrand Guidet, Andreas Valentin and Hans Flaatten. Published by Cambridge University Press. © Cambridge University Press 2016.

# Diagnostic pathways: acute organ dysfunction

Any acute admission to the ICU should immediately have an assessment of organ dysfunction performed. This is primarily a clinical evaluation of the patient using the ABCDE approach [2]:

A. Airway: check for patency; if intubated before admission, confirm correct position of the endotracheal tube.
B. Breathing: see, feel, and listen for signs of breathing; if ventilated, check ventilator settings, in particular tidal volume and $EtCO_2$.
C. Circulation:
   a. First, check for adequate flow (perfusion): skin (mottled, capillary refill time, temperature); patient awake and responding; urinary output.
   b. Second, acquire ABP, HR, and oxygen saturation ($SpO_2$).
D. Disability, using the Glasgow Coma Scale.
E. Exposure, undress and inspect the body.

The outcomes of the clinical examination give the backbone for final evaluation of acute organ dysfunctions. For a formal evaluation it is of great help to use a validated organ dysfunction score (ODS). There are three frequently used ODSs; all have in common that they screen for acute organ dysfunction in six vital organ systems (see also Table 7.1):

1. respiratory
2. circulatory
3. renal
4. CNS
5. hepatic
6. haematology/coagulation.

Using one of the ODSs will give you a 'snapshot' of organ dysfunction status, both the number of organs in failure and their severity. All three systems assign a number from normal function to severe dysfunction using five grades, where 0 indicates a normal function [3]. Although some of the organ screenings require results of blood-chemistry variables, most of the information should be readily available within a short time in the ICU and from the initial clinical assessment.

By using a standardised clinical chemistry screen performed at ICU admittance that also includes the relevant organ dysfunction variables for the ODS assessment, the final calculation can usually be performed within 1–2 hours after ICU admission.

**Table 7.1** Commonly used organ dysfunction scoring systems

| Dysfunction | SOFA | MODS | LODS |
|---|---|---|---|
| Respiration | $PaO_2/FiO_2$ | $PaO_2/FiO_2$ | $PaO_2/FiO_2$ |
| Circulation | MAP and vasopressors | HR × (MAP/CVP) | HR and SBP |
| Renal | Creatinine and urine | Creatinine | Urea and creatinine |
| CNS | GCS | GCS | GCS |
| Hepatic | Bilirubin | Bilirubin | Bilirubin and PT |
| Hematologic | Platelets | Platelets | Platelets and WBC |

MAP = mean arterial pressure, HR = heart rate, CVP = central venous pressure, SBP = systolic blood pressure, GCS = Glasgow Coma Scale, PT = prothrombin time, WBC = white blood cell count

Usual biochemical markers for ODS are:
- Renal function: creatinine and urea
- Hepatic function: bilirubin
- Coagulation: platelets and white blood count (WBC).

Having the ODS at admission makes it possible to follow the development of organ dysfunction during the ICU stay, and hence get a numerical or graphical expression of the burden of OD.

The severity and number of OD have direct impact on the possibility of survival, and in particular an increase in ODS from admittance to day three may indicate a grave prognosis [4].

## Diagnostic pathways: severe trauma

Diagnostic pathways in severe or multi-trauma patients differ somewhat to the process in non-traumatic patients. Initially, most often these patients are handled in the ER, usually by a dedicated trauma team in a trauma centre, which has been shown to improve outcomes [5]. The trauma team is responsible for the initial ABCDE approach, immediate stabilisation, and direct diagnostic work-up. When these patients arrive in the ICU, it is usually after several diagnostic and/or surgical procedures have been performed.

The goal of the initial diagnostic assessment is to reveal any life-threatening injuries and prioritise them. Perhaps diagnostic pathways are most developed and used during the initial phase of severe trauma admission. Such an approach has been a focus for a long time and today there are strict guidelines, dedicated trauma centres, and standardised educational courses available [6]. A strict diagnostic path in this patient group leads to early diagnosis and treatment, and is potentially life saving.

The ABCDE approach as explained previously is used also in this setting, but with some additional diagnostic procedures: usually a chest X-ray will be taken during the initial assessment, and a focused assessment with sonography (FAST; ultrasound) to screen for thoracic and abdominal injuries or fluid (blood) and increasingly a echocardiogram is performed as well.

## Diagnostic pathways: the underlying disease

As illustrated in Figure 7.2, as soon as initial stabilisation of OD is started, the process to identify the underlying disease process also has to be given priority. This work may be difficult, and is an area where we often lack specific diagnostic pathways, but frequently includes evaluation and re-evaluation of the patient.

Some key elements in the diagnostic process of the critically ill patient can be identified:
- past history;
- presentation and symptoms of acute illness prior to ICU admission;
- profile and severity of organ dysfunction;
- arterial blood-gas analysis;
- extended biochemical analysis including electrolytes, infection, and metabolic markers;
- chest X-ray and 12-lead ECG;
- ECHO cardiography;
- microbiology cultures (when indicated).

This process requires experience and cooperation across specialities, and will frequently also necessitate more diagnostic work-up using CT scanning, MRI, and increasingly invasive radiology imaging.

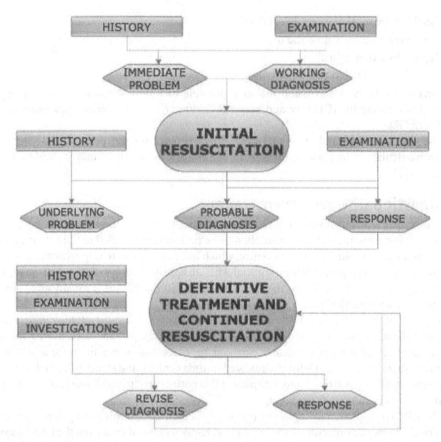

**Figure 7.2** The complex interaction leading to definitive treatment and diagnosis in the critically ill patient.

Bear in mind that the most frequently found disorders of critical illness are also the most often encountered – 'if you hear the sound of hooves, it's usually a horse, not a zebra', at least in Europe.

## Diagnostic pathways: specific diseases

Some important and specific diagnoses and syndromes have received particular attention during the last 20 years. Most notably this includes acute respiratory distress syndrome (ARDS), severe sepsis, and acute kidney injury (AKI). There are several reasons for this:

- Harmonising the understanding of the disease, and hence making therapy more target oriented.
- Getting a more uniform description of what constitutes a disease.
- Making registries and research conform more with regards to these disorders, and hence comparison between centres more reliable

## ARDS

ARDS was first described in 1967, but this specific pulmonary problem had probably been around for a long time. The description led to a focus on the ARDS, and several different definitions were used both clinically and in research. The lack of consensus-based diagnostic

**Table 7.2** Berlin ARDS definition

|  | Mild ARDS | Moderate ARDS | Severe ARDS |
| --- | --- | --- | --- |
| Timing | <1 week since clinical insult or worsening respiratory symptoms | | |
| Chest imaging | Bilateral opacities not fully explained by other defined pathology | | |
| Origin of oedema | Not fully explained by cardiac failure or fluid overload.# | | |
| PaO$_2$/FiO$_2$ ratio* | 40–27.7 kPa | 27.7–13.3 kPa | <13.3 kPa |

#Will need objective assessment (echocardiography).
*with PEEP >5 cm H$_2$O.

criteria led to an American–European consensus conference in 1994, where diagnostic criteria for ARDS were agreed.

The definition was quickly embraced by the intensive care community, and led to several large ARDS trials all over the world. Eighteen years later it was necessary to adjust the definition, partly because the 1994 consensus obviously needed improvement, and new knowledge of the syndrome had emerged. The new definition – the 2012 Berlin definition [7] – has again been adopted by intensivists worldwide.

The Berlin definition of ARDS uses three severities, and four different criteria (Table 7.2).

## Severe sepsis

Since the launch of the Surviving Sepsis campaign in 2004 [1], a particular focus has been on early identification of this syndrome. However, prior to this campaign several consensus conferences had been held, the two most important in 1992 and 2001. The original definition from 1992 still holds its place and defines sepsis as the body's systemic response to a suspected or proven infection. This response is characterised by:

- increased heart rate;
- increased respiratory rate;
- hypo- or hyperthermia; and
- leukopenia/leucocytosis.

Severe sepsis is then understood as sepsis with at least one severe organ dysfunction/failure. Originally, organ failure was poorly defined, and made little room for grading of the organ dysfunction. Hence several investigations have advocated the use of a specific organ failure assessment system, and particularly the SOFA score has been frequently used [8] (see also Table 7.1).

The mortality from severe sepsis has declined steadily since 2000, most probably because of increased awareness, early diagnosis, and using standardised care more than a breakthrough in the treatment of this condition [9]. Early diagnosis and treatment is often presented together in various 'sepsis bundles'.

## Acute kidney injury

Another major diagnostic challenge has been AKI, formerly often named acute renal failure. In contrast to its counterpart, chronic renal failure, the acute form for a long time was ill-defined, and most researchers presented their own set of criteria for its detection. As in all organ dysfunction, this is not an on/off phenomenon and undergoes stages from light, through moderate and severe AKI. Today there are still several different scoring systems, including the SOFA score, which also has stages for level of AKI. The more recently introduced versions are

**Table 7.3** KDIGO staging and definition of AKI [10]

| Stage | S-creatinine | Urine output |
|---|---|---|
| 1 | 1.5 to 1.9 × baseline value OR increase ≥ 26.5 µmol/l (0.3 mg/dl) | <0.5 ml/kg/h 6–12 h |
| 2 | 2.0 to 2.9 × baseline values | <0.5 ml/kg/h ≥ 12 h |
| 3 | ≥3 × baseline value, OR value ≥ 353.6 µmol/l (≥4.0 mg/dl) | <0.3 ml/kg/h ≥ 24 h OR anuria > 12 hours |

AKIN and RIFLE definitions, which are very similar. The network Kidney Disease: Improving Global Outcomes recently launched their definition (Table 7.3), with three stages of AKI according to serum creatinine and urine output.

# Diagnostic pathways: complications

Besides the diagnostic pathways described above, two more diagnoses need to be discussed. These are infrequently present at admission and are usually considered to be a complication or consequence of critical care.

## Ventilator associated pneumonia (VAP)

Pneumonia that develops during invasive ventilation, VAP, is often considered to be a complication from mechanical ventilation or, more precisely, from the endotracheal tube. It is usual to restrict this diagnosis to pneumonia occurring beyond 48 hours of intubation/intermittent positive pressure ventilation (IPPV). Pneumonia occurring prior to this time will often have other explanations. VAP is to a large extent considered to be preventable, and its occurrence is usually measured in number of occurrences (VAP episodes) per 1000 ventilation days, and was recently found to vary from 13 to 51 per 1000 days [11].

Diagnosis of VAP has for a long time been difficult. The intensive care setting frequently obscures the traditional clinical signs and symptoms of pneumonia. However, a likely diagnosis can be performed using clinical data readily available with support from chest X-ray and microbiological cultures of tracheal secretions. Attempts to put these findings into a formalised score (Clinical Pulmonary Infection Score, Table 7.4) have, however, not given a very high sensitivity or specificity in the diagnosis of VAP.

In order to reduce or prevent VAP several quality improvement (QI) programmes have been introduced in ICUs worldwide, and there are several evidence-based procedures shown to reduce the occurrence:

- meticulous hand hygiene;
- sterile techniques during ET manipulations (ex. suctioning);
- use of chlorhexidine oral/dental solutions;
- removal of sub-glottis secretions.

However, since the diagnosis is difficult, and probably varies from unit to unit, it may be difficult to compare VAP across units unless a strict common set of criteria are used.

## ICU delirium

Also called the 'ICU syndrome', acute delirium is a very common occurrence in ICU patients, and is reported in between 30% and 83% of all patients in various types of ICU [13]. Acute delirium is defined in the DSM-IV as [14]:

1. A disturbance of consciousness (i.e. reduced clarity of awareness of the environment) is evident, with reduced ability to focus, sustain, or shift attention.

**Table 7.4** Clinical pulmonary infection score (CIPS)

| Measurement | 0 point | 1 point | 2 point |
|---|---|---|---|
| Temperature | 36.5–38.4 | 38.5–38.9 | >39 or <36 |
| LPK | 4–11 | <4 or >11 | >50% immature |
| Tracheal secretions | None or scant | Non-purulent | Purulent |
| $PaO_2/FiO_2$ kPa | >30 or >ARDS | | <30 w/o ARDS |
| Infiltrates (X-ray) | None | Diffuse or patchy | Localised |
| Existing infiltrates | No change | | Increasing |
| Aspirate growth | None | Moderate to high | = Gram stain |
| If CIPS ≥ 5 points, it is likely that a VAP is present [12] | | | |

2. There is a change in cognition (such as memory deficit, disorientation, language disturbance) or the development of a perceptual disturbance that is not better accounted for by a pre-existing or evolving dementia.
3. The disturbance develops over a short period of time (usually hours to days) and tends to fluctuate during the course of the day.
4. There is evidence from the history, physical examination, or laboratory findings that the disturbance is caused by the direct physiological consequences of a general medical condition.

One of the difficulties with this rather broad definition is to put these four criteria into a meaningful context in everyday life in the ICU. To screen for delirium, more simple and dedicated screening tools have been developed, and one of the most frequently used and translated is the Confusion Assessment Method for the ICU: CAM-ICU [15]. It is dedicated to reveal changes in the four items mentioned above:

1. Is there an acute change from mental status baseline? If YES:
2. Simple tests of inattention (if >2 errors go to 3).
   a. Example: 'squeeze my hand when I say the letter A'.
3. Altered level of consciousness: use the RASS level; if RASS = 0, go to 4.
4. Simple questions for disorganised thinking:
   a. Example 'will a stone float on water?'.

Using these simple methods, ideally one per nurse-shift, will create an effective screening process regarding the development and length of ICU delirium, and will hopefully diagnose patients who would otherwise be left undiagnosed. This is particularly true for hypoactive delirium, where the patient is not agitated.

Use of CAM-ICU (or a similar screening test) at regular intervals and its completeness (i.e. how many of the potential times CAM-ICU was really used) is a frequently used QI (process indicator).

# Diagnostic pathways: conclusions and areas for improvement

If the ICU is to provide systematic diagnostic pathways or not can be considered a process quality indicator for the ICU. The following is a quick checklist that can be used for quality improvement in the ICU:

- Is there a systematic ABCDE approach performed in all acute admissions?
- Does the ICU perform a formal organ dysfunction evaluation using a validated scoring system?

- Is there a standardised (automated) initial haematology-screening at admission including the following?
  - organ dysfunction markers
  - infection markers
  - metabolic markers
  - electrolytes (including Mg, Ph, Ca).
- Is there a standardised severe trauma approach at the hospital?
- Is the following performed within 30–60 minutes after ICU admission?
  - ABG
  - chest X-ray
  - ECG
  - ECCO
  - relevant microbiology cultures.
- Is the ICU using standard diagnostic criteria to document the following?
  - ARDS
  - severe sepsis
  - AKI
  - VAP
  - delirium
- Is there a discussion with relevant specialities performed as soon as possible after acute ICU admission?

# References

1. Dellinger R.P., Levy M.M., Rhodes A., *et al.* Surviving Sepsis campaign: international guidelines for management of severe sepsis and septic shock, 2012. *Intensive Care Med.* 2013; 39:165–228.

2. Thim T., Krarup N.H.V., Grove E.L., Rohde C.V., Løfgren B. Initial assessment and treatment with the Airway, Breathing, Circulation, Disability, Exposure (ABCDE) approach. *Int J Gen Med.* 2012; 5:117–121.

3. Strand K., Flaatten H. Severity scoring in the ICU: a review. *Acta Anaesthesiol Scand.* 2008; 52: 467–478.

4. Flaatten H., Gjerde S., Guttormsen A.B., *et al.* Outcome after acute respiratory failure is more dependent on dysfunction in other vital organs than on the severity of the respiratory failure. *Crit Care.* 2003; 7(4):R72.

5. Demetriades D., Martin M., Salim A., Rhee P., Brown C., Chan L. The effect of trauma center designation and trauma volume on outcome in specific severe injuries. *Ann Surg.* 2005; 242:512–517; discussion 517–519.

6. McCullough A.L., Haycock J.C., Forward D.P., Moran C.G. Early management of the severely injured major trauma patient. *Brit J Anaesth.* 2014; 113(2):234–241.

7. The ARDS definition Task Force TADT. Acute Respiratory Distress Syndrome: the Berlin definition. *JAMA.* 2012; 307(23):2526–2533.

8. Vincent J.L., Moreno R., Takala J., *et al.* The SOFA (Sepsis-related Organ Failure Assessment) score to describe organ dysfunction/failure. *Intensive Care Med.* 1996; 22:707–710.

9. The ARISE Investigators and the ANZICS Clinical Trials Group. Goal-directed resuscitation for patients with early septic shock. *N Engl J Med.* 2014; 371:1496–1506.

10. KDIGO Clinical practice guideline for acute kidney injury. *Kidney Int.* 2012; 2:1–138.

11. Kollef M.H., Chastre J., Fagon J.-Y., *et al.* Global prospective epidemiologic and surveillance study of ventilator-associated pneumonia due to *Pseudomonas aeruginosa*. *Crit Care Med.* 2014; 42:2178–2187.

12. Celik O., Koltka N., Devrim S., *et al.* Clinical pulmonary infection score calculator in the early diagnosis and treatment of ventilator-associated pneumonia in the ICU. *Crit Care* 2014; 18 (suppl 1): P304.

13. Young J., Murthy L., Westby M., Akunne A., O'Mahony R. Diagnosis, prevention, and management of delirium: summary of NICE guidance. *BMJ.* 2010; 341:c3704.

14. American Psychiatric Association. *Task Force on DSM-IV. Diagnostic and Statistical Manual Of Mental Disorders.* 4th edition. Washington, DC: American Psychiatric Association, 2009.

15. Ely E.W., Inouye S.K., Bernard G.R., *et al.* Delirium in mechanically ventilated patients: validity and reliability of the confusion assessment method for the intensive care unit (CAM-ICU). *JAMA.* 200(286):2703–2710.

# Chapter 8

# Transport of ICU patients

Carole Schwebel, Claire Fossard, and Clémence Minet

## Introduction

Moving from a stationary safe ICU is a common procedure in critical care daily practice required for diagnostic or therapeutic procedures not available at bedside, so half to two-thirds of ICU patients will experience at least one transport during their ICU stay [1–3].

Local organization and regionalized critical care induces an increase in the number of intra- and also inter-hospital transports [4]. Transport of ICU patients is challenging and comes with a risk of incidents and adverse events with considerable parallels between inter- and intra-hospital transfers of the critically ill patient [2,4–7].

Numerous studies in different ICU settings – adults, children, or neonates – have reported intra-hospital-related adverse events as early per-procedural complications or secondary late insults [1,7,8]. The ongoing multicenter multinational study initiated in fall 2014 on patient safety during intra-hospital transport of ICU patients endorsed by the European Society of Intensive Care Medicine highlights interest in and the importance of this field [9]. Contributing factors are identified, and many of them are preventable [10–12]. As part of an ICU stay, quality and safety also apply to transport periods. High incidence and impact of transport-related adverse events justify a dedicated policy using preventive strategies to ensure safe and secure procedures inside and outside ICUs, as well as – especially – during transportation of critically ill patients [13,14].

Quality issues targeting transport should comprise: (1) basic medical skills in critical care for caregivers involved in transport; (2) selection and preparation of the patient, including an appropriate escort for the patient's condition and equipment; (3) knowledge of transport equipment and monitoring; (4) anticipation of possible medication shortages and ruptures; (5) documentation of any incident complication or intervention during transport for feed-back analysis in a continuous quality improvement program [13,14].

## Transport of ICU patients: a core element of critical care practice

Transport of critically ill patients is required in daily practice for diagnostic or therapeutic or any additional procedure, including surgery not available at bedside. Advanced diagnostics and procedures and access to specialized care are routinely needed during ICU stays in emergency or elective situations for clinically stable or unstable patients, potentially carrying complex equipment. Patients requiring transport have significantly higher severity scores at

*Quality Management in Intensive Care*, ed. Bertrand Guidet, Andreas Valentin and Hans Flaatten. Published by Cambridge University Press. © Cambridge University Press 2016.

admission into ICU, and greater use of vasopressors and mechanical ventilation, describing linkage between ICU transports and severity of illness [1,2]. Need for transport occurs early in the ICU stay; half of all first transports occur during the first 24 hours of ICU admission [2]. Reported diagnoses triggering transports are mostly respiratory failure, coma, and sepsis [1,4]. Feasibility of complex transports requiring extensive logistic support (e.g., ECMO, intra-aortic balloon) has been studied [15].

In 100 consecutive surgical patients requiring intra-hospital transport (IHT), 84% of those transports were for abdominal CT scan, head CT scan, or angiography [16].

In a large multicenter cohort study, 28.5% of ICU ventilated patients experienced $1.7 \pm 1.3$ intra-hospital transports and up to 17 transports per patient were required during the ICU stay. Excluding the operating room, the most frequent destinations are the CT scan room (93.6%), MRI department (5.52%), and the nuclear medicine or interventional radiology suite (0.5%). Few procedures have concerned combined transportation (0.65%) [1].

As the radiology suite is the major destination, use of portable CT scans have been proposed as an alternative to transport of ICU patients, despite previously reported inferior radiological quality compared to conventional stationary imaging. Feasibility and safety of portable equipment has been assessed in the ICU population. Important diagnostic information with subsequent therapeutic impact without requiring patient transport outside the ICU has been reported either in routine follow-up or emergency procedure [17,18]. However, numerous complex clinical situations require advanced diagnostics procedures not available at bedside, making transport unavoidable.

# Transporting ICU patients: a risky procedure

During transport, the secure surroundings of the ICU are replaced by an unfavorable environment that may be more or less controlled than the ICU, leading to potential mishaps from various origins in respect of the severity of illness and clinical features at departure, typology, and equipment of patients, and transport pattern itself [3,14]. As part of the ICU stay, the same level of care – including physiologic monitoring, ongoing delivery of organ support, prompt recognition and emergency intervention for life-threatening conditions – is expected during transport.

Numerous studies on out-of-ICU patient transports have reported adverse events in adult, children, and neonates populations following procedural complications or delayed injuries [1–3,6–8].

Removal of patients from ICU during IHT is associated with an overall complications rate of up to 70% [3,6], depending on different classifications and definitions for adverse events. Reported events range from physiological changes with no clinical relevance to life-threatening situations and to death [1,3,14].

The impact of IHT on patient outcome has been documented in literature through various study designs. A cross-sectional analysis of 191 incidents during IHT identified 55 (31%) serious adverse events, including physiological derangement (15%), patient/relative dissatisfaction (7%), prolonged hospital stay (4%), physical/psychological injury (3%), and death (2%) [10].

IHT was associated with a significant risk for development of VAP in an exposed/non-exposed matched monocenter cohort study [8]. In a two-year retrospective monocenter study in a critically ill cancer-based population, authors reported higher hospital mortality rates in transported patients than in non-transported ICU patients [2].

In a large, unselected ICU population, IHT was associated with a significant increase in the risk of experiencing at least one incident (OR 1.85, 95% CI [1.62–2.22], $p < 0.0001$).

**Table 8.1** Complications of intra-hospital transport from the time of transport (d0) through day four (d4) post-transport and outcome of transported ICU patients

| | Exposed patients $n = 1659$ | Unexposed patients $n = 3344$ | | | |
|---|---|---|---|---|---|
| | No. (%) | No. (%) | OR* | 95%CI** | p value |
| Severe bleeding (d0–d1) | 33 (1.99) | 30 (0.90) | 2.292 | [1.34;3.93] | 0.003 |
| Myocardial infarction (d0–d1) | 3 (0.18) | 11 (0.33) | 0.598 | [0.16;2.30] | 0.45 |
| Deep vein thrombosis (d0–d1) | 22 (1.33) | 8 (0.24) | 4.474 | [1.90;10.56] | 0.0006 |
| Extubation (d0) | 13 (0.78) | 22 (0.66) | 1.446 | [0.69;3.03] | 0.33 |
| Cardioversion (d0–d1) | 19 (1.15) | 53 (1.59) | 0.684 | [0.38;1.22] | 0.20 |
| Pneumothorax (d0–d1) | 27 (1.63) | 18 (0.54) | 2.603 | [1.37;4.94] | 0.004 |
| Nosocomial pneumonia (d1–d4) | 142 (8.56) | 146 (4.37) | 1.387 | [1.06;1.82] | 0.02 |
| Atelectasis (d0–d1) | 25 (1.51) | 14 (0.42) | 2.859 | [1.40;5.85] | 0.004 |
| Hypoglycemia (d0) | 56 (3.38) | 51 (1.53) | 2.270 | [1.49;3.46] | 0.0001 |
| Hyperglycemia (d0) | 394 (23.75) | 385 (11.52) | 2.287 | [1.93;2.71] | <0.0001 |
| Hypernatremia (d0–d1) | 259 (15.61) | 321 (9.60) | 1.550 | [1.28;1.88] | <0.0001 |
| Patients experiencing at least one adverse event | 621 (37.43) | 744 (22.25) | 1.852 | [1.62;2.12] | <0.0001 |
| ICU mortality | 428 (25.8) | 1069 (32.0) | 0.876 | [0.75;1.02] | 0.09 |
| Day-28 mortality | 470 (28.3) | 1157 (34.6) | 0.874 | [0.75;1.02] | 0.08 |
| Post-transport SOFA | | | | | 0.89 |
| Increase | 632 (38.1) | 1231 (36.8) | 1 | | |
| Decrease or no change | 1027 (61.9) | 2113 (63.2) | 0.991 | [0.87;1.13] | |
| Post-transport LOS, median [IQR] | 7 [3; 16] | 3 [0; 9] | | | <0.0001 |
| [0–4] | 580 (34.96) | 1955 (58.46) | 1 | | |
| ]4–11] | 501 (30.20) | 728 (21.77) | 1.527 | [1.29;1.81] | |
| ]11–27] | 374 (22.54) | 439 (13.13) | 1.264 | [0.99;1.61] | |
| >27 | 204 (12.30) | 222 (6.64) | 0.886 | [0.56;1.41] | |
| Adapted from [1]. | | | | | |

Transported patients were at higher risk of deep venous thrombosis and respiratory and metabolic events occurring up to four days after transport. Transportation was also associated with significant higher post-transport ICU length of stay (Table 8.1) [1].

Even though direct association of IHT and mortality cannot be convincingly established, a targeted quality program is required [1,2].

## Transport-related incidents and adverse events are preventable

Of 900 contributing factors identified, 46% were system-based and 54% human-based. Communication problems, inadequate protocols, in-servicing/training, and equipment were prominent equipment-related incidents. Errors of problem recognition and judgment, failure to follow protocols, inadequate patient preparation, haste, and inattention were common management-related incidents. Rechecking the patient and equipment, skilled assistance, and prior experience were important factors limiting harm [10].

After reviewing records, 70% of experienced adverse events could have been avoided by better preparation prior to transport, communication, and use of checklists and protocols [12].

# How to prevent adverse transport events and achieve safe transports

As contributing factors for incidents and adverse events during transport are identified, dedicated preventive strategies can be developed. As transport is a complicated and multifaceted process, a comprehensive approach addressing key issues is required to mobilize all staff and the ICU team. In a clinical quality improvement audit using a prospective pre- and post-intervention design, an interdisciplinary preventive program resulted in significant reductions for the "technical problems" category of incidents (25% vs. 7.5%, $p < 0.001$), as well as problems related to the patient's mobilization category (14.4% vs. 7.5%, $p = 0.05$) [11].

Key issues to address for smooth transport of ICU patients must include the following.

## Appropriate training

Despite the high risk for patient harm during transport, critical care providers receive little to no training on how to perform safe and effective transport. Being an outstanding intensivist in ICU does not necessarily mean being qualified for transporting the critically ill. A critically ill patient prepared and accompanied by an inexperienced escort is a risky combination [13,14]. Minimizing transport-related risks requires specific training for healthcare providers involved in ICU transport, targeting medical competencies in life-threatening situations and efficient team working to provide a safe continuum of critical care during transport. The same level of monitoring, care, and intervention should be provided outside the ICU as it is inside, without the benefit of additional manpower in narrow, unfamiliar, and often distant environments [13,14].

Training for transport has been pointed out in various working groups and professional societies and is now recommended as a specific objective in basic intensive care courses for students and juniors [19].

As simulator-based training can mimic medical, logistic, and technical problems commonly faced during ICU patient transportation, training sessions for intensivists and ICU nurses can be useful and helpful for addressing safety risks. Even if simulation originally targeted inter-hospital transfer, application for IHT is relevant and suitable for all care providers involved in transport of critically ill patients [20].

Recommendations based on published evidence and expert opinion have been established to enhance patient safety [13,14].

## Checklists and other transport tools

Experience from other high-risk settings may also apply to IHT. Checklists and do-it lists addressing patient and equipment preparation may anticipate technical problems and prevent equipment-related incidents. The effectiveness of checklists widely used in aviation, medical, or nuclear industries indicate they can be useful for patient and equipment pre-transport assessment and evaluation. Routine checklist completion by caregivers may detect operational safety omissions and represent a first step in training [21]. A checklist is of interest because of various and complex patient equipment requirements; a transport team needs also to anticipate, prevent, and resolve technical problems [20]. Pre-transport checklists or other formats of directed forms, like scorecards, have previously been suggested [4,14,21]. A scorecard may help healthcare providers in patient assessment prior to transport by orienting staff to the complexity of transport, and may trigger subsequent actions [22].

Transport tools should include a pre-transport checklist, a patient assessment form, a destination checklist, an observation chart, and sections for documentation of transport results and complications, as well as a reminder to re-check equipment [21].

Various devices developed and implemented in critical care setting to avoid disconnection or disruption of tubes and drains in daily ICU practice are useful tools applicable during transportation to handle lines, therapeutic tubes, and wires.

## Appropriate escort and transport equipment

Adequate provision of highly qualified staff and transport is an important factor limiting harm during transportation [13,14]. Specialist retrieval teams commonly used for IHT are made up of clinicians trained in intensive care able to provide a continuum of critical care during transport. They are associated with reduced preventable adverse events and reduced risk-adjusted mortality in pediatric ICU [23]. Applied to IHT, the overall rate of clinically significant adverse events is relatively low, as reported recently in a monocenter retrospective study [24]. At least two persons trained in transport (nurse, physiotherapist, resident, fellow, or senior physician) are required, depending on the patient's clinical conditions and equipment. Standard equipment includes: a cardiac monitor with defibrillator; airway management equipment and a resuscitation bag (to allow for emergency intubation and manual ventilation via mask and tube); sufficient gas supplies; standard resuscitation drugs and intravenous fluids; and specific essential medications required by the patient transported and a portable ventilator for patients receiving mechanical ventilation [13,14]. Caution should be used regarding portable ventilators' performance as important differences have been demonstrated in a bench study. Turbine ventilators seem to offer better operational performance when tested in normal, ARDS, or obstructive conditions. The most recent turbine ventilators outperformed pneumatic ventilators and proved comparable to modern ICU ventilators [24].

## Miscellaneous

Functional communication between the ICU and transport team, and between the ICU and destination location is expected to avoid/mitigate incidents, maintain continuity of care, and improve patient outcome. In a prospective audit of the quality of IHT, pre-transport recommendations given by the intensivist of the ICU were ignored in 50% of transports with evidence of adverse events [12].

Finally, basic principles related to respect of the patient's dignity, privacy, and standard of hygiene precautions apply during transport periods.

## Quality applied to transport of ICU patients: how to proceed in practice

Different steps targeting pre-transport, transport itself, and post-transport must be distinguished.

### Step 1: pre-transport planning and organization

1. *Benefit/risk of transport*: to be evaluated by medical staff and a senior physician, weighing the anticipated benefit against inherent risks of transport with back-end discontinuity of care, especially for unstable patients.

**Table 8.2**  Checklist for intra-hospital transport

- Identify patient according to local standards.
- Notify mobilization precaution if needed.
- Check authorization for IV contrast use (document allergy and renal function).
- Provide medical chart and blood group documentation in case of surgery or interventional procedure at risk of bleeding.
- Secure various lines, cords, drains, tubes, dressings.
- Secure properly airways and endotracheal tube.
- Identify specific line for emergency IV access.
- Empty all collecting bags (nasogastric, urine, stomy).
- Perform tracheal and oro-tracheal suction.
- Limit ongoing medications with medical supervision/agreement.
- Provide sufficient reserves of treatments in respect of anticipated transport duration.
- Provide sufficient dextrose intake if artificial nutrition support is withdrawn to prevent hypoglycemia.
- Check eligibility of patient (patient's weight, portable pace-maker, and defibrillator) and appropriateness of equipment for MRI department if required.
- Check patient's vital signs and parameters (MAP, SAP, HR, $SpO_2$, consciousness, comfort) prior to transport as baseline documentation.
- Adapt sedation protocol for uncomfortable patients or planned invasive procedure.
- Check patient adaptation and oxygenation to dedicated transport ventilator: observe patient's ventilation in ICU room for at least ten minutes prior to starting transport.
- Inform destination location about patient's clinical features, including hygiene precautions (e.g., isolation) if needed.
- Ensure monitoring at the same level available and required in ICU with, at a minimum, continuous EKG, pulse oxymetry, non-invasive blood pressure, heart and respiratory rate, capnography for ventilated patients. More complex monitoring may occur depending on patient's condition (e.g., neurosurgical patients, cardiovascular patients).

**Table 8.3**  Transport equipment verification

- Check for sufficient autonomy of various batteries (monitor, ventilator, pumps).
- Check for sufficient oxygen supply.
- Test portable defibrillator.
- Set appropriate alarms for various monitoring devices.
- Provide a portable suction device.
- Provide drugs for basic and advanced resuscitation in case of emergency life-threatening situations.

2. *Patient preparation and conditioning for transport*: use a checklist, to be completed by the registered nurse in charge of the patient (Table 8.2).
3. *Transport equipment verification* (Table 8.3).
4. *Call for adequate transport team* to provide appropriate care based on underlying diagnosis, clinical status, and anticipated problems.

# Step 2: during-transport assessment and record
Record vital signs at ICU departure, on-site arrival, and during the journey: record incidents, complications, or adverse events during the round trip and on-site for exhaustive traceability.

# Step 3: post-transport management
- Control the patient's vital signs.
- Recheck equipment of the patient.
- Restore all treatments withdrawn before transport.

- Reconnect transport equipment and devices.
- Analyze incidents that occurred during transport to adjust future local practice and protocols.

An integrated transport tool is a double-sided document that encompasses these major areas of transport processes, which appears relevant and useful, and is recommended at each unit to improve patient safety in a continuous quality improvement program targeting transport of ICU patients [21].

## Conclusion

Transportation is a pivotal aspect in management of critically ill patients in daily practice. However, transport of ICU patients is a risky procedure even though it occurs routinely. The quality policy that applies to an ICU also applies for transport periods. In this era of safety culture in the ICU, a dedicated quality improvement program targeting transport is required to minimize the risks and provide the same level of care inside and outside the ICU.

## References

1. C. Schwebel, C. Clec'h, S. Magne *et al.* Safety of intra-hospital transport in ventilated critically ill patients: a multicenter cohort study. *Crit Care Med* 2013;41:1919–1928.

2. L.P. Voigt, S.M. Pastores, N.D. Raoof, *et al.* Review of a large clinical series: intrahospital transport of critically ill patients: outcomes, timing, and patterns. *J Intensive Care Med* 2009;24:108–115.

3. C. Waydhas. Intrahospital transport of critically ill patients. *Crit Care* 1999; 3:R83–R89.

4. T.C. Blakeman, R.D.Branson. Inter-and intra-hospital transport for critically ill. *Respir Care* 2013;58:1008–1021.

5. J.P.N. Papson, K.L. Russell, D.M Taylor. Unexpected events during the intrahospital transport of critically ill patients. *Acad Emerg Med* 2007;14:574–577.

6. L.T.S. Zuchelo, P.A. Chiavone. Intrahospital transport of patients on invasive ventilation: cardiorespiratory repercussions and adverse events. *J Bras Pneumol* 2009;35(4):367–374.

7. J.M. Droogh, M. Smit, J. Hut, *et al.* Inter-hospital transport of critically ill patients: expect surprises. *Critical Care* 2012; 16:R26.

8. N. Bercault, M. Wolf, I. Runge, *et al.* Intrahospital transport of critically ill ventilated patients: a risk factor for ventilator-associated pneumonia – a matched cohort study. *Crit Care Med* 2005; 33:2471–2478.

9. SEE 3 (Sentinel Events Evaluation 3). Multinational study on patient safety during intrahospital transport of ICU patients. www.see3.org

10. U. Beckmann, D.M. Gillies, S.M. Berenholtz, *et al.* Incidents relating to intra-hospital transfer of critically ill patients: an analysis of the reports submitted to the Australian Incident Monitoring Study in Intensive Care. *Intensive Care Med* 2004;30:1579–1585.

11. M. Berube, F. Bernard, H. Marion *et al.* Impact of a preventive programme on the occurrence of incidents during the transport of critically ill patients. *Intensive Crit Care Nurs.* 2013;29(1):9–19.

12. J.J. Ligtenberg, L.G. Arnold, Y. Stienstra, *et al.* Quality of interhospital transport of critically ill patients: a prospective audit. *Crit Care* 2005;9(4):R446–R451.

13. J. Warren, R.E. Fromm Jr., R.A. Orr, L.C. Rotello, *et al.* Guidelines for the inter-and intrahospital transport of critically ill patients. *Crit Care Med* 2004;32: 256–262.

14. B. Fanara, C. Manzon, O. Barbot, *et al.* Recommendations for the intra-hospital transport of critically ill patients. *Crit Care* 2010;14:R87.

15. P. Prodhan, R.T. Fiser, S. Cenac, *et al.* Intrahospital transport of children on extracorporeal membrane oxygenation: indications, process, interventions and effectiveness. *Pediatr Crit Care Med* 2010;11(2):227–233.

16. J.M. Hurst, K. Davis, D.J. Johnson, *et al.* Cost and complications during in-hospital transport of critically ill patients: a prospective cohort study. *J Trauma* 1992;33(4):582–585.

17. K. Peace, E.M. Wilensky, S. Frangos, *et al.* The use of a portable head CT scanner in the intensive care unit. *J Neurosci Nurs* 2010;42(2):109–116.

18. M.M. Maher, P.F. Hahn, D.A. Gervais *et al.* Portable abdominal CT: analysis of quality and clinical impact in more than 100 consecutive cases. *Am J Roentgenol* 2004 183(3):663–670.

19. COBATRICE: Competency-based training in intensive care medicine in Europe. www.cobatrice.org

20. J.M. Droogh, H.L. Kruger, J.J. Ligtenberg, *et al.* Simulator-based crew resource management training for interhospital transfer of critically ill patients by a mobile ICU. *Jt Comm J Qual Patient Saf* 2012; 38:554–559.

21. R.J. Jarden, S. Quirke. Improving safety and documentation in intrahospital transport: development of an intrahospital transport tool for critically ill patients. *Intensive Crit Care Nurs* 2010; 26:101–107.

22. R. Esmail, D. Banack, C. Cummings, *et al.* Is your patient ready for transport? Developing an ICU patient transport decision scorecard. *Healthc Q* 2006;9:80–86

23. P. Ramnarayan, K. Thiru, R.C. Parslow, *et al.* Effect of specialist retrieval teams on outcomes in children admitted to paediatric care units in England and Wales: a retrospective cohort study. *Lancet* 2010;376:698–704

24. R. Kue, P. Brown, C. Ness, *et al.* Adverse clinical events during intrahospital transport by a specialized team: a preliminary report. *Am J Crit Care* 2011;20:153–162.

25. S. Boussen, M. Gainnier, P. Michelet. Evaluation of ventilators used during transport of critically ill patients: a bench study. *Respir Care.* 2013;58(11):1911–1922.

# Mortality and morbidity conferences

Iris Pélieu and Christophe Faisy

## Introduction

Through its activity, the intensive care unit (ICU) is an important source of life-threatening adverse events (AEs) despite the monitored environment and the high density of caregivers. Indeed, ICUs are identified as high-risk structures due to the complexity of the diagnostic or therapeutic procedures, the multiplicity of actors involved in decision management, and the multiple severe organ failures in ICU patients. Since the publication of the Institute of Medicine's groundbreaking report, *To Err is Human, Building a Safer Health Care System* in 1999, prospective studies have shown a highly variable rate of AEs in ICUs, according to the type of AE reported, most of which were medication administration errors [1–6]. Medical error occurs during the implementation phase of healthcare procedures in about three-quarters of all cases in the ICU, and there would be a cumulative effect on the risk of error [1,6]. Ways of improving the systems for preventing and limiting the effects of in-ICU AE have become a major concern in the last two decades. Efficiency of medical practices founded on evidence-based medicine fits into the methods recognized by the healthcare authorities to promote quality of care. However, the efficiency and continuous improvement of the quality of care is insufficient for a full understanding of the concept of patient safety. Indeed, patient safety includes the effort to reduce or eliminate potentially preventable AEs [7]. Automation, computerization, double-checking, and bundles of care also reduce human errors, but have limitations [8,9]. A system-based approach in which the determination of how the error occurred is the key question, as is the case in standardized mortality and morbidity conferences (MMCs), supports quality improvement and safety culture in the ICU [8–11].

## Toward standardized MMCs in the ICU

Methods for improving patient safety have been developed, like the mandatory reporting of AE or the comparison of results with standards (for instance, the *Standardized Mortality Ratio*). However, these procedures preclude determination of the causes of AE, require additional work, need sometimes significant resources, and do not address the problems associated with individual guilt, fear of retaliation, or the loss of professional reputation involved by the individual error. Mortality rates are included in performance scorecards or dashboards, and actively engage with national patient safety improvement initiatives. The measurement of mortality as an outcome parameter confronts caregivers with the problem

*Quality Management in Intensive Care*, ed. Bertrand Guidet, Andreas Valentin and Hans Flaatten. Published by Cambridge University Press. © Cambridge University Press 2016.

of monitoring the follow-up on the results. Indeed, when proven structure and process interventions are already applied, the cause of a suboptimal performance cannot be deduced easily. One approach is to evaluate the causes of death or AE and to judge their preventability. To confront this important healthcare problem, high-risk specialties, like surgery or anesthesiology, have successfully improved the quality of care they provide and the safety of their patients by systematizing MMCs [12,13]. MMCs are a tool for evaluating care management and improving patient care (Figure 9.1). During the MMCs, caregivers need to elicit input from all staff involved in the incident, use a structured framework to investigate underlying contributing factors, and assign responsibility for management and follow-up on recommendations. Furthermore, the MMCs determine the preventability of the AE. However, an interdisciplinary approach may also emphasize how MMCs can be useful in addition to their educational value, with respect to debate of clinical management and alternative treatments. Increasingly, hospitals integrate MMCs into their governance processes. To support this, healthcare authorities have produced guidance for case analysis. Traditionally, adverse outcomes discussed at MMCs have been attributed to individual competence in treating patients rather than the system or process failures [13]. Although both contribute to errors, the focus on individuals has led clinicians to fear embarrassment and loss of reputation, making them reluctant to speak openly about errors at meetings. This defensive behavior is thought to be counterproductive to eliminating AEs and ensuring patient safety [14]. In light of this fact, we will explain implementing systematized MMCs in the ICU and avoiding the pitfalls of defensive behavior.

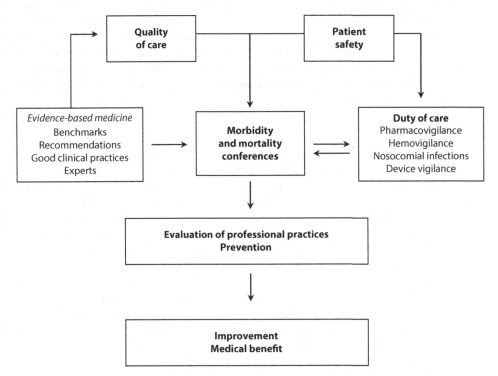

**Figure 9.1** Role of mortality and morbidity conferences in the governance of patient safety and quality of care.

# MMCs procedure

## MMCs rules

The aim of the MMCs is to identify collectively the latent errors (design or planning actions, management organization, organizational, and training) representing about 90% of the preventable part of AEs rather than the errors attributable to individuals. Before implementing regular MMCs, it seems essential to hold an informal meeting with the medical and nursing staff to present the goals and structures of this process and to clarify the introspective aspect of the MMCs: implementing an open peer discussion among physicians and nurses to review individual and team interventions and practices without intimidation, shame, or guilt. It is important to develop a safe and non-critical environment before considering any other aspect of the meeting. These rules can be formally stated in a charter signed by the head of department and the MMC coordinators. A permanent group of coordinators, including a head nurse, a nurse, and a staff physician (the MMC moderator) is established and is always present at every MMC. To facilitate improvement, MMCs need to be structured and systematic in reviewing and discussing deaths, directing discussions toward improving system and process variations. There are seven steps in MMC procedure: case identification, case preparation and review, case analysis, case discussion, case classification, recommendations, and follow-up (Figure 9.2).

## Who, when, and where

Establishing regular MMCs monthly encourages attendance, reduces forgetting details, and limits individual guilt. MMCs are a resource for learning, improvement, and accountability, so the presence of residents and junior doctors is indispensable in order to present and discuss the cases. The participation of an outside auditor experienced in chairing such discussions could provide a more objective perspective than caregivers directly responsible for the patient and could contribute to improving the quality and usefulness of MMCs. The participation of nurses in MMCs is a way to better balance the organizational culture in the ICU [15].

## Case identification

MMCs are designed to analyze preventable AEs, but it is not essential that they be exhaustive. Indeed, the rate of exhaustively reported AEs is not necessarily a better safety or quality indicator than selected AE or sentinel events [15]. Sentinel events retained for MMCs should be consensually chosen during the preliminary informal meeting because they were considered potentially preventable in optimal ICU practice (possible markers of dysfunction) [5]. In our experience, the sentinel events eligible for MMC analysis are unexpected cardiac arrest during an ICU stay, unplanned extubation, need for reintubation within 24–48 hours after planned extubation, and readmission to an ICU within 48 hours after ICU discharge. This list is voluntarily restrictive and can evolve over time. It is not recommended to select a patient's chart if there is a judicial indictment, although it has never been demonstrated that MMCs enhance the prosecution of medical injury and malpractice litigation. Sentinel events can be collected by different methods, such as the use of an "incident book" to which caregivers always have access or the collection of pre-filled forms filed in inboxes [16]. The limitations of these techniques is that they are voluntary and confidentiality must be respected. The selection of the AEs (usually 1–3 cases) that will be analyzed during the MMC takes into account the objectives of improving patient safety and quality of care without forgetting the educational value of the cases.

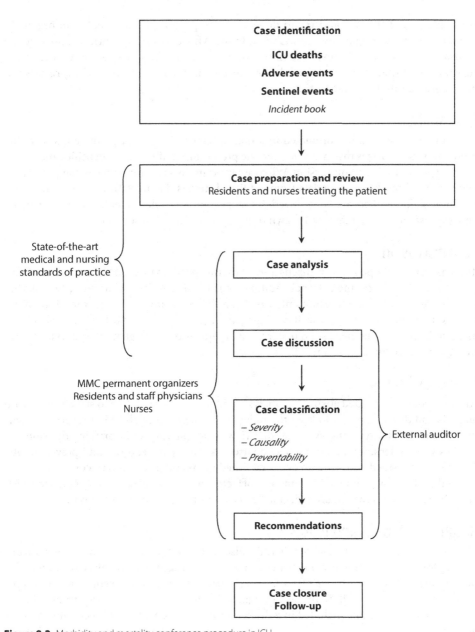

**Figure 9.2** Morbidity and mortality conference procedure in ICU.

## Case preparation and review

Under the supervision of a senior intensivist, residents and nurses directly involved in patient care prepare the presentation of the case on the basis of the following criteria: educational value, improvement of quality of care, preventable outcome, and medical or nursing management critique. To enhance the overall learning experience, these staff members also should complete the patient's history, chronology of the facts, and consequences of the AE, and try to determine the personal, contextual, and organizational aspects that might have contributed to the AE. Such a framework can provide the assurance that all AEs are reviewed in the same way [10]. When necessary, a short literature review on specific subjects can also be presented. When available, autopsy results can be integrated into the presentation.

## Case analysis

The conference should be conducted in a non-judgmental and non-punitive manner. The moderator summarizes the case, and then the presenting staff member identifies and develops the specific topics for discussion. When appropriate, local performance is compared with external benchmarks by using data from published studies (Figure 9.2). The moderator and/ or senior staff members are encouraged to report similar or relevant errors they have made and lessons/benefits that they had drawn from reflecting upon those errors.

## Case discussion

The case is then opened for discussion with the participants. MMC attendees (staff physicians, nurses, and the external auditor) focus the discussion on the severity, causality (institutional and ICU environment, work conditions, team-related factors, individual factors, task-related factors, and staff management), and preventability of the event [17]. The aim is to examine the system of care and organization management and to find ways to prevent the recurrence of the AE.

## Case classification

An anonymous preprinted abstract or analysis grid serves as a guideline to structure the case analysis and discussion and to keep the reflection focused on establishing severity, causality, and preventability of the event. With a view to simplifying and clarifying decisions by the MMC attendees, a Likert scale may be used to classify AE severity and preventability. Causality is classified according to pre-established items and discussion to consensus determines the hierarchy (primary or secondary) of factors when several have contributed to an AE [17]. Primary cause is considered the main causal factor contributing to an event.

## Recommendations and follow-up

The moderator and external auditor close the discussion by developing a case summary from the employed analysis. Finally, all participants are encouraged to help devise recommendations to prevent the recurrence of a similar AE. Each consensually accepted action of prevention is subjected to follow-up by a designated staff member or working group with an implementation schedule included in a drafted protocol. The number of recommendations must be limited to allow the system to work with efficiency. A national survey assessing the implementation of MMCs in French ICUs has shown that MMCs lead to drafting of new procedures in 83% of cases, revision of procedures in 63%, plan training programs in 50%, and change in organizational management in 72% [18]. Writing a summary record of MMCs according to the rules of anonymity and insisting on analyzing the causes and prevention decisions is the responsibility of the leaders of the group committee. The distribution of this report summary to the ICU team is also a good way to increase staff awareness of the risks of AE and their prevention without forcing functions/constraints. Data archiving (analysis summaries and minutes grids) obeys the rules governing administrative archives and part of the record for running the service. These data, as well as those on the record collection of AEs, can later be used for the purpose of evaluation of prevention.

## Learning from MMC experiences

Few data are available on the feelings of the nurses who are involved in the MMC process. This may seem paradoxical, since a prospective study has shown that 59% of AEs were reported by nurses, 27% by residents, and less than 3% by senior doctors [16]. Another study reported that over 80% of MMC participants were doctors [19]. However, a recent survey indicates that there is currently a higher rate of participation of ICU nurses in MMCs [18]. Furthermore, MMCs improve communication between nurses and physicians, sometimes more so than classical staff meetings [1]. Doctors' feelings regarding MMCs seem to be different from those experienced by nurses. In terms of practice, junior doctors and residents feel the educational benefit from these meetings and this confirms the results of the surveys published on this topic. However, we can see through their opinions the tangible expression of fear of disapproval and the achievement of their image within the paramedical team. This fear may explain why doctors in training seem to have a less positive image of MMCs [20]. Senior doctors, even though they recognize the educational role of MMCs, sometimes have difficulty explaining medical errors and are less accepting than younger colleagues when the care they provide is questioned, and may be concerned about the potential effect on their leadership within the healthcare team [5,13]. Absenteeism from meetings could be a symptom of this difficulty with such situations. It is clear that a radical change of mindset requires a lot of time and persuasion. The attitude of the head of department is critical to make a successful transition in attitude and behavior. Education about changes induced by the communication of errors is the first step for improving performance in the ICU. In this way, it has been demonstrated that implementation of regular MMCs in the ICU enhances the emergence of a team satisfaction oriented culture in which norms emphasize achieving self-expression, cooperation, and staff development [15]. This point is an important one, because the cultural values shared by an ICU team play a key role in improving performance. Indeed, MMCs stimulate doctors and nurses to discuss informally their organizational problems more often and without fear. Lastly, the holistic evaluation of MMCs in the ICU showed that AEs analyzed by caregivers during MMCs are influenced by their organizational culture, questioning their ability to handle problems and find corrective actions regarding an AE [15].

## Conclusion

MMCs are an established part of medical education, offering a broad platform for discussions and exchanges between caregivers working in the ICU. MMCs may enhance ICU performance by changing organizational culture. Their potential for improving quality of care and patient safety depends on there being a global assessment approach with structural and systematic analysis. Indeed, MMCs that adopt a standardized and systematic review process can focus on system and organizational failures, provide a record of meeting outcomes and follow-up for corrective actions, and facilitate the reporting of meeting outcomes and assurance to the hospital board. MMCs can make a difference to patient care and to critical care practices by refocusing the management of medical and nursing care on the patient. In this way, MMCs contribute to the governance of patient safety [10].

# References

1. J.M. Rothschild, C.P. Landrigan, J.W. Cronin, *et al.* The Critical Care Safety Study: the incidence and nature of adverse events and serious medical errors in intensive care. *Crit Care Med* 2005; 33: 1694–1700.

2. A. Valentin, M. Capuzzo, B. Guidet, *et al.* Errors in administration of parenteral drugs in intensive care units: multinational prospective study. *Br Med J* 2009; 338: 1–8.

3. A. Valentin, M. Capuzzo, B. Guidet, *et al.* Patient safety in intensive care: results from the multinational Sentinel Events Evaluation (SEE) study. *Intensive Care Med* 2006; 32: 1591–1598.

4. A. Pagnamenta, G. Rabito, A. Arosio, *et al.* Adverse event reporting in adult intensive care units and the impact of a multifaceted intervention on drug-related adverse events. *Ann Intensive Care* 2012; 2: 47.

5 H. Ksouri, P.Y. Balanant, J.M. Tadié, *et al.* Impact of morbidity and mortality conferences on analysis of mortality and critical events in intensive care practice. *Am J Crit Care* 2010; 19: 135–145.

6. D. Bracco, J.B. Favre, B. Bissonette, *et al.* Human errors in a multidisciplinary intensive care unit: a 1-year prospective study. *Intensive Care Med* 2001; 27: 137–145.

7. T.A. Brennan, A. Gawande, E. Thomas, *et al.* Accidental deaths, saved lives, and improved quality. *N Engl J Med* 2005; 353: 1405–1409.

8. M. Garrouste-Orgeas, F. Philipart, C. Bruel, *et al.* Overview of medical errors and adverse events. *Ann Intensive Care* 2012; 2: 2.

9 S.R. Ranji, K.G. Shojania. Implementing patient safety interventions in your hospital: what to try and what to avoid. *Med Clin N Am* 2008; 92: 275–293.

10. J. Higginson, R. Walters, N. Fulop. Mortality and morbidity meetings: an untapped resource for improving the governance of patient safety. *BMJ Qual Saf* 2012; 21: 576–585.

11. Y.L. Nguyen, H. Wunsch, D.C. Angus. Critical care: the impact of organization and management on outcomes. *Curr Opin Crit Care* 2010; 16: 1–6.

12. G.J. Annas. The patient's right to safety: improving the quality of care through litigation against hospitals. *N Engl J Med* 2006; 354: 2063–2066.

13. E. Pierluissi, M.A. Fischer, A.R. Campbell, *et al.* Discussion of medical errors in morbidity and mortality conferences. *JAMA* 2003; 290: 2838–2842.

14. A.T. Cunningham, E.C. Bernabeo, D.B. Wolfson, *et al.* Organisational strategies to cultivate professional values and behaviours. *BMJ Qual Saf* 2011; 20: 351–358.

15. I. Pélieu, J. Djadi-Prat, S.M. Consoli, *et al.* Impact of organizational culture on preventability assessment of selected adverse events in the ICU: evaluation of morbidity and mortality conferences. *Intensive Care Med* 2013; 39: 1214–1220.

16. S. Osmon, C.B. Harris, W.C. Dunagan, *et al.* Reporting of medical errors: an intensive care unit experience. *Crit Care Med* 2004; 32: 727–733.

17. C. Vincent, G. Neale, M. Woloshynowych. Adverse events in British hospitals: preliminary record review. *Br Med J* 2001; 322: 517–519.

18. K. Kuteifan, P.M. Mertes, C. Bretonnière, *et al.* Implementation of morbidity and mortality conferences in French intensive care units: a survey. *Ann Fr Anesth Reanim* 2013; 32: 602–606.

19. H.J. Aboumatar, C.G. Blackledge, C. Dickson, *et al.* A descriptive study of morbidity and mortality conferences and their conformity to medical incident analysis models: results of the morbidity and mortality conference improvement study, phase 1. *Am J Med Qual* 2007; 22: 232–238.

20. S.P. Harbison, G. Regehr. Faculty and resident opinions regarding the role of morbidity and mortality conference. *Am J Surg* 1999; 177: 136–139.

# Chapter 1

# Intensive care unit triage

Czarina C.H. Leung and Charles D. Gomersall

## Introduction

Triage is the process of determining critically ill patient prioritization for ICU admission when vacancies are scarce [1]. Absolute ICU resource deficiency relative to demand is a worldwide phenomenon to varying degrees [2–4] and future demands will continue to rise due to an aging population and prolongation of survival with chronic disease. In some developed territories such as Hong Kong and the United Kingdom, with only 3.5–4 ICU beds per 100,000 population, considerable triage pressure exists in routine practice [5]. Conceivably, in developing countries, the triage pressure is more intense. Even countries with a higher supply of ICU beds are not immune to the need for triage, especially when faced with disasters resulting in overwhelming numbers of critically ill patients. The experience of severe respiratory syndrome (SARS) and the H1N1 epidemic highlighted the need for pre-emptive development of triage policy, a framework for effective triage and contingency planning for rapid adaptive expansion of critical care resources in order to ensure maximal and fair provision of care [6]. In order to ensure population-wide distributive justice, ICUs in the same geographical region should collaborate and employ uniform triage processes, especially during crisis. Triage scores and protocols theoretically can also be utilized as a decision-support system, but in practice they are not yet fully developed to assist in clinical judgment [7]. Both the American Thoracic Society (ATS) and the Society of Critical Care Medicine (SCCM) state that admission should be reserved for patients with sufficient medical need and potential benefit, i.e., reasonable prospects of substantial recovery [1,8]. Currently, there is a paucity of prognostication data related to ICU triage and lack of general consensus on the most appropriate resource allocation strategy. This chapter will examine the ethical issues and common approaches, and highlight important difficulties associated with ICU triage.

## Ethics

The four *prima facie* moral principles for medical provision are beneficence, non-maleficence, autonomy, and distributive justice [2]. Triage considers patients with substantial critical care needs who are not excluded on grounds of autonomy or non-maleficence. (In this context, autonomy refers to the patient's informed choice to refuse ICU admission. Non-maleficence

*Quality Management in Intensive Care*, ed. Bertrand Guidet, Andreas Valentin and Hans Flaatten. Published by Cambridge University Press. © Cambridge University Press 2016.

dictates that futile life-sustaining measures that may cause suffering to the patient should not be applied, although futility is difficult to define and difficult to identify with certainty.) Thus, distributive justice is the key principle to be considered when making triage decisions. It is imperative that the triage process is based on a decision-making framework that is ethical, equitable, transparent, consistent, and clinically sensible [1].

The principle of distributive justice in ICU triage is aimed at equitable allocation of valuable critical care resource without prejudice against an individual's non-medically relevant characteristics such as religion, gender, social, or financial status. There are various divergent views on what justice or equitable means – their interpretation will be influenced by local culture and social standards. There are at least two schools of thought regarding the application of distributive justice. One focuses on an individual's fair opportunity to welfare (egalitarian) and the other on ways to achieve maximal societal benefit (utilitarianism).

## Egalitarian

The egalitarian approach promotes equal opportunity for ICU admission on a "first come, first served" basis when resources must be rationed. In this way, each patient who meets the threshold for critical care need is regarded as equal and has an equal chance of admission in the "natural lottery" determined by the relative time of presentation. This approach has been praised for circumventing triage officers' biases. The caveat is that patients who are admitted may not be the ones with the greatest need or derive the most benefit from ICU admission. Admission indiscriminant of potential benefit may incur inadvertent societal cost by occupying beds with patients who derive minimal benefit while foregoing the opportunity to save the lives of those who may benefit most. Furthermore, the timing of presentation and the source of referral may be confounded by social issues, such as pressures applied by influential patient's relatives and clinicians. Therefore, the egalitarian approach may not achieve truly equal opportunity in clinical practice.

The ATS recognizes the merits of assessing potential benefit but endorses the egalitarian approach to circumvent the difficulty with accurately predicting benefit [8].

## Utilitarian

The utilitarian approach aims at achieving "maximal benefit for the greatest number". Prioritization for ICU admission is based on estimated benefit that may be derived from ICU admission. This approach is recommended by the Society of Critical Care Medicine and is most commonly encountered in clinical practice. However, the metrics of "benefit" are not explicitly defined. While hospital or short-term survival were the focus of many previous studies, "benefit" should also encompass longer-term outcomes such as post-ICU quality-adjusted life years (QALY) – i.e., the arithmetic product of life expectancy multiplied by quality of life – as achieving these targets will translate to greater overall societal gains. Benefit can therefore be conceptualized as:

Potential benefit = (Probability of survival with intensive care – Probability of survival without intensive care) × quality-adjusted life expectancy

To achieve maximal benefit for the greatest number under resource constraints, priority for ICU admission should go to those with a substantial predicted increase in survival as well as a reasonable number of post-ICU QALY. This is consistent with common approaches such as categorizing patients as too well or too ill. Patients labeled as "too well" are typically those with low risk of mortality. In this group of patients the benefit resulting from ICU admission must be low even if it results in mortality being reduced to zero. For example, a patient with a 2% risk of mortality without ICU cannot derive more than a 2% reduction in mortality risk by being admitted to the ICU. Conversely, a patient who is "too ill," with a mortality risk of 98% with intensive care, cannot derive more than a 2% reduction in risk even if the mortality without intensive care is 100%. Outside these extremes the survival benefit from intensive care is the same, whether mortality is reduced from 90% to 70% or 30% to 10%. However, as previously mentioned, ICU survival is not the only issue. There is little benefit if the patient dies shortly after discharge or the patient has a poor quality of life. Thus patients with diminished life expectancy such as those with advanced age and poor premorbid health or functional states receive low ICU admission priority [9]. Multiple studies have shown that, in practice, advanced age is associated with greater chance of refusal of ICU admission, especially during resource constraints [10,11]. A 2014 consensus statement published by the Task Force for Mass Critical Care suggests that during a crisis ICU admission should be refused if potential life expectancy is less than one year or estimated mortality is 90% or more [7].

The likely benefit to an individual patient should, however, not be the only consideration. In order to maximize the benefit to society as a whole it is necessary to also consider the likely cost, in terms of resources, of treating the patient. In an ICU with limited resources relative to demand, an increased expenditure of resources on one patient reduces the resources available to others.

Thus, triage usually requires complex decisions, involving multiple estimates, a process complicated by the absence of data on which to base estimates. As a result, predictions may be inaccurate; for example, in one study, while the mortality of those admitted was 64%, that of patients deemed "too well" was surprisingly high, reaching 8% [12]. To address this issue, attempts have been made to devise triage scores. Unfortunately these scores have largely been based on a prediction of low or high mortality if admitted to ICU and therefore do not give an estimate of survival benefit. Furthermore, their performance may be setting-dependent. The Eldicus prospective observational study developed an initial rejecting score for predicting mortality despite intensive care, and final triage score for predicting survival without intensive care. However, out of 6796 patients triaged, only 114 patients (91 and 23, respectively) would have been refused (1.7%), making the clinical application of the score limited [13]. A triage protocol involving a SOFA score advocated by Christian and colleagues triaged patients into different groups, including: high and intermediate priority for ICU admission; do not admit but reassess if need arises; and expectant/palliative management. Although this approach appeared to predict mortality well in one setting, it performed poorly in another [14–16]. It is sometimes argued, on a conceptual basis, that scoring systems should not be used for triage as group data should not be applied to individuals. This ignores the fact that the whole basis of Western medicine is the application of group data to individuals and that the basis for a Utilitarian approach to triage is to maximize benefit for society (a group), not for an individual. It is further argued that the calibration of scoring systems is too poor. However, the real question is not whether the calibration is good or poor, but their performance relative to triage officers' estimates. The future direction of triage score development, as PREEDICCT Group states, may be to calibrate to different disease processes and to produce comparable predictions on a spectrum of outcome metrics including survival, quality of life, and resource consumption [17].

Prediction of post-ICU quality of life is equally difficult, although there are increasing data on quality of life after intensive care. Assessment of pre-ICU quality of life is important as it is almost inconceivable that intensive care will result in an improved quality of life after discharge. This assessment is made difficult by the fact that patients are often unable to communicate their perceptions of their quality of life. However, there are data suggesting concordance between close relative surrogates and a patient's assessment of their own quality of life before admission to ICU [18,19].

## Accountability for reasonableness

Triage decisions are complex and intertwined with ethical dilemmas. Regardless of which approach is chosen, the triage decision should be morally justifiable, clinically reasonable, transparent, and clearly documented [2]. The triage approach should reflect society's interpretation of distributive justice, metrics of benefit, and the most appropriate utilization of limited healthcare resources. A process advocating open discussion of these important issues as well as the consensus on agreeable triage approach and transparency on rationale of triage decision is termed *accountability for reasonableness* [20]. This practice is likely to enhance credibility and consistency with societal expectations. It is a pragmatic move away from a practice heavily reliant on moral defenses or unilateral triage decision process. The rationale for a triage decision leading to refusal of ICU admission and discussions with relevant parties should be clearly documented. As critically ill patients' conditions can change over time, triage decisions also need to be dynamic. Furthermore, re-consultations and appeals of decision should be expected and encouraged, as we need to pool our clinical experience and make the best decisions for the patients.

## Reverse triage

When a newly referred patient has a higher potential for benefit than another who is already on life support in the ICU, should the latter be transferred out of ICU so that the newly referred patient can receive ICU care? In practice, an ICU doctor's fiduciary duty to patients already admitted makes justification of care withdrawal difficult as early ICU discharge may be associated with increased mortality [21]. According to the SCCM Ethics Committee and ATS [1,8], the obligation to patients already admitted and requiring continued ICU care outweighs the justification of admitting new patients during non-crisis and non-battlefield triage. In reality, it is likely not feasible to remove patients from life-sustaining therapies to facilitate care for others even though it has been suggested that during pandemics or other critical care crises that withdrawal of therapy to free a bed for a patient with a better prognosis should be considered [7]. Regulations on end-of-life care exist in many countries. In Hong Kong, for example, the Medical Council stipulates that withdrawal of life-sustaining support requires patient or surrogate assent. Therefore, reverse triage is limited by patient and surrogate wishes – making it very unlikely to be practically feasible.

## Undertriage and overtriage

Undertriage and overtriage are related to the accuracy and threshold of triage process, local policies, and degree of resource constraints relative to demand for ICU service [22]. However, their definitions are confusing and counterintuitive. Undertriage occurs when the severity of illness and needs of patients are not recognized, leading to refusal or delay of ICU admission and, ultimately, worse outcome. Overtriage results from over-liberal admission, which may lead to depletion of resources and subsequent survival reduction [22]. When ICUs over-admit, the costs and workload of the healthcare system escalates, leading to overall reduction of cost-effectiveness.

## Cultural/social/legal framework

Triage approaches and outcome targets should be in line with societal and legal standards. Inclusive, ethical, pragmatic approaches like accountability for reasonableness should be encouraged. Cultural and societal expectations have major influences on the interpretation and enactment of distributive justice. For example, in surveys done in Israel, a high proportion of physicians indicated that they would admit a patient whose quality of life would be poor, whereas in Hong Kong, China, and many European countries, it is widely accepted that only patients with substantial potential for benefit improvement would be admitted [23]. Societal acceptance of triage practice is not universal – in some regions of the world, anecdotal evidence suggests triage officers commonly face physical and social pressures to admit certain patients, threatening the impartiality and ideals of distributive justice.

Institutional triage policies must be put in place to facilitate doctors' triage decision-making. The policies should be explicit and realistic recommendations on resource allocation, with legal limitations clarified in advance. In a pluralistic society, open and inclusive discourse among the stakeholders should be encouraged in order to generate societally endorsed triage policies. This facilitates compatibility with societal views on distributive justice, agreeable targets for outcome (mortality alone or QALY), and preferred triage approaches, e.g., egalitarian, utilitarian. Through this process the public and referring units would also learn the rationale of triage in advance, reducing the uncertainties and distrust when individual needs arise. The concept of prioritization of collective good over individual benefit must also be explicit; the public and healthcare providers should be forewarned that ICU admission and even life-sustaining therapies may be rationed under resource constraints to benefit society as a whole. It should be emphasized that triage must occur before the ICU has been filled to capacity, as once full, the decision is inevitably to refuse admission as there is no possibility of admitting the patient. When the supply of ICU resources is chronically surpassed by demands, the society and institutions have the responsibility to either provide more resources – e.g., increase ICU resources, provide intermediate care services – or reduce demands by reviewing programs that generate high ICU needs or accept a chronic inability of ICUs to take in patients who are eligible for admission. For acute surges in critical needs, contingency plans should also be established in advance. Triage policies should be reviewed and updated as disease prognosis changes following advances in medical therapeutics and as more prognostication data emerge. Committees should oversee the performance of such guidelines [1].

## Conclusion

Triaging critically ill patients with resource constraints is one of the most difficult and stressful elements of ICU duty [24,25]. The triage process is intertwined with ethical and practical dilemmas, contributed by escalating critical care demands, complexity of medical treatments, prognostic uncertainty, and the paucity of data to inform evidence-based triage strategies. There is currently no perfect solution for this complex problem. Whether an egalitarian or utilitarian approach is selected, the process must be consistent, transparent, and compatible with local cultural, societal, and legal framework. Accountability for reasonableness offers a framework for open discussion and safeguards against inconsistencies in the triage process. It is important to have societal endorsement of triage approaches and target outcomes – whether the society believes that the dichotomous survival–mortality outcome or QALY gained should guide the prioritization practice. Triage criteria and decision support tools such as triage scores should also undergo updates to reflect changes in outcome from advancing medical treatments and emerging prognostication data. Data regarding disease-specific outcome with and without ICU admission is crucial for the development of more accurate triage strategies – for example, it was through a previous comparative study of those accepted and refused ICU admission that we came to understand the flaws in the common practice of admitting the most severely ill patients during times of resource constraints, while it is in fact those in the middle range of critical illness severity who would derive the greatest incremental benefit. Our approach (Figure 10.1) undergoes constant recalibration through audits, contestation, or re-consultations, and updates with emerging data in order to move closer to an accurate and informed triage process that maximizes overall societal benefit.

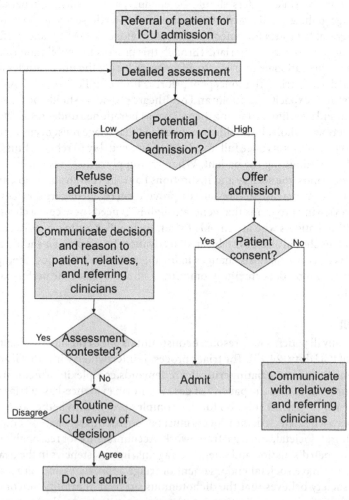

**Figure 10.1** Our approach to the triage decision-making process.

# References

1. Society of Critical Care Medicine Ethics Committee. Consensus statement on the triage of critically ill patients. *JAMA*. 1994;271(14):1200–1203.

2. Joynt G.M. Gomersall C.D. Making moral decisions when resources are limited: an approach to triage in ICU patients with respiratory failure. *SAJCC*. 2005;21(1):34–44.

3. Adhikari N.K., Fowler R.A., Bhagwanjee S., Rubenfeld G.D. Critical care and the global burden of critical illness in adults. *Lancet*. 2010;376(9749):1339–1346.

4. Wunsch H. Is there a Starling curve for intensive care? *Chest*. 2012;141(6):1393–1399.

5. Wunsch H., Angus D.C., Harrison D.A., *et al*. Variation in critical care services across North America and Western Europe. *Crit Car Med*. 2008;36(10):2787–2793.

6. Gomersall C.D., Loo S., Derrick J.L., *et al*. Expanding ICU facilities in an epidemic: recommendations based on experience from the SARS epidemic in Hong Kong and Singapore. *Int Care Med*. 2006;32:1004–1013.

7. Christian M.D., Sprung C.L., King M.A., *et al*. Triage: care of the critically ill and injured during pandemics and disasters: CHEST consensus statement. *Chest*. 2014;146(4 Suppl):e61S–74S.

8. Force ATSBT. Fair allocation of intensive care unit resources. *Crit Care Med*. 1997;156:1282–1301.

9. Bagshaw S.M., Webb S.A., Delaney A., *et al*. Very old patients admitted to intensive care in Australia and New Zealand: a multi-centre cohort analysis. *Crit Care*. 2009;13(2):R45.

10. Sinuff T.K.K., Cook D.J., Luce J.M., Levy M.M. Values, ethics and rationing in critical care task force: rationing critical care beds – a systematic review. *Crit Care Med*. 2004;32(7):1588–1597.

11. Sprung C.L.A.A., Kesecioglu J., Pezzi A., *et al*. The Eldicus prospective, observational study of triage decision making in European intensive care units: Part II – intensive care benefit for the elderly. *Crit Care Med*. 2012;40(1):132–138.

12. Joynt G.M., Gomersall C.D., Tan P., Lee A., Cheng C.A., Wong E.L. Prospective evaluation of patients refused admission to an intensive care unit: triage, futility and outcome. *Int Care Med*. 2001;27(9):1459–1465.

13. Sprung C.L., Baras M., Iapichino G., *et al*. The Eldicus prospective, observational study of triage decision making in European intensive care units: Part I – European Intensive Care Admission Triage Scores. *Crit Care MEd*. 2012;40(1):125–131.

14. Shahpori R.S.R., Doig C., Boiteau P., Zygun D. Sequential organ failure assessment in pandemic planning. *Crit Care*. 2010;14(Suppl 1):477.

15. Christian M.D., Hamielec C., Lazar N.M., *et al*. A retrospective cohort pilot study to evaluate a triage tool for use in a pandemic. *Crit Care*. 2009;13(5):R170.

16. Christian M.D., Hawryluck L., Wax R.S., *et al*. Development of a triage protocol for critical care during an influenza pandemic. *CMAJ*. 2006;175(11):1377–1381.

17. Christian M.D.F.R., Muller M.P., Gomersall C., *et al*. Critical care resource allocation: trying to PREEDICCT outcomes without a crystal ball. *Crit Care*. 2013;17(1):107.

18. Hofhuis J., Hautvast J.L., Schrijvers A.J., Bakker J. Quality of life on admission to the intensive care: can we query the relatives? *Int Care Med*. 2003;29(6):974–979.

19. Capuzzo M., Moreno R.P., Alvisi R. Admission and discharge of critically ill patients. *Curr Op Crit Care*. 2010;16(5):499–504.

20. Daniels N. Accountability for reasonableness. *BMJ* 2000;321:1300–1301.

21. Daly K., Beale R., Chang R.W. Reduction in mortality after inappropriate early discharge from intensive care unit: logistic regression triage model. *BMJ*. 2001;322(7297):1274–1276.

22. Christian M.D., Sandrock C.E., Devereaux A., Geiling J., Amundson D.E., Rubinson L. Ethical issues and the allocation of scarce resources during a public health

emergency. *Ann Intern Med.* 2009;150: 890–891.

23. Einav S., Soudry E., Levin P.D., Grunfeld G.B., Sprung C.L. Intensive care physicians' attitudes concerning distribution of intensive care resources: a comparison of Israeli, North American and European cohorts. *Int Care Med.* 2004;30(6):1140–1143.

24. Sprung C.L., Geber D., Eidelman L.A., *et al.* Evaluation of triage decisions for intensive care admission. *Crit Care Med.* 1999;27(6):1073–1079.

25. Giannini A., Consonni D. Physicians' perceptions and attitudes regarding inappropriate admissions and resource allocation in the intensive care setting. *Brit J Anaesth.* 2006;96(1):57–62.

# End-of-life care

Wai-Tat Wong and Gavin M. Joynt

## Introduction: ethical and moral issues at the end of life

End-of-life (EOL) care in the intensive care unit (ICU) is concerned with ensuring optimal care for patients with terminal disease. The focus of EOL care is thus to provide the patient with the best quality of life possible for the limited period they are predicted to survive. Life support therapy (LST) in the ICU has reached a high level of technical sophistication such that it has become possible to continue to support the organs of patients and sustain life, even when meaningful recovery from the condition is no longer possible. Continuation of LST in such patients does not provide net medical benefit to the patient. In modern ICU practice, spontaneous deaths are now uncommon, with 60–70% of ICU deaths occurring after withholding or withdrawal (WH/WD) of such non-beneficial LST [1,2]. Timely "goal of care" discussions, that aim to clarify prognosis, and delineate patient and family expectations of short- and long-term health outcomes, are key to ensuring that patients' best interests are served. Based on the outcome of these discussions, initiation of EOL decision-making may begin. Both processes are crucial to optimizing the delivery of ICU care. Continuing inappropriate LST at the EOL potentially violates healthcare workers' duty of care, and increases suffering both for patients and their families. It also contributes to stress and conflict within the ICU healthcare team.

Ethical and moral justifications for common practices at the EOL are complex, culturally influenced, and driven by individual values. A detailed exploration of these issues is beyond the scope of this chapter; we attempt to synthesize a reasonably acceptable approach to practice while recognizing that one universally acceptable approach does not exist.

Briefly, it is generally accepted that LST should be WH/WD when the patient's best interest is no longer served by LST. This condition is met when the burden of ongoing treatment outweighs the net health benefit the patient is likely to derive in terms of length of time of survival or quality of life. The LST in this instance could be considered "non-beneficial treatment."

Many have used the "principled" approach of ethical reasoning to justify the limitation of LST once it has been identified as "non-beneficial." Briefly, the moral principles that are weighed and balanced are beneficence, non-maleficence, autonomy, and justice. Beneficence must be assessed on the basis of likely prognosis – for survival, functionality, and quality of life. Burdens are composed of immediate suffering/discomfort caused by life support in the ICU, as well as future suffering and loss of quality of life in the long term. Thus at EOL, when LST

---

*Quality Management in Intensive Care*, ed. Bertrand Guidet, Andreas Valentin and Hans Flaatten. Published by Cambridge University Press. © Cambridge University Press 2016.

no longer serves to substantially benefit patients by failing to meet a positive benefit–burden criterion, physicians are obliged to weigh the principle of beneficence and non-maleficence, and thus consider limitation of LST when beneficence is not sustained.

The influence of autonomy, or "self-rule" in final decision-making varies with regions and countries and leads to different models of decision-making. Some take the view that the healthcare team best makes final decisions, others that patients/surrogates should make such decisions independently, and yet others that the decision should be shared. In reality, in the absence of advanced directives or a durable power of attorney, ICU patients are frequently unable to exert their autonomy because of reduced mental capacity caused by the underlying critical illness, usually compounded by the necessary use of sedative drugs. In this setting surrogate decision-makers, usually family, are used to assess what the patient's autonomous views might be. Whatever model of decision-making is used, the primary objective at EOL is always to provide patients a dignified, pain-free life prior to death.

Justice refers to fair and appropriate distribution of limited resources within a society. While inappropriate prolongation of scarce and costly ICU care may be considered to violate the ethical principal of justice by indirectly impacting other potential ICU patients with better prognoses, its application at the EOL in ICU is complex, and in high-income countries is rarely directly considered in decision-making that may lead to WH/WD LST.

## Establishing early "goals of care" in a patient/surrogate conference

For most patients, admission to ICU heralds a life-changing event. It is important to establish a relationship with the patient/family/surrogate as early as possible, so that they can be provided with appropriate medical information as well as emotional and psychological support. Usually critically ill patients at EOL are incapable of participation in complex discussions, and communication is often with family or surrogates. A goal of care discussion within 24–48 hours should ensure that a meaningful connection is forged between the healthcare team and the surrogate/family. This discussion should enhance the family's understanding of intensive care, provide information such as medical facts, options for treatment, and *prognosis*, and set the scene to provide emotional support. Most importantly, it should also elicit the patient's values from the family/surrogate, and establish expected "goals of care." As cure is often the initial expected goal of care, early discussions do not necessarily lead to the discussion of palliation or limitation of LST.

## Shifting goals of care from cure to palliation

### Initiation of WH/WD discussions

Because they are familiar with the features of terminal illness and aware of the burdens of LSTs, physicians are most likely to trigger EOL discussions. In principle, WH/WD discussions should be triggered when the physician recognizes that the LST cannot provide sufficient net medical benefit and are no longer in the patient's best interest (i.e., non-beneficial treatment). Net medical benefit is usually weighed against the burden of ongoing treatment. The benefit of treatment should be derived in terms of both length of survival and resultant quality of life [3]. A lengthy survival with poor quality of life may not be considered as a beneficial outcome. The burden of treatment should include physical discomfort associated with ongoing treatment, the possibility of institutionalization, and impact on social roles in the case of survival. What constitutes quality of life is subjective, and dependent upon a patient's religious and cultural values. Hence, an open and honest discussion with the family is necessary before one can ascertain a treatment to be non-beneficial.

On the premise that the following circumstances create the condition such that benefits are unlikely to outweigh burdens of LST, commonly accepted practical factors that may trigger WH/WD discussions include: a limited expected length of survival (days or weeks), severe brain injury with expected poor neurological recovery, multi-organ failure with more than three organs involved and lasting for over one week, and any illness demonstrating persistent unresponsiveness to maximal therapy in ICU [7]. Advanced age and a severe illness, in isolation, may not warrant WH/WD discussions as severe illness may still be reversible, and outcomes in elderly patients may not always be poor, especially when measured in terms of quality of life [3]. Prognostication uncertainty is common at EOL. With agreement and consensus among various competent specialists, the healthcare team who initiate EOL decision-making should be able to prognosticate with more confidence, potentially making subsequent WH/WD decisions more objective and consistent [3]. Occasionally, EOL discussions are initiated by patients' families or by the patient him/herself. This may occur through contact during "goal of care" discussions or routine conferences. Written advance directives may give specific instructions on when WH/WD should be triggered, but are variably utilized around the world.

## Autonomy in decision-making

Key components that are essential for decision-making capacity are possession of a set of values and goals necessary for evaluating different options, the ability to receive and understand information, and the ability to communicate, reason, and deliberate one's choice [4]. For obvious reasons, ICU patients frequently lack decision-making capacity, and in this setting the patient's values and preferences can be made known by three means: (1) a prior advanced directive; (2) previous opinions made known to family/surrogates; (3) family/surrogate's substituted judgment based on their understanding of the patient.

An advanced directive is a written document made by a person with decisional capacity stating his/her preferences for medical care if or when he/she loses decision-making capacity. Although there is in general consensus regarding the need to respect an advance directive, the legal status of this document varies in different countries [2]. When implementing advanced directives, the content should be interpreted carefully to ensure that the patient's wishes and best interests are served. In the absence of a formal directive, surrogates' substituted decisions on EOL care should be gathered. The patient's known or presumed thoughts and feelings with regard to serious illnesses, death, or dying, and views on acceptable future quality of life, should be elicited from the family. Surrogates/family members are often expected to make such decisions and ought to be reminded to make decisions based upon the patient's values and preferences, not their own. The weight given to the role of autonomy in decision-making varies within and between regions and countries, and this largely determines the basic model of decision-making.

## Models of decision-making

Decision-making at the EOL is a complex process involving the patient and/or patients' families as surrogate decision-makers, ICU physicians, primary care clinicians of other specialties, nurses, and, when appropriate, other healthcare professionals. Depending largely on how much autonomy in healthcare decision-making is expected within societies in different parts of the world, different models of decision-making are used. The paternalistic model and shared management decision-making models are most common. In paternalistic models, management decisions become the primary responsibility of the healthcare team, and are sensitively communicated to patients/surrogates to ensure they understand the rationale for decisions. The patient's autonomy in this setting is relatively restricted. The paternalistic approach is the more common model used in many Northern European countries. Shared decision-making is a dynamic process where different stakeholders all share responsibility for EOL decisions [4]. The aim is to reach consensus with the patient/surrogate on a process that is primarily in accordance with the patient's desires and values. Shared decision-making is an increasingly recommended model in North America, where the individual's autonomy is highly valued. This model is also utilized in parts of Asia, where autonomy is extended to include the family unit, as family involvement in healthcare decision-making is expected and highly valued.

## Limiting life-support: practical implementation

### Communication

Effective communication and avoidance of unnecessary LST at the EOL are increasingly recognized as important components in quality of EOL care outside the ICU setting [5], and are associated with better family bereavement outcomes. Family/surrogate conferences are important palliative care intervention in EOL in the ICU setting. A well-planned and structured family conference can improve family satisfaction and resource utilization, whereas a poorly conducted conference potentially inflicts emotional harm upon a family [6,7].

The primary purpose of EOL family conferences usually involves re-orienting the treatment goal from cure to palliation. To best achieve this, the conference ought to be well planned and structured according to the family's needs, taking extra care with important issues (Table 11.1). Multiple family meetings may be required for clarification, information gathering, discussion of treatment options, and final EOL management decisions. A consensus among professional teams is a prerequisite for a family meeting for EOL decision-making. Information provided about the patient's medical condition, management plan, and prognosis should be accurate and consistent between teams. This may require additional research and/or obtaining expert opinion, so that the rationale for determining appropriate EOL care for individual patients is unambiguously and explicitly communicated and documented.

The quantity and complexity of information provided to family members should be individualized based upon their educational background, culture, and their perceived understanding from previous family conferences. A summary of the content should be repeated at the end of the interview. Especially in Western cultures, directly discussing death and dying is deemed more appropriate than use of euphemistic terms [8]. Most families disbelieve physicians' prognostication; and trust from the family can be improved by consistent information from different clinicians [9]. All treatment options, including continuation of LST, with anticipated benefits and burdens should be discussed. While there is evidence that most surrogates prefer complete honesty with regard to prognostic information, it remains important that poor prognoses are transmitted with sensitivity. Some surrogates/family respond with anger or denial of bad news, especially during the early stage of admission, and repeated, sensitive communication is necessary.

Common verbal empathetic strategies include acknowledging emotion, encouraging expression, paraphrasing, apologizing, affirming adaptive coping, and keeping silent to allow listening. Non-verbal strategy can be provision of a gentle touch, or offering a tissue to a crying family member, or a drink in an appropriate time in a comfortable and quiet environment within ICU [10]. Physicians commonly dominate the discussion, using up to 70% of the time

**Table 11.1** Example of patient/surrogate communication plan in ICU at end of life; ICU patients generally lack decision-making capacity and family members are usually placed in the position of surrogate

| | | |
|---|---|---|
| On ICU admission | Goal of care meeting (within 24–48 hours of ICU admission) | • Assess surrogate understanding<br>• Share information (medical facts, options of treatment, prognosis)<br>• Provide emotional support<br>• Elicit patient's goals and values from surrogate<br>• Establish goals of care |
| Patient has terminal illness | Healthcare team consensus on prognostication and management plan | • Continue LST, or WH/WD LST<br>• May consider time-limited trial of LST with predefined criteria of success or failure |
| Conduct surrogate interview | Assess family understanding and perception of illness | • Allow time for surrogate expression of understanding, and give appropriate clarification |
| | Assess family emotions and their needs | • Demonstrate verbal and non-verbal empathy |
| | Provide prognostic information and treatment options | • Expected length of survival<br>• Quality of life after survival<br>• Possible institutionalization<br>• Impact on social role<br>• Aggressive support or WH/WD LST with palliation<br>• Physical and psychological burden |
| | Gather information about the patient's views of death and dying | • Check the availability of an advance directive<br>• Specifically ask for previous expressions about death or dying |
| | Physician recommendation | • Provide a balanced recommendation on EOL care based on available personal and clinical information, and estimated prognosis<br>• Reassure surrogate of goal of comfort and dignity for patient in dying phase |
| | Finalized action plan | • LST to be WH/WD if appropriate<br>• Timing of WH/WD<br>• Anticipated effect<br>• Palliation/symptom management |
| Follow-up after EOL decision | Avoid abandonment feelings | • Arrange follow-up meeting<br>• Referral to social worker, religious or spiritual support |

to deliver what they perceive as important clinical information and treatment options. They may neglect the surrogate/family's need to talk about their loved one's illness, clarify their understanding and express their concerns and emotions. The proportion of time allowed for the family to talk has been positively associated with family satisfaction at EOL care [11]. Allowing family to talk is not necessarily time consuming as it may save time having to deal with conflict caused by misunderstanding. A follow-up interview should be offered in most circumstances.

In addition to explaining and establishing the decision to proceed with EOL care, by sensitively informing the surrogate (paternalistic approach), or achieving consensus (shared decision-making), measures to be taken to ensure patient comfort, respect, and dignity during the ICU stay should also be conveyed to the family. Surrogates/relatives should be reassured that symptoms, if any, will be controlled by the use of medications and that the patient will die a comfortable and "naturally predestined" death, usually within hours of withdrawal of LST. As the intention of limitation of LST is comfort and not shortening of the dying process in most instances, the family should also be prepared for the possibility of a prolonged dying process.

Short communication skills training courses have been shown to improve the process and outcome of care [12]. Communication skills training courses should be offered to potential communicating healthcare team members. Physicians experienced in dealing with emotions and conflict should be delegated based on particular patient and/or family needs.

## Withholding and withdrawing life support treatments

Withholding and withdrawing LSTs are generally considered ethically identical, although some ICU physicians distinguish the two. "Withholding support" (WH) is defined as not initiating or escalating LST, including CPR. "Withdrawing support" (WD) is defined as actively discontinuing LST, including CPR. All LSTs may be WH/WD, provided the goal is patient comfort. This includes, but is not limited to WH/WD of inotropes, vasopressors, renal replacement therapies, blood products, and mechanical ventilation. Parenteral fluids are generally continued, but to be discontinued if medically indicated [13].

Irrelevant monitoring and observation should be discontinued to avoid unnecessary discomfort and stress both to the patient and their relatives.

Mechanical ventilator support (including pre-set pressure, volume, and respiratory rate) can be reduced by around 50% every few minutes, followed by symptom reassessment and medication adjustment [14]. Some patients respond to reduction of ventilator support with an increase in rate and depth of breathing (especially if acidemic), and this "air hunger" is uncomfortable to the patient and distressing for relatives to witness. When necessary, analgesia and sedation should be adjusted to ensure a comfortable, pain, and stress-free environment for the patient. "Death rattle" caused by accumulation of broncho-pulmonary secretions in the upper airway may be relieved by subcutaneous or intravenous hyoscine hydrobromide injection. Dependent on the patient's response and comfort levels, the entire withdrawal process may take from as little as ten minutes to a few hours. In summary, LST is usually withdrawn progressively, allowing sufficient time to treat patient's symptoms, or family distress, but not so slowly as to unnecessarily prolong suffering. Family should be interviewed after completion of the withdrawal process.

## Analgesia and sedation

The goal of quality EOL care is ensuring maximal comfort during the dying process. The use of powerful analgesics and anxiolytics to control pain and anxiety may also potentially hasten death by inhibiting respiration and producing hypotension. While there is little evidence that when used for symptom control the use of opioid or benzodiazepine hastens death in the ICU setting [15], it remains an ethical concern. Most ethicists and doctors rely on the principle of "double effect" to justify the use of sedatives and analgesics in this setting. Double effect states that if the primary reason for drug use is justified pain control and enhanced comfort, the possible associated shortening of time to death is an acceptable side-effect [16].

It is recommended to moderately escalate opioid doses in anticipation of discomfort after initiating WH/WD of LST. In addition, during WH/WD LST, drugs should be carefully but effectively titrated to achieve the relief of the patient's symptoms. Opioids, usually morphine, offer good pain relief, and decrease central respiratory drive. This effect is particularly helpful in reducing air hunger that may occur during mechanical ventilation withdrawal. Morphine is usually given intravenously (loading dose of 1–5 mg and maintenance infusion of 1–2 mg per hour, which can be titrated incrementally by 50–100% until symptoms are relieved; each increment in infusion rate should be accompanied by a bolus of 1–5 mg to ensure the new effect is rapidly achieved). Alternatively, or in addition, anxiolytics such as a benzodiazepine can be administered to enhance comfort. Midazolam is commonly used (intravenous loading dose of 1–2 mg and maintenance infusion of 0.5–2 mg per hour, titrated to symptoms). At the EOL "terminal sedation" is defined as deliberately inducing and maintaining deep sleep for control of intractable symptoms [13]. This approach may be applicable to selected ICU patients.

For cultural or religious reasons, surrogates/relatives sometimes request that patients be allowed to "wake up" prior to death. Interruption of sedation/comfort care is rarely appropriate, as patients rarely regain full consciousness because of the critical illness, organ failure, and drug accumulation, and interruption is likely to cause pain and discomfort. It is usually sufficient to carefully communicate this reality to the surrogates/relatives.

Palliative care specialty involvement in the management of EOL in ICU may be useful to deal with patients who have difficult physical symptoms, but has not been shown to be universally useful in this setting [17].

## Documentation

Clear documentation is a legal safeguard for patients, family, and healthcare professionals. Clear documentation of goals of EOL care is also a simple and effective means of communication among different healthcare teams.

Medical record documentation should include the rationale for decision-making, key agreements reached with patient/surrogates, and all planned and implemented interventions. Compared to other treatment modalities in the ICU, EOL care documentation has been found to be incomprehensive. Most clinicians document "do not resuscitate" (DNR) orders, and orders for "withholding or withdrawing mechanical ventilator support," but often neglect documenting the limitation of other invasive treatments, including renal replacement therapy, vasopressor support, or artificial nutrition. Vague terms including "comfort care," "terminal care," and "no further active intervention" provide a general instruction, but should be accompanied by clear, specific instructions [18]. Research suggests that details during family conferences are only documented about half of the time; the role of substituted decisions by family is frequently omitted, up to one-quarter of records omit documentation of the exact date and time of withdrawing treatment [19].

A suggested checklist for documentation is provided in Table 11.2. Printed or computerized data entry forms that help document and remind physicians about key components of EOL care may improve processes in the ICU, and ensure complete documentation. Intermittent audits of the documentation processes are useful to identify inadequacies that can be improved.

## Dealing with conflict

The intensely emotive nature of EOL decision-making means that conflict among healthcare workers or between family/surrogate and healthcare workers is not uncommon, and exacerbated by poor communication. Attempts to sincerely communicate usually resolve the problem, but some situations may warrant an ethics consultation to help clarify and resolve conflicts [20]. Occasionally, transfer of the patient's care to another team may be useful. Rarely, the use of legal avenues may be required.

## Healthcare worker stress

While dealing with EOL issues can be challenging, it has also been demonstrated that providing inappropriate LST to dying patients can aggravate stress for ICU healthcare providers. Persistent stress from witnessing and providing inappropriate LST is associated with increased fatigue, burn-out syndrome, and staff resignations from the ICU.

**Table 11.2** Suggested brief template for developing a documentation process for EOL decision-making (WD/WH) and implementation

| | |
|---|---|
| Preconditions to decision-making at EOL | Patient's decision-making capacity present?<br>Written medical advance directive present?<br>Initiation of WD/WH discussion<br>• Physician<br>• Family (surrogates)<br>• Patient<br>• Other<br>Trigger of WD/WH discussion?<br>• Pre-morbid status/conditions<br>• Present illness<br>• Response to treatment<br>Consensus among different HCW for WD/WH discussion with family<br>• Healthcare providers in ICU (doctors, nurses, other relevant carers)<br>• Relevant healthcare providers from attending specialties |
| Content of EOL family meeting | Explanation of physician initiation and trigger (if initiated by physician)<br>Explanation/exploration of patient initiation and trigger (if initiated by patient)<br>Explanation/exploration of initiation and trigger (if initiated by family)<br>Checking previous expressed values and preferences<br>Explanation of concept of decision-making process (region determined)<br>If necessary (autonomous or shared decision-making model)<br>• clarification of consensus among surrogates, or with patient<br>• confirmation of patient decision, or substituted decision by surrogate<br>Explanation of process to patient/surrogate<br>• LST to be withheld<br>• LST to be withdrawn<br>• Timing of withdrawal<br>• Explanation of possible symptoms during process<br>• Explanation of management plan of possible symptoms |
| Implementation after EOL decision | LST withheld<br>LST withdrawn<br>Timing of withdrawal<br>Comfort medication including dosage |
| Follow-up | Social worker, religious and spiritual support referral<br>Arrangement of follow-up meeting with surrogate<br>Adjustment/changes to original decision-making |

# Conclusion

Initiation of EOL care should be recognized as a therapeutic intervention in ICU, and warrant proper planning, anticipation of problems, prior explanation to family, and stepwise implementation. Clear documentation of the EOL decision and implementation process is important for communication and quality assurance. Importantly, limitation of LST should not be interpreted as a limitation of care, but rather a refocusing of care, with the objective of ensuring that ongoing medical care is in the patient's best interest.

# References

1. Buckley TA, Joynt GM, Tan PY, Cheng CA, Yap FH. Limitation of life support: frequency and practice in a Hong Kong intensive care unit. *Crit Care Med.* 2004;32:415–420.

2. Sprung CL, Cohen SL, Sjokvist P, *et al.* End-of-life practices in European intensive care units: the Ethicus Study. *JAMA.* 2003;290:790–797.

3. Joynt GM, Lipman J, Hartog C, *et al.* The Durban World Congress Ethics Round Table IV: health care professional end-of-life decision making. *J Crit Care.* 2015;30:224–230.

4. Sprung CL, Truog RD, Curtis JR, *et al.* Seeking worldwide professional consensus on the principles of end-of-life care for the critically ill: the consensus for Worldwide End-of-Life Practice for Patients in Intensive Care Units (WELPICUS) Study. *Am J Respir Crit Care Med.* 2014;190:855–866.

5. Heyland DK, Dodek P, Rocker G, *et al.* What matters most in end-of-life care: perceptions of seriously ill patients and their family members. *CMAJ.* 2006;174:627–633.

6. Lilly CM, De Meo DL, Sonna LA, *et al.* An intensive communication intervention for the critically ill. *Am J Med.* 2000;109: 469–475.

7. Lilly CM, Sonna LA, Haley KJ, Massaro AF. Intensive communication: four-year follow-up from a clinical practice study. *Crit Care Med.* 2003;31:S394–S399.

8. Billings JA. The end-of-life family meeting in intensive care part I: indications, outcomes, and family needs. *J Palliat Med.* 2011;14:1042–1050.

9. Zier LS, Burack JH, Micco G, *et al.* Doubt and belief in physicians' ability to prognosticate during critical illness: the perspective of surrogate decision makers. *Crit Care Med.* 2008;36:2341–2347.

10. Levin TT, Moreno B, Silvester W, Kissane DW. End-of-life communication in the intensive care unit. *Gen Hosp Psychiatry.* 2010;32:433–442.

11. McDonagh JR, Elliott TB, Engelberg RA, *et al.* Family satisfaction with family conferences about end-of-life care in the intensive care unit: increased proportion of family speech is associated with increased satisfaction. *Crit Care Med.* 2004;32: 1484–1488.

12. Roter DL, Hall JA, Kern DE, Barker LR, Cole KA, Roca RP. Improving physicians' interviewing skills and reducing patients' emotional distress: a randomized clinical trial. *Arch Intern Med.* 1995;155: 1877–1884.

13. Kompanje EJ, van der Hoven B, Bakker J. Anticipation of distress after discontinuation of mechanical ventilation in the ICU at the end of life. *Intensive Care Med.* 2008;34:1593–1599.

14. Curtis JR, Vincent JL. Ethics and end-of-life care for adults in the intensive care unit. *Lancet.* 2010;376:1347–1353.

15. Chan JD, Treece PD, Engelberg RA, *et al.* Narcotic and benzodiazepine use after withdrawal of life support: association with time to death? *Chest.* 2004;126:286–293.

16. Trankle SA. Decisions that hasten death: double effect and the experiences of physicians in Australia. *BMC Med Ethic.* 2014;15:26.

17. Cheung W, Aggarwal G, Fugaccia E, *et al.* Palliative care teams in the intensive care unit: a randomised, controlled, feasibility study. *Crit Care Resusc.* 2010;12:28–35.

18. Melltorp G, Nilstun T. Decisions to forego life-sustaining treatment and the duty of documentation. *Intensive Care Med.* 1996;22:1015–1019.

19. Kirchhoff KT, Anumandla PR, Foth KT, Lues SN, Gilbertson-White SH. Documentation on withdrawal of life support in adult patients in the intensive care unit. *Am J Crit Care.* 2004;13:328–334.

20. Aulisio MP, Chaitin E, Arnold RM. Ethics and palliative care consultation in the intensive care unit. *Crit Care Clin.* 2004;20:505–523.

Chapter

# 12

# Tools to improve patient safety and adverse events

Andreas Valentin

The notion of a nearly error-free intensive care medicine was challenged over the last years through growing evidence confirming weak points in patient safety. The classic medical principle of 'first do no harm' refers primarily to the balance of risks and benefits of a specific treatment, but reflects at the same time a basic approach to patient safety. In a more advanced concept, patient safety is considered as the assurance that a course of medical treatment will proceed correctly and provide the best possible chance to achieve a desired outcome. The very complex process of intensive care for the most severely ill patients is accompanied by a not unexpected accumulation of risk for error and adverse events. The intrinsic risk of a critically ill patient (disease, pathophysiologic derangements, etc.) adds to an extrinsic risk created by the process of care itself. The ultimate goal in terms of patient safety consists of reducing this extrinsic risk. Of note, there will never be a completely error-free process of care, but every possible effort must be made to approach this goal. It is of utmost importance to realise that individual failures are not completely preventable, nor the clue to improving quality of care. Instead, the design of the process of care, structures, and other system factors are considered as key elements in building a safer environment for the most vulnerable patients.

## Patient safety in intensive care: the scope of the problem

Intensive care is characterised by a complex course of interaction among several medical specialties and professions, use of sophisticated healthcare technology, and significant time pressure. Considering the tight coupling between the complexity of the system and the high potential for harm, most intensive care units (ICUs) seem to function very well. But over the last decades, several studies have revealed a serious safety problem in intensive care medicine. In a landmark study, Donchin recorded an average of 178 activities per patient per day and an estimated 1.7 errors per patient per day [1]. Subsequent research in large national or multinational cohorts of ICUs has confirmed that intensive care patients are frequently exposed to error, and flaws in patient safety are a common problem in ICUs worldwide [2]. In an observational study involving 205 ICUs from 29 countries, 38.8 errors per 100 patient days related to (1) medication, (2) lines, catheters, and drains, (3) equipment failure, (4) artificial airway, and (5) alarms, were observed [2].

Research in patient safety is frequently based on a broad definition of error as an occurrence that harms or could have harmed a patient. An error does not necessarily lead to patient

*Quality Management in Intensive Care*, ed. Bertrand Guidet, Andreas Valentin and Hans Flaatten. Published by Cambridge University Press. © Cambridge University Press 2016.

harm, but highlights weak and unsafe steps in the process of care. From this perspective, every error carries the chance to gain an insight into an unsafe practice or even into the defensive barrier that has prevented actual harm.

## Can we measure patient safety? What do we need to know?

To assess the current status of development constitutes an important starting point in the task of improving patient safety [3]. While a method using observers will likely be restricted to scientific purposes, the use of self-reporting systems or chart reviews has been shown to be practicable in clinical settings. Of note is that different methods will retrieve different findings. A considerable advantage of self-reporting systems is that contextual information is provided by the medical staff directly involved. Another important advantage is the creation of a team culture that relies on an atmosphere of assurance instead of the conventional approach of 'blame and shame'. It is therefore of utmost importance that medical staff be assured that they can report errors without fear of reprisal.

Incidents without subsequent harm are estimated to happen 3–300 times more frequently than harmful events, and they provide insight into the defensive barriers that prevent actual damage. An approach aimed to detect common characteristics behind the evolution of errors and to concentrate on systems which are most often the proximal cause of error requires exploration of opportunities for error, incidence rates, causes, and contributing factors, as well as preventive factors.

To measure advances in safety is a difficult undertaking. A valid measurement of advances in safety would require knowing the denominator (e.g. opportunities for harm) and the numerator (actual events). Actual harm is not always obvious and may only be detected by active screening (e.g. device-related infection, deep venous thrombosis).

## From risk assessment to risk reduction

The actual risk of an unfavourable outcome in critically ill patients depends not only – but to a considerable extent – on the quality of the care process. Any in-depth analysis of critical incidents soon reveals that two components are present when an error turns into an actual incident: human factors and system factors combine to reduce patient safety. Human errors are estimated to be involved in approximately 70% of medical errors. But while human factors play a major role, they are clearly less amenable to change than are system factors. The capabilities of human beings are limited and subject to many environmental influences. It is therefore of utmost importance that systems and work environments be designed in such a way as to prevent error or to mitigate the consequences when error occurs.

Although recognising an error after the fact is an important prerequisite for making improvements, it is obviously preferable to catch safety concerns in advance. A system in which one drug can be easily confused with another is certain to bring harm to a patient at some point. An anticipatory approach would require identifying and reviewing the look-alike and sound-alike drugs and taking action to prevent them being administered erroneously.

Several interventions have been shown to reduce errors or even to decrease the rate of adverse events associated with particular ICU activities. A number of domains have been identified in which changes in infrastructure, process, and culture can result in a substantial risk reduction.

## Human errors and ergonomic nightmares

With respect to human factors, the ICU has been described as a 'hostile environment' [4]. Diffuse or flashy lighting, difficult access to the patient and/or equipment, a lack of space, and chaotic background noise are examples of environmental conditions with which most healthcare workers in ICUs are familiar. The negative impact of such an environment may become even greater when requirements for multitasking coupled with information overload are present. In many instances, physicians and nurses need to act like an integrated clinical database, but often without the support of a properly structured information flow and an environment designed with adherence to ergonomic principles [5].

## System factor: workload and staffing

Excessive workload and working hours, shortness of sleep, and fatigue reduce the performance of healthcare personnel, and hence most likely patient safety [6]. Most of the studies in this field rely on neurocognitive and neuropsychiatric tests, rather than assessing real-life clinical performance. Although evidence from clinical studies is limited, in particular with respect to intensive care medicine, available information suggests that continuous working hours should be restricted to a maximum of 24 hours.

While working hours of nursing staff are usually strictly limited to not more than 12 hours, it has been observed that inappropriate high nursing workload is associated with an increased risk of hospital-acquired infections [7] and medication errors [8].

Working hours in the ICU and ICU staffing models are closely related to each other. Similar to regulations on working hours, ICU staffing models vary widely around the world. While evidence that involvement of intensivists in the care of critically ill patients improves outcomes is broadly accepted, the need for 24-hour in-house coverage by intensivists and, in particular, the impact of night-time intensivist coverage on ICU patient outcomes is still debated.

Demanding tasks, time pressure, and emotional stress add an additional burden for medical staff in ICUs. Burn-out and excessive job strain are common and can affect the quality of patient care. Although a clear association between burn-out among ICU personnel and the causation of error has not been demonstrated, the reported numbers are of concern. Knowing these facts, it is indisputably the duty of ICU managers and hospital administrators to optimise schedule design and ensure appropriate levels of staffing.

## Safety climate: a key factor

While recognising that system design is the major source of error, the question then arises: what is the culture behind these systems? A major change is necessary to overcome a culture of blame and shame and to create a new attitude toward learning. The steps in such a development will often evolve from a culture of denial ('We don't have that kind of incident'), to a reactive culture (reaction only after things have already gone wrong), to a general attitude of risk management as an integral part of the thinking of all professionals and managers. As a prerequisite, it is necessary to abandon the unrealistic goal of perfection, to accept the limitations of human nature, and to expect errors.

The very basis of such an approach can be described by the term *safety climate*, which has been defined as 'the shared perception of employees concerning the degree to which safety is a top priority for employees within the organization' [9]. For intensive care medicine the importance of a positive attitude towards safety issues was demonstrated in a study involving 57 ICUs from Austria, Germany, and Switzerland [10]. Whereas a higher workload was

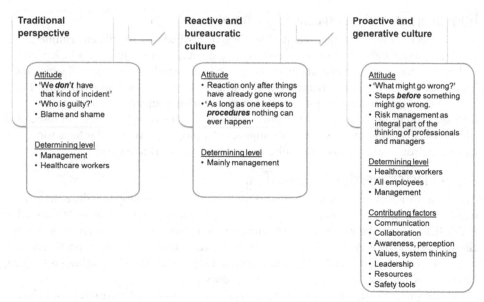

**Figure 12.1** Framework for the development of an advanced approach to patient safety.

associated with a higher occurrence of medication and dislodgement errors, a higher developed safety climate apparently contributed to a reduction of medical errors. The transformation of traditional patterns of behaviour, including the assignment of blame, into a new culture focused on systemic improvements in patient safety relies on an atmosphere of trust and respect that allows open communication. Such an open communication is the prerequisite for a helpful error-reporting system. The implementation of an adverse event reporting system in ICUs was included in a list of nine safety indicators recommended by a task force on quality and safety of the ESICM [11]. In this context it is of utmost importance that responsible leaders foster teamwork, trust, and individual commitment to patient care. The impact of such cultural changes is difficult to measure, but should not be underestimated and constitutes an essential key to improved patient safety (see Figure 12.1).

## Education and training

Considering ICUs as complex systems for the management of complex situations, it becomes clear that the actions of operators in these systems require a high level of knowledge, skill, and competence [12]. Education and training need to be seen as a continuum ongoing throughout the practice of intensive care. The safety of patient care depends on it. For instance, a multicentre study by Pronovost *et al.* showed an impressive and sustained reduction in catheter-related bloodstream infections after an intervention with strong educational elements [13].

The use of simulation exercises and team training has been encouraged in a recently published list of patient safety strategies considered as ready for adoption in clinical practice [14]. While simulation-based team training is an indispensable part of educating resuscitation teams and is increasingly used in anaesthesia and surgical disciplines, it has not yet attracted intensive care teams in the same way. Nevertheless it seems unlikely that beneficial effects of team training already demonstrated in other disciplines will not apply to intensive care medicine as well. One of the few studies with critical care teams demonstrated significant improvements in measures of teamwork and team behaviour after a simulation-based training intervention [15].

## Key elements: routine situations and continuity of care

Contrary to popular belief, errors occur most frequently in routine situations, not in unforeseeable events. As an example, the second multinational Sentinel Events Evaluation study revealed that 69% of parenteral medication errors at the administration stage took place in routine situations [8]. But a simple organisational factor such as the routine check of perfusors and infusion pumps at nurses' shift changes was associated with a decreased risk for a medication error. Fortunately, every routine procedure in an ICU carries the potential to minimise the causes or at least the consequences of error. Several studies have demonstrated that a routine procedure such as the insertion and maintenance of a central venous line is amenable to considerable improvement. Routine procedures are therefore a major starting point when looking systematically at opportunities to improve patient safety.

Other important areas of concern are gaps in the continuity of care. Obviously, standard situations such as patient transport, information transfer, and shift changes are important targets for anticipatory safety strategies. Handoff by different disciplines (particularly physicians and nurses) occurs frequently and represents a routine procedure, but at the same time a most vulnerable step. Interplay between team members and quality of information transfer among ICU staff has a profound impact on the occurrence of medical error. Appropriate and concise communication is the cornerstone of any attempt to prevent loss of information and a diminishing continuity of care in a fast-paced ICU environment. Since this process is characterised by the communication of complex information under time pressure, a structured approach focused on leadership, task allocation, rhythm, standardised processes, checklists, awareness, anticipation, and communication will support a comprehensive and safe handover.

## Medication errors: a particular safety concern

The process of getting the right drug to the right patient at the correct point in time via the appropriate route is much more complex than it first appears. This process can be divided into several stages, including prescription, preparation, dispensation, administration, and monitoring, with each of these steps carrying a particular risk for error. Prescription and time-related errors are the most frequent, but their potential impact should not be underestimated (e.g. delayed antibiotics in septic shock). Strategies to decrease medication errors refer to the above-mentioned specific stages in the process of medication use.

### Prescription stage

Probably one of the most promising strategies for reducing medication errors during prescription and transcription is the implementation of a computerised physician order entry (CPOE). But while elimination of transcription errors and ambiguous orders are a clear advantage of this expensive technology, results from studies in terms of patients' outcome are still inconclusive. A highly structured paper form and carefully designed process for documentation of orders, preparation, and administration might still be seen as an equivalent alternative.

Different from the common approach, CPOE systems have the potential to integrate interactive tools like allergy warnings or to enable clinical pharmacists to review electronic orders and provide subsequent recommendations. Potential drug–drug interactions are rarely recognised during the prescription process but may compromise patient safety by leading to toxicity or a decreased therapeutic effect. Computerised algorithms for the identification of unsafe prescriptions or potential drug–drug interactions are considered as promising tools when properly integrated in electronic prescribing systems. Although many of these problems during the medication prescription stage might also be mitigated by the involvement of pharmacists in daily rounds, results from studies involving pharmacist intervention in ICUs are still mixed [16].

## Preparation stage

Standardisation of drug infusions and drug labelling are important areas of interest during the prescription stage. In a study simulating the management of a patient with septic shock, medication errors were 17 times less likely when prefilled syringes were used. Even more interesting, infusions that were prepared during the actual management of the simulated patient were significantly less likely to contain the expected concentration than drug infusions prefilled by pharmacists or pharmaceutical companies [17].

Standardised drug labelling has beneficial effects in terms of optimised legibility and display of information and is an evidence-based strong recommendation when using agreed standards.

## Administration stage

Pertinent to different definitions about 30–45% of all medication errors occur during the administration stage. While a simple routine check of infusion pumps during nurses' shift changes has been associated with an error reduction of 30% [8], other more sophisticated measures like the integration of information technologies (e.g. bedside barcoded medication) are still more promise than reality. In intensive care the use of so-called smart pumps has gained considerable interest. These infusion pumps contain integrated features including drug/dose calculations, programmable volume and time calculations, alarms, and drug-specific libraries with a safe dosing range for each drug. This technology represents an attempt to intercept possible human errors at the bedside but might cause new problems, like a reduced ability to react quickly and be flexible in emergency situations.

## Bundles and multifaceted programmes

A system approach in terms of patient safety means to design structure and processes of a given ICU in a way to protect patients from preventable harm and to assure timely, appropriate care. This approach requires not the sequential implementation of single interventions, but rather a balanced interdisciplinary effort directed to process characteristics and execution of several measures in parallel. Care bundles and multifaceted programmes combine different components and measures, not least including an educational domain [18]. Such bundles and programmes have been shown to be effective in preventing insulin errors, accidental tube/catheter removal, catheter-related blood-stream infections, and drug-related adverse events. For example, a successful multifaceted intervention to reduce drug-related adverse events consisted of: (1) a change from handwritten to electronic prescription; (2) standardised labelling of continuously infused medications; (3) implementation of identical models of perfusors and infusion pumps; and (4) partial involvement of a pharmacist [19].

## Safe care requires more than avoiding errors

Increased awareness and recent research have triggered a movement in which patient safety is considered as a top priority in most ICUs worldwide. It is important to recognise that patient safety does not pertain only to the prevention of error. Safe care means the assurance that every patient will receive medical care that is timely, appropriate, and evidence-based. There are several examples of how patient safety is assured not only by the absence of error but by the reliable use and safe practice of processes in ICUs. For instance, many processes in the care of critically ill patients are highly time-sensitive and thus highlight the need for proper handling at the patient site as well as in secondary areas such as the delivery of medications.

Tools and measures to increase patient safety include new healthcare technologies, multifaceted programmes, standardisation, and adaptation of working conditions to human limits. To develop a culture of safety based on open communication, anticipation of risks, and effective teamwork constitutes the key element in this challenging, but no longer ignorable, evolution.

# References

1. Donchin Y., Gopher D., Olin M., et al. A look into the nature and causes of human errors in the intensive care unit. *Crit Care Med.* 1995;23(2):294–300.

2. Valentin A., Capuzzo M., Guidet B., et al. Patient safety in intensive care: results from the multinational Sentinel Events Evaluation (SEE) study. *Intensive Care Med.* 2006;32(10):1591–1598.

3. Vincent C., Burnett S., Carthey J. Safety measurement and monitoring in healthcare: a framework to guide clinical teams and healthcare organisations in maintaining safety. *BMJ Qual Saf.* 2014;23(8):670–677.

4. Donchin Y., Seagull F.J. The hostile environment of the intensive care unit. *Curr Opin Crit Care.* 2002;8(4):316–320.

5. Sevdalis N., Brett S.J. Improving care by understanding the way we work: human factors and behavioural science in the context of intensive care. *Crit Care.* 2009;13(2):139.

6. Endacott R. The continuing imperative to measure workload in ICU: impact on patient safety and staff well-being. *Intensive Care Med.* 2012;38(9):1415–1417.

7. Penoyer D.A. Nurse staffing and patient outcomes in critical care: a concise review. *Crit Care Med.* 2010;38(7):1521–1528.

8. Valentin A., Capuzzo M., Guidet B., et al. Errors in administration of parenteral drugs in intensive care units: multinational prospective study. *BMJ.* 2009;338:b814.

9. Naveh E., Katz-Navon T., Stern Z. The effect of safety management systems on continuous improvement of patient safety: the moderating role of safety climate and autonomy. *Qual Manag J.* 2011;18:54–67.

10. Valentin A., Schiffinger M., Steyrer J., Huber C., Strunk G. Safety climate reduces medication and dislodgement errors in routine intensive care practice. *Intensive Care Med.* 2013;39(3):391–398.

11. Rhodes A., Moreno R.P., Azoulay E., et al. Prospectively defined indicators to improve the safety and quality of care for critically ill patients: a report from the Task Force on Safety and Quality of the European Society of Intensive Care Medicine (ESICM). *Intensive Care Med.* 2012;38(4):598–605.

12. COBATRICE. International standards for programmes of training in intensive care medicine in Europe. *Intensive Care Med.* 2011 Mar;37(3):385–393.

13. Pronovost P.J., Goeschel C.A., Colantuoni E., et al. Sustaining reductions in catheter related bloodstream infections in Michigan intensive care units: observational study. *BMJ.* 2010;340:c309.

14. Shekelle P.G., Pronovost P.J., Wachter R.M., et al. The top patient safety strategies that can be encouraged for adoption now. *Ann Intern Med.* 2013;158(5 Pt 2):365–368.

15. Frengley R.W., Weller J.M., Torrie J., et al. The effect of a simulation-based training intervention on the performance of established critical care unit teams. *Crit Care Med.* 2011;39(12):2605–2611.

16. Manias E., Williams A., Liew D. Interventions to reduce medication errors in adult intensive care: a systematic review. *Br J Clin Pharmacol.* 2012;74(3):411–423.

17. Adapa R.M., Mani V., Murray L.J., *et al.* Errors during the preparation of drug infusions: a randomized controlled trial. *Br J Anaesth.* 2012;109(5):729–734.

18. Marsteller J.A., Sexton J.B., Hsu Y.J., *et al.* A multicenter, phased, cluster-randomized controlled trial to reduce central line-associated bloodstream infections in intensive care units. *Crit Care Med.* 2012;40(11):2933–2939.

19. Pagnamenta A., Rabito G., Arosio A., *et al.* Adverse event reporting in adult intensive care units and the impact of a multifaceted intervention on drug-related adverse events. *Ann Intensive Care.* 2012;2(1):47.

# Chapter 3

# Clinical data management

**Chapter 13**

Olaf L. Cremer and Casper W. Bollen

## Introduction

As the implementation of electronic medical record (EMR) systems is evolving across hospitals worldwide, new concepts and applications are being developed at a rapid pace. Reports by the Healthcare Information and Management Systems Society [1] show that by 2014 over 50% of US hospitals will have reached an advanced stage of EMR implementation that includes the use of computers not only for scheduling, billing, and document management, but also for clinical reporting, physician order entry and decision support – tasks that are critical to safe and efficient patient care (Figure 13.1).

Despite these advances in implementation, there remains a general lack of systematic testing and validation of the safety and efficacy of EMR systems. Most of the studies that have been performed have focused on "easy" performance metrics, such as data accuracy and completeness, but more complex aspects such as the granularity, timeliness, and interoperability of data remain poorly studied [2]. More importantly, user satisfaction of doctors and

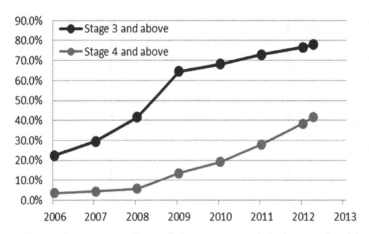

**Figure 13.1** HIMSS EMR adoption rates in US hospitals. Stage 3 systems include electronic clinical documentation, medication administration, basic decision support (error checking), and medical image access outside the radiology department. Stage 4 systems include computerized order entry and more advanced decision support (clinical protocols). HIMSS = Healthcare Information and Management Systems Society; EMR = electronic medical record.

*Quality Management in Intensive Care*, ed. Bertrand Guidet, Andreas Valentin and Hans Flaatten. Published by Cambridge University Press. © Cambridge University Press 2016.

nurses working with these systems on a daily basis has not been sufficiently addressed. In fact, physician experiences documented by the American Medical Association and the RAND Corporation demonstrate that most EMRs fail to support efficient and effective clinical work, and that many clinicians feel demoralized rather than supported by EMR technology [3]. The biggest gripes that were noted involved poor usability and time-consuming data entry, a lack of health information exchange within and between systems, distraction from face-to-face patient care, a degradation of the quality of clinical documentation due to misuse of templates, and general inefficiencies and less fulfilling work content.

Against this backdrop, this chapter will discuss some of the challenges of efficient clinical data management in general, and in an intensive care unit (ICU) in particular. For this we will primarily adopt the perspective of the end-user (as opposed to that of, e.g., the hospital administrator or systems engineer). We will provide considerations regarding the user interface design, the preferred data model, and the technical implementation of EMRs in a critical care setting.

## Challenges of data management

A patient data management system (PDMS) in the ICU integrates the information that is generated by the patient monitoring system, various bedside equipment, and the hospital information system (Figure 13.2), and as such it represents a specialized form of the general-purpose EMR. This integration of vast amounts of data entails special consideration of the functional requirements and information management challenges that must be met by a PDMS.

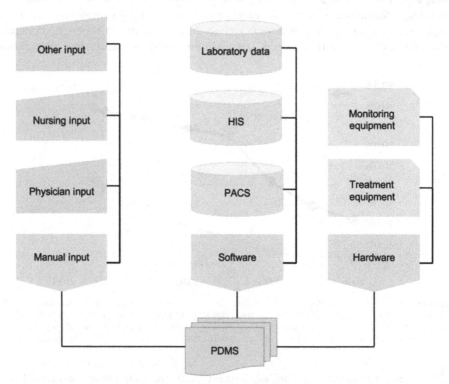

**Figure 13.2** PDMS data interfaces. A patient data management system (PDMS) has three types of data interface. First, the graphical user interface that allows manual input by users. Second, the software interface to send and receive data to/from other information systems. Third, the hardware interface obtains data from monitoring or other bedside equipment. HIS = hospital information system; PACS = picture archiving and communications system.

Functional requirements will likely vary by user type. For instance, hospital administrators may have a principal interest in the collection of billing data and quality-of-care indicators; pharmacists may need support for their logistical processes; and scientists may want to mine structured, research-quality data. But from a clinical point of view there are really only two primary demands. First, among the wealth of data that are available in a critical care environment, a PDMS must reduce the time to meaningful clinical data synthesis while avoiding information overload. Second, a PDMS must help avert medical error and support protocol adherence while avoiding alerting overload.

Difficulties in information management that are specific to a PDMS also primarily relate to the large amounts of data that become available at the bedside and need to be processed, displayed, and interpreted in real time. These data enter the PDMS either automatically as they are generated by bedside devices, or can be manually recorded, e.g., in the case of nursing observations. Furthermore, patients in the ICU exhibit a large diversity of diagnoses and clinical presentations. They typically also have a large number of concurrent problems, requiring multiple simultaneous interventions. As a result, a PDMS must accommodate a clinical dataset that is not only larger, but also more diverse and complex than is the case for a general-purpose EMR. Finally, the ICU environment is special with respect to the large number of caregivers that may simultaneously be involved in the management of individual patients, and the frequent interruptions that typically occur during the daily care process. Consequently, an efficacious PDMS design must be flexible with respect to user authorizations, and must support multitasking and non-linear workflows. Taken together, this is not a small challenge.

## Design considerations

As an information system, the fundamental operations of a PDMS amounts to data entry, data retrieval, and data processing. Data entry relates not only to the storage of clinical data generated by end users, bedside equipment, and other information systems, but also to programming and configuration of the system itself by application specialists. Data retrieval involves both the simple reproduction of information on an individual patient level as well as the generation of knowledge on an aggregate level, either for management or scientific purposes. Finally, data processing is required to transform raw data into intelligible information concepts in order to generate true added value, for instance by offering decision support. For all these operations, the quality of data contained in the system is the pivotal aspect by which the clinical value of a PDMS should be determined. Therefore, design considerations should center on offering possibilities to record and communicate data in a rich variety of formats (completeness), provide context for the user to assess the validity of information (correctness), perform cross-checks between different sources of data (concordance), analyze how information relates to other information (plausibility), and support means for reliable entry and retrieval of data in real time (currency). To accomplish this, a PDMS design must encompass both a user-friendly interface as well as suitable underlying data models that allow comprehensive data processing. In addition, there are several technical requirements concerning the dependability of the system, data security, and event logging that should be taken into consideration.

## The application interface

Usability and acceptance of any application will ultimately be determined by the ergonomics of its interface. This principle applies not only to the human–application interface but is also of relevance to any application–application interfaces (Figure 13.2). Typically, most

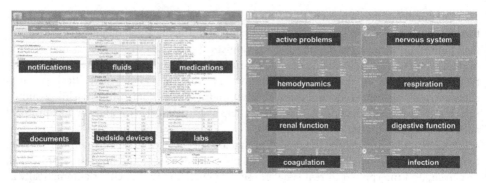

**Figure 13.3** Database-centered versus patient-oriented information views. Database-centered views display information organized by data source, whereas patient-oriented views display information organized by clinical concepts.

**Table 13.1** Success factors for acceptance of electronic health records by physicians

| | |
|---|---|
| User acceptance | Access to local FAQ lists; friendly user interfaces; notification message systems; context-aware user interfaces; automatic bookmarks based on recurrent search paths. |
| Workflow impact | Access to electronic workflow and process documentation. |
| Interoperability | Access to documents about standards; access and compatibility with other information systems. |
| Technical support | Support directories; knowledge directories, technical report hyperlinks. |
| Peer support | Electronic bulletin boards; collaborative filtering; skill directories. |

charting will require humans to manually enter information regarding bedside observations. However, monitoring devices, respirators, and other bedside equipment increasingly connect to the PDMS as well. Furthermore, several other information systems will typically be used in hospitals and these will also generate (and accept) information. This complex interplay between systems mandates the use of, and compliance to, standardized open interface definitions.

With regard to the human–application interface, a number of key factors have been identified that will ultimately determine user acceptance. Among these factors, ease of use is principal (Table 13.1). Ease of use primarily relates to the perceived complexity of the graphical user interface (GUI) and the extent to which its concepts appeal to the mindset of the user. First of all, the GUI should hide complexity rather than confront the user with convoluted views and disregard of context. Second, the GUI should provide patient-oriented and concept-oriented information views rather than force the user into a database-centric mindset (Figure 13.3). The data model (i.e., the format by which information is stored in the database) is irrelevant in this respect. Third, the user interface should facilitate rather than dictate clinical workflow. This requirement calls for a PDMS that is highly configurable and rapidly adaptable to changes in local workflow, and is one of the main reasons why hospital-wide all-purpose EMRs are poorly accepted in many ICUs today. Lastly, the user interface should respect the experience levels and working contexts of the various types of users. This is particularly true for computerized order entry, where these issues are of prime importance. Disrespect for differences in workflow between the various stakeholders involved in the medication cycle (i.e., physician, nurse, and pharmacist) as well as fragmented decision support are common failures in this domain. Of note, poor design and implementation of a computerized physician order entry system has been associated with adverse clinical outcome [12].

With regard to the application–application interface, interoperability between systems can generally be maintained by one of three strategies. The first strategy is to commit to a single vendor and fully adapt to its all-purpose system to cover all aspects of hospital information technology, ranging from general accounting to highly specialized clinical documentation. The alternative strategies comprise a best-of-suite and a best-of-breed strategy. With a best-of-suite strategy, a single core information system is selected to which modular special-purpose applications are appended if, and only if, those systems offer functionalities that the primary system cannot deliver. With a best-of-breed strategy there is essentially no core system, and for every distinct aspect of data management the best possible application is used. The former approach has generally been identified to be the most profitable [9]. However, both strategies require that different information systems can readily interconnect, which underlines the need for a standardized data interface. Even within a single application, lack of modularization may result in code that is error prone and difficult to maintain. Indeed, consistent partitioning of code and the use of standard application programming interfaces have been identified as important quality metrics of large-scale software systems [13].

## The data model

By definition, a data model is an abstraction of real-life concepts, observations, and perceptions that are typically very complex. The simplest and most straightforward way to model a data entity, therefore, is to put it in a string of free text. However, as this clearly impedes any further processing of data, clinical documentation systems in use today increasingly utilize highly structured forms for data entry, forcing end-users into the confines of predefined questions and responses. Yet clinical practice involves documentation of multiple types of information, many of which contain elements of uncertainty that need to be updated or corrected later. Failure to acknowledge this "fuzzy" aspect of clinical data inevitably leads to loss of information and user dissatisfaction. Furthermore, a complex and overly structured data model may impede the highly variable and demanding workflows in the ICU, where time can be of the essence. Therefore, in the abstraction and modeling of clinical data a natural trade-off exists between the preservation of freedom of expression and the need to categorize and process data. Failure to successfully address these challenges is likely to result in suboptimal documentation and loss of information [10].

A closely related and equally important aspect of data modeling relates to explicit consideration of the context in which the information is to be used. Computerized order entry makes for a clear example in this domain. Historically, prescribing has been modeled around the concept of individual drug products. This was largely determined by a pharmacist's point of view. However, perceived benefits of computerized order entry for physicians primarily relate to getting appropriate decision support when selecting treatment for a particular disease or symptom. The generation of a flawless electronic drug order will be merely considered as a by-product, and the technicalities involved a nuisance. In contrast, nursing staff will be mainly interested in computerized support for the planning, preparation, and administration of drugs. Lack of a data model that adequately supports these varying functional requirements will fail to adequately support the complete medication cycle in the ICU, which includes timely identification of problems, proper selection of drug therapies, and subsequent application and evaluation of treatment [11].

## Technical implementation

Nothing can degrade user confidence and erode acceptance more than poor dependability and performance of software. Therefore, reliability of the PDMS should be made as predictable and transparent as possible by subjecting the application to extensive software and hardware testing (which should preferentially be done on-site and involve end-users). After the system "goes live" performance of the client software and database servers should also be carefully monitored. Preferentially, PDMS vendors should provide the tools to do so. In addition to continuous performance monitoring and periodic systems checks, technical and peer support should be readily available to end-users at all times (Table 13.1).

As integration of information originating from different sources is mostly necessary, a uniform protocol for the transfer of data between various system components is mandatory. Clearly, well-defined application programming interfaces that are HL7 compliant may enhance technical interoperability. Furthermore, in addition to stationary computer terminals using keyboard, mouse, and screen, modern clinical environments may entail the use of a large variety of system-independent, highly responsive, mobile user interfaces. Indeed, tablet computers and even smartphones have already become ubiquitous tools to access patient data in many hospitals today. PDMS vendors should embrace these new opportunities and offer web-based user interfaces in their systems. The ability to access patient data on a mobile platform may have advantages for ICU departments in particular, given their high-tech, real-time, monitored environments. However, as wireless technologies for data access become increasingly widespread, any technical malfunction will disrupt clinical work even more easily.

## Big data

With the advent of ever increasing amounts of high-resolution data, new strategies for processing and storage need to be developed. Despite the fact that hospital information systems in general, and PDMS applications in particular, will produce huge quantities of data, many such system vendors do not provide the necessary tools to partition or otherwise upscale their databases. Notorious data producers like Amazon and Google have already devised innovative answers to deal with the problems that are inherently associated with access to and scalability of their large data bulks. These solutions favor data stores distributed over a large numbers of servers as opposed to a classical SQL database running on a single server. Unfortunately, medical software developers seriously lag behind in adopting these new technologies.

## Data security

With the advent of mobile computing and ubiquitous internet access, the safeguarding of medical data is becoming ever more important. On the one hand, optimal security will demand restricted user access accompanied by stringent authorization procedures. On the other hand, overly strict security protocols may significantly hamper clinicians working in an ICU environment that entails shared responsibilities, numerous workflow interruptions, and frequent switching of attention between patients. Single sign-on technologies that implement the clinical context object workgroup HL7 standard protocol (CCOW) may be used to alleviate the burden imposed by security procedures under such circumstances. In addition, automated logging of user access to individual patient files is mandatory to enable audits of appropriate use and to abide by general privacy guidelines.

## Future developments

Until recently, the focus of PDMS developers has been on the display of data from multiple sources (e.g., labs, imaging, bedside medical devices, pharmacy orders, nursing observations) in clinically meaningful ways. Significant progress within this area has been made, although the ergonomy of the graphical user interface that has been adopted by vendors to obtain such data integration has clearly not yet been optimized in many cases. However, major unaddressed deficiencies in PDMS functionality remain due to the limited organizational structure that is implemented for note taking, as well as the relatively primitive methods that are used to code medical information into structured data elements.

Currently, medical notes mostly consist of unstructured, narrative texts with many duplications of information (and inconsistencies as a consequence thereof). This practice imposes significant barriers to searching, summarization, and statistical analysis of such information, as well as to the implementation of decision-support systems. Unfortunately, extraction of structured information from narrative documents is still used in experimental settings only. Furthermore, the organizational framework that is adopted for such documents typically consists of little more than time-oriented (chronological) and/or source-oriented structures – the latter meaning that records are simply arranged by where and how the information was entered into the system (e.g., by medical specialty, visit, procedure type, etc.).

In order to overcome these limitations, future PDMS designs should adopt new concepts with respect to the organization of medical notes. The development stages proposed in Table 13.2 provide a useful framework in this regard. First-stage objectives are to ensure that patient encounters are recorded only once in the system, that note generation is organized around clinical problems, and that key findings of history and physical examination are coded for later use. In the second stage of development, physicians continue to record most clinical information as a free text narrative. However, they start formatting these notes with the use of structured headings and classifications, in order to enable transcription software to subsequently generate coded entries for core data elements. The feasibility of such an approach is supported by a Finnish study, which found that a large proportion of the medical narratives presently recorded by neurologists and surgeons in response to consultation requests already contain a number of standard headings, nomenclatures, and classifications [4]. Headings may be varied and can create all kinds of structure, including patient history (medical, family, social), functional status, risk factors, health problems, preventive measures, medications, reason for care, treatment goals, outcomes of care, tests and examinations, vital signs, diagnoses, surgical procedures, technical aids, living will, tissue donor will, etc. Similarly, terminologies that can frequently be found in medical narratives already include such elements as diagnostic classifications, standard nomenclatures of surgical procedures, comorbidity and disease severity scores, functional outcome scales, etc. Third-stage objectives then become to further the development of natural-language processing techniques for automatic information extraction and retrieval. Finally, as a fourth-stage objective, full semantic interoperability within and across electronic health records must be achieved. However, this can only be done by the use of clinical archetypes, invoking formal definitions of specific clinical concepts which are constructed by using generic information models. A well-known example in this domain is the Systematized Nomenclature of Medicine Clinical Terms (SNOMED-CT) [5].

**Table 13.2** Development framework for the documentation of medical narrative

| Stage 1 | • Information is recorded only once<br>• Notes are organized around clinical problems<br>• Key findings are coded for later use |
|---|---|
| Stage 2 | • Physicians record patient data as free text but with structured headings<br>• Limited transcription occurs to generate coded data entries |
| Stage 3 | • Natural language processing for information extraction and retrieval |
| Stage 4 | • Semantic interoperability across systems using clinical archetypes |

As the ability to extract accurate and meaningful clinical information from a PDMS improves, so will the possibilities for decision support. At present, such technology is limited mainly to model-driven (rule-based) systems, implying that all solutions are preprogrammed by algorithms. This approach allows for relatively simple applications, such as promotion of cost awareness, alerting for drug–drug or drug–allergy interactions, and support of guideline adherence (e.g., by providing care bundle checklists, vaccination reminders, etc.). However, much more advanced concepts for clinical decision support using data-driven (self-learning) methodologies have already been conceived, more than a decade ago [6]. By using neural networks, fuzzy logic, machine learning, case-based reasoning, Bayesian belief networks, and similar techniques that allow for ambiguity in the data, decision-support systems become capable of arriving at novel, unexpected solutions. They may then begin to act as intelligent assistants to clinical experts. Examples of successful deployment of artificial intelligence into clinical practice is still scarce at present [7]. However, future PDMS applications will likely include increasingly advanced clinical decision-support systems to assist with diagnosis, prognostication, antibiotic stewardship, and (other) therapeutic decision-making – domains where providing accurate probabilistic estimates of patient outcomes may offer genuine guidance to attending doctors and nurses.

# References

1. HIMSS Analytics. Healthcare Information and Management Systems Society. www.himssanalytics.org/home/index.aspx (accessed 15 May 2014).

2. Chan K.S., Fowles J.B., Weiner J.P. Review: electronic health records and the reliability and validity of quality measures – a review of the literature. *Med Care Res Rev.* 2010;67(5):503–527.

3. Friedberg M.W., Chen P.G., Van Busum K.R., *et al. Factors Affecting Physician Professional Satisfaction and Their Implications for Patient Care, Health Systems, and Health Policy.* Santa Monica, CA: Rand Corporation, 2013.

4. Häyrinen K., Harno K., Nykänen P. Use of headings and classifications by physicians in medical narratives of EHRs: an evaluation study in a Finnish hospital. *Appl Clin Inform.* 2011;2(2):143–157.

5. SNOMED CT: The Global Language of Healthcare. The International Health Terminology Standards Development Organisation. www.ihtsdo.org/snomed-ct (accessed 13 November 2014).

6. Hanson C.W., Marshall B.E. Artificial intelligence applications in the intensive care unit. *Crit Care Med.* 2001;29(2):427–435.

7. Williams C.N., Bratton S.L., Hirshberg E.L. Computerized decision support in adult and pediatric critical care. *World J Crit Care Med.* 2013;2(4):21–28.

8. Moore G. Integrated suites vs best of breed–advantage 2013. YouTube, 12 February 2014.

9. Ford E.W., Huerta T.R., Menachemi N., Thompson M.A., Yu F. Health information technology vendor selection strategies and total factor productivity. *Health Care Manage Rev.* 2013;38(3): 177–187.

10. Meystre S., Shen S., Hofmann D., Gundlapalli A. Can physicians recognize their own patients in de-identified notes? *Stud Health Technol Inform.* 2014;205: 778–782.

11. Maat B. Optimization of electronic prescribing in pediatric patients. Diss. U Medical Center Utrecht, 2014.

12. Han Y.Y. Unexpected increased mortality after implementation of a commercially sold computerized physician order entry system. *Pediatrics.* 2005;116(6):1506–1512.

13. Sarkar S., Kak A.C., Rama G.M., Metrics for measuring the quality of modularization of large-scale object-oriented software. *IEEE T Software Eng.* 2008;34(5):700–720.

# Electronic ICU management systems

John C. O'Horo, Ronaldo A. Sevilla Berrios, and
Brian W. Pickering

## Introduction

The modern framework for quality improvement in healthcare dates back to 1966, with the Donabedian model. This model assesses healthcare in terms of structure, processes, and outcomes of care. In his original paper, Donabedian discusses the benefits and costs of several different methods of gathering information. These methods include direct observation (thorough but costly, and prone to the Hawthorne effect) and survey data (simple for inferring, but offers little direct information). However, Donabedian dedicated the majority of his discussion of information sources to the medical record. Donabedian noted that this is necessarily the main source of information on quality, but is subject to several limitations, including:

1. lack of ready access;
2. variable documentation practices and quality;
3. veracity and verifiability of statements in the record.

Donabedian opined that:

[M]uch discussion has centered on the question of the completeness of clinical records and whether, in assessing the quality of care based on what appears in the record, one is rating the record or the care provided. What confuses the issue is that recording is itself a separate and legitimate dimension of the quality of practice, as well as the medium of information for the evaluation of most other dimensions. [1]

Beyond these limitations, data from this era took significant time to gather, analyze, and process. This means most quality improvement (QI) data are retrospective, and carry the limits inherent to such studies.

Around the same time, electronic medical records began to emerge. Lawrence Weed (inventor of the SOAP note) introduced the Problem Oriented Medical Record in Vermont. This early system allowed for improvement of documentation quality and standardized input [2]. Separately, G. Octo Barnett invented a similar program for Massachusetts General Hospital. This system, COSTAR, directly assessed quality assurance by querying for fallouts from care, such as determining when positive *Strep* throat cultures did not have follow-up [3]. Despite being hailed as revolutionary, relatively few hospitals outside of government institutions and a handful of academic centers adopted this new technology. In the 1990s, EMRs were still not implemented in the majority of healthcare settings.

*Quality Management in Intensive Care*, ed. Bertrand Guidet, Andreas Valentin and Hans Flaatten. Published by Cambridge University Press. © Cambridge University Press 2016.

The now infamous Institute of Medicine "To Err is Human" report highlighted the impact of medical errors in terms of morbidity and mortality, and the extent to which healthcare lagged behind other major industries in risk management and quality improvement. The report identified several key reasons, including communication problems and a lack of transparency. However, the slow rate of adoption of technology in healthcare received special mention [4]. Medical records had not advanced much in the preceding decades, and Donabedian's vision of adoption of better records as a quality improvement tool in and of itself was more or less ignored.

In his 2004 address to the world healthcare congress, then Secretary of Health and Human Services Tommy Thompson asked:

> Why is it that when you go into a grocery store, a high school freshman can check out all of your groceries without making a single mistake? But doctors still haven't learned how to write. Doctors have terrible handwriting, and they scribble prescriptions that nurses and pharmacists misread or mis-transcribe. If a nurse reads a script "UG" as an "MG" she could administer a thousand doses instead of one-milligrams instead of micrograms. [5]

The fact that healthcare lagged behind grocery stores in using technology to prevent errors was an embarrassment. The adoption of electronic technology in healthcare incentivized via the HITECH Act [6] has increased significantly in the last decade. This has allowed for novel approaches to quality assessment and improvement.

Beyond addressing the weaknesses Donabedian cites, the EMR provides novel tools for quality improvement. Content is easier to verify through queries of objective data also stored in the record in the form of "digital signatures" [7]. Computers can provide up-to-date care models and information better to physicians. As Dr. Weed said:

> In the 1950s, when computers came along, the engineers and the physicists they caught on right away. You use the computer to do what the human mind can't do. If you want to go to the moon, you can't have humans doing the calculations…. When are [medical schools] going to wake up and stop moving knowledge through heads and start moving knowledge through tools? [8]

Finally, and perhaps most significantly, electronic systems can provide information in real time about both technical processes of care and outcomes. Data about daily goals of care, discharges, mortality, and length of stay can be queried as they become available, ensuring relevant and accurate information to guide organizational decisions [7].

## A case study in implementation of a clinical informatics quality improvement tool: the smart electronic checklist

Electronic medical records (EMRs) have an intrinsic potential to directly impact and improve patient care delivery. Initially, this was achieved through superior documentation of medical plans of care and events [9]. But more recently, an alternative pathway has been explored, medical decision-support tools. Point-of-care information aids can enhance physicians' ability to provide high-quality care [10], and considering that EMRs already contain a large volume of patient data, it is possible to use this information to personalize care recommendations [11].

What follows is a case study in implementation of a quality improvement tool using an informatics approach in a medical intensive care unit (ICU). The key phases in the development, implementation, and sustainability of quality improvement tools integrated in the

EMR are outlined in Table 14.1. A novel EMR interface which presents information in a manner directly applicable to ICU care was already established in the ICU and was used as the platform for developing the quality improvement tool [12,13]. This interface organizes data by organ systems and highlights laboratory and vital data critical to providing timely critical care interventions; it also minimizes end-user data overload, improves efficiency of data gathering, and reduces medical decision-making errors [14].

A key target for quality improvement was rounding. In the pre-intervention period, morning rounds began with clinicians collecting information from the medical record, and reorganizing and summarizing it for discussion among members of a multidisciplinary care team (MDCT). The end goal of MDCT rounds is to delineate a working plan for the day, complete with goals and objectives for advancing patient care. This process had inherent inefficiencies and potential sources of error, such as time spent gathering data, difficulty in identifying missing process-of-care information, or tasks written on paper and not shared across the entire team. After extensive discussion with local clinical practice, a smart electronic rounding tool was designed and built. Using rapid cycle iterative prototyping the tool was optimized with practice to automatically extract and display process information already available in the electronic medical record, including vital signs, patient medications, certain laboratory results, and ventilator data. This information was used to generate a customized checklist for each patient based on common "best practices" pertinent to their care. This smart checklist was displayed within the existing novel user interface to address all routine medical care processes on a daily basis.

**Table 14.1** Steps in the development and integration of electronic quality improvement tools into the clinical environment

| Development phase | Strategy |
| --- | --- |
| Stakeholder engagement | Identify the quality improvement target with key stakeholders. |
| | Determine the workflow integration point(s) for decision support and alerts. |
| | Identify the data requirements for point-of-care decision support and alerts. |
| | Clinical site visit with project champions and potential super-users. |
| Technical development | Integrate the key required data into a central data repository with a rules engine. |
| | Refine developed rules and test rule performance against the gold standard of clinical review. |
| | Use a rapid prototype process such as AGILE to develop iterations of the quality improvement tool which can be tested in safe clinical environments. |
| Implementation | Review by key stakeholders with approval to proceed to live clinical environment. |
| | Develop education materials and tailored implementation plans with key stakeholders. |
| | Train champions and super-users in the use of the quality improvement tool. |
| | Launch a day event with emphasis on stakeholder goals and clarification of any education gaps. |
| Sustainability | Quality improvement dashboard which track key success metrics. |
| | Formal error reporting or enhancement request mechanism linked to rapid turnaround of request. |
| | Stakeholder appreciation days and workshops. |
| | Leadership or externally mandated compliance with quality metric. |

Examples of processes represented on the smart checklist include; sedative medications break/discontinuation; low tidal volume ventilation strategy; ventilator-associated pneumonia prevention bundle compliance; spontaneous breathing trials patient safety for transfer; glucose monitoring and control; deep venous thrombosis (DVT) prophylaxis; delirium evaluation and treatment and evaluation of antibiotic therapy appropriateness. An example of the type of rules embedded in the rounding tool is that developed for the detection of potentially injurious mechanical ventilation. The ventilator-induced lung injury sniffer uses the patient's height to calculate an ideal tidal volume for the patient and compares this value to the ventilator set tidal volume. Any set tidal volumes >6 ml/kg of ideal body weight are displayed as an alert on the rounding dashboard. The clinical team is prompted to address highlighted processes of care and record their actions within the rounding tool. Similar sniffers have been effectively deployed as research strategies and as administrative tools; however, they are challenging to implement in clinical practice, with few examples to draw upon for real-time clinical support [15].

Challenges, both anticipated and unanticipated, arise when translating quality improvement tools into routine clinical practice. In the case of the ICU checklist discussed above, initial implementation was slow; a small number of users adopted the tool very quickly, a larger group adopted later, and there remained a small group of committed non-adopters. A pilot implementation phase was used to work out bugs and troubleshoot workflow integration issues. Figure 14.1 illustrates a typical implementation and adoption cycle for quality improvement projects integrated into clinical practice.

After the pilot implementation, clinical "champions" on the unit – persons familiar with the workflow of that particular ICU who were early adopters and enthusiastic about the potential benefits – were engaged as key drivers of the broader implementation process. The "on the ground" perspective of the clinical champions was key to the success of the broad implementation system. Insights and changes made to implementation which derived from the champions perspective included: a revised education schedule to coincide with the start date of new clinical learners coming on service – this resulted in all physicians receiving a refresher training session before the end of their first day in the ICU; and the addition of a prompter to morning rounds to periodically remind clinicians to address rounding tool items when rounding tool checklist completion was low. These and other interventions resulted in an overall improvement in utilization of the checklist tool from 40% completion at base line to 60–70% compliance rate. These provider-centered, on-the-ground efforts were supplemented

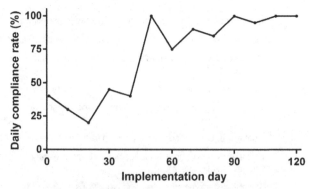

**Figure 14.1** A sample of daily checklist completion compliance rates following the introduction of an electronic checklist and quality improvement administrative dashboard.

with the development of an administrative dashboard which gave direct and indirect supervisors of clinical teams access to real-time checklist compliance rates. The implementation team, in conjunction with clinical leadership, reviewed daily the administrative dashboard and provided direct feedback to the clinician team. These mixed strategies, relying on both human efforts and electronic surveillance [16,17], pushed compliance to 95% or higher on any given day of the implementation period. The impact of these efforts on checklist compliance is illustrated in Figure 14.1.

## Conclusion

The widespread adoption of EMRs has significant implications for quality improvement in the ICU setting. Ready access to large quantities of structured data offers many potential advantages over traditional manual chart review. Once validated, these data can be utilized to generate real-time performance reports. Integration of such reports into the workflow offers bedside clinicians the opportunity to address potential quality-of-care lapses before they occur. The development of such integrated tools requires significant investment in time and effort and is currently beyond the scope of many ICU practices. As the EMR infrastructure matures it is likely that both academic and commercial partners will offer ready-made quality improvement tools for the ICU. The challenge for providers will be to evaluate the claims made for these tools and to choose one which will work for their particular practice needs. While the authors are optimistic that the emerging widespread adoption of the EMR is a positive development, the fundamental observation of Donabedian, that quality improvement is highly reliant on data contained within the medical record, is even more relevant when human pattern recognition is replaced with the informatics approach outlined above. The medical record will always remain only as useful as the data entered into it. Any quality improvement process dependent on the automated extraction of data from the EMR must pass a corresponding clinical validation step in which the signal derived from the extracted data is compared to the clinical reality. To inadequately invest in this step is to risk chasing inappropriate targets and will have unintended consequences for clinical care.

## References

1. Donabedian A. Evaluating the quality of medical care. 1966. *Milbank Q.* 2005;83(4):691–729.

2. Stratmann WC, Goldberg AS, Haugh LD. The utility for audit of manual and computerized problem-oriented medical record systems. *Health Serv Res.* 1982;17(1):5–26.

3. Barnett GO, Winickoff R, Dorsey JL, Morgan MM, Lurie RS. Quality assurance through automated monitoring and concurrent feedback using a computer-based medical information system. *Med Care.* 1978;16(11):962–970.

4. Kohn LT, Corrigan J, Donaldson MS. *To Err is Human: Building a Safer Health System.* Washington, DC: National Academy Press, 2000.

5. Thompson T, ed. Address of Tommy G. Thompson Secretary of Health and Human Services to the World Health Care Congress. World Healthcare Congress; 27 January 2004, Washington, DC.

6. Health Information Technology for Economic and Clinical Health (HITECH) Act, Pub. L. No. 111–115, Stat. 226 (2009).

7. Alsara A, Warner DO, Li G, Herasevich V, Gajic O, Kor DJ. Derivation and validation of automated electronic search strategies to identify pertinent risk factors for postoperative acute lung injury. *Mayo Clinic Proceedings.* 2011;86(5):382–388.

8. Wright A, Sittig DF, McGowan J, Ash JS, Weed LL. Bringing science to medicine: an interview with Larry Weed, inventor of the problem-oriented medical record. *J Am Med Inform Assoc.* 2014;21:964–968.

9. Rector A, Nowlan W, Kay S, Goble C, Howkins T. A framework for modelling the electronic medical record. *Methods of Inf Med*. 1993;32(2):109–119.

10. Shortliffe EH, Buchanan BG, Feigenbaum EA. Knowledge engineering for medical decision making: a review of computer-based clinical decision aids. *Proceedings of the IEEE*. 1979;67(9):1207–1224.

11. Weiss SM, Kulikowski CA, Amarel S, Safir A. A model-based method for computer-aided medical decision-making. *Artificial Intelligence*. 1978;11(1):145–172.

12. Pickering BW, Herasevich V, Ahmed A, Gajic O. Novel representation of clinical information in the ICU: developing user interfaces which reduce information overload. *Appl Clin Inform*. 2010;1(2):116–131.

13. Herasevich V, Pickering BW, Dong Y, Peters SG, Gajic O. Informatics infrastructure for syndrome surveillance, decision support, reporting, and modeling of critical illness. *Mayo Clinic Proceedings*. 2010;85(3):247–254.

14. Ahmed A, Chandra S, Herasevich V, Gajic O, Pickering BW. The effect of two different electronic health record user interfaces on intensive care provider task load, errors of cognition, and performance. *Crit Care Med*. 2011;39(7):1626–1634.

15. Herasevich V, Tsapenko M, Kojicic M, *et al.* Limiting ventilator-induced lung injury through individual electronic medical record surveillance. *Crit Care Med*. 2011;39(1):34–39.

16. McDonald CJ. The barriers to electronic medical record systems and how to overcome them. *J Am Med Inform Assoc*. 1997;4(3):213–221.

17. Hunt DL, Haynes RB, Hanna SE, Smith K. Effects of computer-based clinical decision support systems on physician performance and patient outcomes: a systematic review. *JAMA*. 1998;280(15):1339–1346.

# Chapter 5

# ICU staff
## Needs and utilization

### Gaetano Iapichino and Dinis dos Reis Miranda

Every intensive care unit (ICU) has different care requirements depending on its type, volume, and severity of patients admitted, and the unit's standing practice/policies of care [1,2]. Most of the resources available to the ICU are fixed, comprising the number of beds, the technological environment, and the permanent staff. The largest part of the fixed resources allocated to the ICU is the nursing staff.

## Nursing staff

Intensive care (IC) is mainly provided by nurses. It is therefore logical that the nursing staff serves as a reliable benchmark for evaluating the match between provision and use (seen here as demand) of ICU resources.

When planning an ICU, the number of nurses required depends mainly on three decisions/ factors: (1) the number of beds; (2) the expected level of complexity of care to be provided per bed or, in other words, the mean daily amount of nursing work per bed; (3) the expected/ planned annual occupancy/availability. In ideal circumstances, these three decisions should be preceded by a thorough survey of the medical activities in the hospital delivering patients to the ICU (annual number, type, and complexity), and of the general wards receiving the patients afterwards, so that the ICU can establish clear discharge policies.

In 1990, we recommended a useful formula for calculating the nursing staff in the ICU [1] (Table 15.1). However, there may be constraints in planning a new ICU: for instance, the

**Table 15.1** Formula for calculating the nursing staff in an ICU

No. of professionals = A × B × C × D × E / F × G, in which:

A. No. of shifts per day (usually three)
B. No. of beds in the unit
C. No. of days the unit is operative per week (usually seven)
D. Desired occupancy rate (85% recommended)
E. Extra manpower for holidays, illness, etc. (usually 20%)
F. No. of patients (beds) to be assisted by one professional
G. No. of days/week each professional works.

Making the necessary re-arrangements (F) can also be worked out if the number of professionals staffing the unit is known [1].

*Quality Management in Intensive Care*, ed. Bertrand Guidet, Andreas Valentin and Hans Flaatten. Published by Cambridge University Press. © Cambridge University Press 2016.

number of beds (space constraint) and/or the number of nurses (budget constraint) may have already been decided. Two approaches are presented here: theoretical and pragmatic.

# The theoretical approach

Knowing the nursing tasks required, the ICU staffing can be calculated from the requirements per patient, alone, or can also take account of the effect of the work required on the wellbeing of the worker.

*The patient-based theoretical approach* assumes a direct, proportional relation between severity of illness and the intensity and complexity of the care required: therapeutic interventions, technologic and human resources, etc. This approach considers two methods: the "dependency method" and the "activity method."

## The dependency method

The rationale behind this method lies in the advantages of optimizing the provision of resources and demand in the care of the critically ill, in terms of effectiveness and efficiency. These were the reasons why ICUs were created, as this level of care (LOC) could not be provided *ad hoc* in general wards. This approach aims at the better use of resources (particularly staff) while maintaining the same quality of care. The dependency method assumes that IC can be provided effectively at different LOCs, provided the requirements of each patient are matched by the resources made available: a "fixed" nurses per bed (B:N) ratio for each level.

LOCs were initially defined in 1983 by the Bethesda Consensus Conference, supported by the use of the Therapeutic Intervention Scoring System (TISS) [3], and by a 1990 report of the European Society of Intensive Care Medicine (ESICM) [1]. In 1997, an ESICM task force [4] considered the following LOCs: Level 1 (lowest) with a B:N ratio of 3:1; Level 2 with a B:N ratio of 1.6:1; and Level 3 (highest) B:N ratio of 1:1. The recommended ratios were revisited on various occasions [5]. In 2001 LOCs were described simply based on the presence of six of the nine items [6] used in the Nine Equivalents of Nursing Manpower Use Score (NEMS) rating system [7].

In 2011 the ESICM Working Group on Quality Improvement redefined LOCs [8]. This time, severity of illness (involving a set of clinical conditions) was linked to B:N ratios and the professional mastering of particular technologies. The highest (LOC III, B:N ratio 1:1) comprised patients with multiple (two or more) acute vital organ failures of an immediate life-threatening nature. LOC II (B:N ratio 2:1) grouped patients requiring monitoring and pharmacological and/or device-related support (e.g., hemodynamic support, respiratory assistance, renal replacement therapy) for only one acutely failing vital organ system that could be life-threatening. The lowest level (LOC I, B:N ratio 3:1) comprised patients with organ dysfunction needing continuous monitoring and minor pharmacological or device-related support; or because of clinical instability or shortage of nursing staff in a regular ward.

Quantification is the strength of this method. However, it has some major weaknesses: (1) it is often hard to confirm the clinical conditions on which decisions are to be based at admission/discharge; (2) the method does not provide any actual quantification for distinguishing the levels; (3) the method can only be assessed by IC professionals, and is not open to hospital managers; (4) the "competence criterion" regarding the use of IC technologies makes the method difficult to manage correctly, considering that IC medicine is a recognized specialty both for physicians and nurses.

## The activity method

With the "activity method" the allocation of nursing staff depends on what work is required for each patient [9]. Several tools have been devised and validated for measuring nursing workload; however, we will only examine the systems whose use has attracted the general attention of professionals.

Quantifying the work of nurses, these tools help assess operative LOCs per patient, i.e., the number of patients assisted by one nurse (P:N ratios). The first rating system was the TISS, published in 1974 [3]. This version comprised 57 items, chosen by a panel of experts, describing medical and related nursing activities in the ICU. It was initially proposed as a severity score, but its use declined as specific severity scores were developed. The TISS has been updated several times to clinical practice in the ICU, and the number of items reduced: in 1983, the TISS had 76 items; in 1996, 28 (TISS-28) [10]; in 1997, TISS-28 was further compressed into nine items – the NEMS [6]. All these scores take 40–50 cumulative points as corresponding to the work of one experienced ICU nurse in each shift. TISS-28 and NEMS are both still currently used in many ICUs for clinical and research purposes.

Although these instruments reflect the nursing workload, the TISS has been criticized [11–13]. Briefly: (1) the weights to the items, attributed by consensus, were related to the notion of severity of illness and the use of technology. For example, "mechanically ventilated" was assigned lower weight than "mechanical ventilation under muscle relaxation"; but the nursing time and workload are roughly the same; (2) the assumed correlation between workload and the type and number of therapeutic interventions in the ICU does not reflect the nursing work as it overlooks many nursing tasks not strictly related to the patient's condition (e.g., communications among staff, support for patient or relatives, administrative tasks) [14,15]; (3) because the TISS items focus on diagnosis, medical interventions, and the related technologies used, the score only covers 43% of all nursing tasks (all the others are considered to be equally distributed over all patients). Understandably, although the TISS correlates very well with severity of illness and overall cost, it has only weak discriminative power for the nursing workload among patients.

Finally, the Time-Oriented Score System (TOSS) published in 1991 [12] and the Canadian Project for Research (PRN) in Nursing developed in 1980 – with a version for the ICU – have introduced the novelty of rating the time required by a nurse to complete the tasks involved with the patient.

TOSS was validated on a general adult ICU population. In addition to tasks related to the level of patient acuity or severity of illness, it considers some nursing interventions not in direct contact with the patient. The score provides a measured figure for the time required for each of 82 tasks in a list of 12 categories of nursing jobs. The overall nursing workload (in minutes) per shift or day is based on the rate of execution of all scored tasks.

The PRN lists eight categories of procedures. Each category is composed of 35 tasks and 87 modalities that are described and weighted. A fixed score is assigned to each task (one point equals five minutes). The time needed to complete each task correctly is determined by Delphi consensus. However, the use of the PRN system has rarely been reported in the last two decades, perhaps because it is too complex to be practical, and not stable enough for use in comparative studies.

The Nursing Activities Score (NAS) [11], developed and primarily validated in ICUs with a general adult population, was published in 2003. Consisting of 23 items, the NAS measures the average time it takes a nurse to complete each nursing task. The items (and sub-items), selected by an international panel of experts (Delphi method), describe all nursing activities in the ICU, independent of patient conditions, diagnosis, or the interventions to which the activities might be related. For example, washing was itemized instead of incontinence, monitoring and/or presence at bedside instead of Swan-Ganz catheter, etc. The activities itemized remain therefore independent of any changes in the strategies of care, such as the adoption of new technologies. Time was determined by the "work-sampling" technique, a somewhat complex statistical method that replaces real clocking.

The NAS covers 81% of nursing activities in the ICU. The other approximately 19% not itemized are personal activities, such as personal care, eating, resting, etc. These were proportionately accounted for in the scored activities. In the NAS, 100 points equals the work of one nurse around the clock.

Use of the NAS is increasing rapidly around the world. Several studies have shown that this score is also applicable in non-general ICUs, and in pediatric ICUs [16], and its suitability for measuring nursing workload in ICUs with different LOCs has been demonstrated on several occasions. The robustness of the NAS has drawn the attention of ICU managers eager to match provision and demand of nursing care during the daily shifts [17]. These studies suggest that the NAS could serve to survey the *de facto* B:N ratios in all wards and services where patients are cared for in hospital: this could lead to a comprehensive, knowledge-based policy of patient transfers among the various hospital departments.

Keeping appropriate records of the performance of the items around the clock may prove cumbersome. However, these scores can be almost completely recorded online. The NAS was proposed for the online monitoring of costs in the ICU [18].

## The worker-based theoretical approach

Workload can be measured from the worker's perspective [9]. This measure, developed 20 years ago for aviation (NASA_TLX), has been used to measure the ICU nursing workload [19]. The aim of this approach is to define the nursing impact of each activity (six domains: mental, physical, temporal demand, frustration, effort, and performance) to encompass the complexity of the ICU nursing workload. It is always problematic for ICU management to quantify day-by-day nursing workloads and take decisions on the numbers of nurses needed.

## The pragmatic approach

One important point concerns the dual terminology used in the literature to define ICU nursing staffing: number of beds per nurse (B:N ratio) and number of patients per nurse (P:N ratio). Though at first glance they look similar, they can in fact depict different situations. The "dependency methods" define LOCs in terms of B:N ratios, assuming that all beds are equal and the total number of nurses for the ICU is calculated using one formula, such as in Table 15.1. In principle, B:N ratios indicate a recommendation or guideline, whereas P:N ratios express a measurement: a P:N of 3, for example, does not mean that all those patients receive the same amount of nursing care (it might be 60%, 25%, and 15%, or any other figure; the beds are obviously not equal as regards consumption of resources). It is therefore quite possible that in daily practice the recommended LOC (B:N ratio) will not correspond to the LOC actually provided (P:N ratio).

Indeed, these LOCs are rarely respected on account of various admission/discharge constraints or inadequacies [2,5,20]. In 75% of the ICUs examined in the EURICUS studies, there was a major mismatch between resources made available and those used. This concerned the use of beds and the use of nursing manpower (72% of work available). In many situations the mismatch may be caused by the "recovery function of the ICU," reserving empty beds for post-operative admissions. Another common reason is that other staff members in the unit may do work usually done by registered nurses (aides or student nurses, therapists, technicians). This releases manpower for assisting more complex cases or for dealing with more patients without having to raise the number of nurses. If this is not the case, however, there is a "waste" of nursing manpower and ICU resources [5,20,21].

In Europe, ICUs very rarely employ scoring systems to measure the use of nursing manpower. In addition, the "dependency methods" of staffing (produced by panels of experts) may not have been based on quantification studies, and therefore do not always work properly. Consequently, every ICU needs to engage in the exercise of detecting inappropriate use of resources in terms of both nurse workload and provided vs. planned LOC [14].

### Inappropriate use of nursing work

This exercise can be best accomplished by applying the NAS for a reasonable length of time (say, 6–12 months); this is the only published scoring system covering all nursing activities in the ICU. All the NAS scores can be summed up to give the amount of nursing work consumed, which can then be compared to the total available nursing work in the same period. Dividing the total NAS points actually scored by the total available number of NAS points (depending on the number of nursing full-time-equivalents in the ICU) gives the work utilization rate [2,5].

Summarizing, in an existing or a new ICU, whatever the method employed to determine the nursing staff, scoring systems must be used to measure nursing manpower: for the daily adjustment of provision and demand of nursing care; to fine-tune admission and discharge decisions; for auditing management policies regarding the nursing staffing of the ICU; for online monitoring of costs.

### Inappropriate delivery of levels of care

Usually, ICUs are designed to provide one LOC (including beds, technology, and staffing). Most units are intended for high-level care, with only a minority for lower levels (intermediate, step-down units). Indeed, when a high-level patient is improving but is not yet ready to be transferred to a ward, this may block the admission of a more severe patient [22]. The absence of step-down units/facilities has deleterious effects on the cost and quality of care [23].

We designed a simple, easy-to-use approach to monitor practice patterns and determine the rate and appropriateness of human and fixed resource use on a shift or daily basis [7]. To optimize staff and equipment utilization with a fixed number of nurses, we simply have to overcome the notion of the ICU having a fixed number of beds. The number of operative beds should be established starting from a minimum – when all patients require the planned LOC – up to a maximum – when all patients only require a lower LOC [20,21].

This fits in with the important idea that staffing must be flexibly matched to need throughout each patient's stay [24]. It can safely increase the use of resources in a high-level ICU, allowing admission of a new high-risk patient while avoiding too early discharge. This means implementing a post-intensive step-down flexible section inside the high-level ICU without increasing staffing. The practicability of this project depends on the structure of the unit (e.g., space for the planned number of beds with technology and staff at LOC 3 and space and technology (no nurse) for additional (say, one-third of beds) at LOC 1) [21].

# Medical staff

No score like the one for nurses has yet been devised for physicians. There are two possible reasons for this: the nature of medical work and how it is organized.

As the distribution of tasks is organized by the hospital, the level of "abstract" as opposed to "concrete" issues of patient care in the ICU is quite different for the medical and the nursing staff. Nursing work is primarily focused on provision of care. Therefore, nursing staff spend almost all their time in the ICU. The medical staff are specifically responsible for the planning of care. Therefore, they frequently do not spend all their time close to patients and quite often work outside the ICU. Consequently, in the ICU the physicians' tasks are often more abstract and nurses' mainly concrete. This makes it harder to rate the physicians' tasks using a score.

The medical staff in the ICU are organized quite differently from the generally accepted and practiced professional standardization of the nursing staff. Particularly among non-university ICUs, there are still big differences in medical staffing: (1) the ICU may not have its own medical staff; (2) in those ICUs with an open organization, for example, the medical staff, when there are any, are not primarily responsible for the care of the patients; (3) the number of physicians staffing the ICU varies and is not centrally controlled. Some studies indicate that there are too few physicians to staff all the ICUs properly and that the shortage will persist for some time to come [25]. Optimal medical ICU staffing may depend on the type, size, and case-mix of the unit, among other factors [16,21,26].

Medical presence in the ICU is a key factor in providing proper high-level care. Their presence has been significantly associated with the reduction of complications and mortality in the ICU.

The medical organization in each ICU is the director's managerial choice. If an ICU wants to treat high-LOC patients, continuous medical attention during nights, weekends, and holidays by experienced physician(s) with IC medicine, certification must be guaranteed. For 6–8 high-level beds there must be no fewer than one fully dedicated physician on a round-the-clock basis.

# References

1. D. Reis Miranda, D. Langrehr. National and regional organisation. In: Miranda D.R., Williams A., Loirat P., eds. *Management of Intensive Care: Guidelines for Better Use of Resources*. Dordrecht and Boston, MA: Kluwer Academic Publishers, 1990; 83–102.

2. D. Reis Miranda, D. W. Ryan, W. B. Schaufeli, V. Fidler. *Organisation and Management of Intensive Care: A Prospective Study of 12 European Countries*. Berlin, Heidelberg: Springer, 1998; 13–36.

3. D.J. Cullen, J.M. Civetta, B.A. Briggs, *et al.* Therapeutic Intervention Scoring System: a method for quantitative comparison of patient care. *Crit Care Med* 1974; 2: 57–60.

4. P. Ferdinande. Recommendation on minimal requirements for intensive care departments: Members of the Task Force of the European Society of Intensive Care Medicine. *Intensive Care Med* 1997; 23: 226–232.

5. R. Moreno, D. Reis Miranda. Nursing staff in intensive care in Europe: the mismatch between planning and practice. *Chest* 1998; 113: 752–758.

6. G. Iapichino, D. Radrizzani, G. Bertolini, *et al.* Daily classification of the level of care: a method to describe clinical course of illness, use of resources and quality of intensive care assistance. *Intensive Care Med* 2001; 27: 131–136.

7. D. Reis Miranda, R. Moreno, G. Iapichino. Nine equivalents of nursing manpower use score (NEMS). *Intensive Care Med* 1997; 23: 760–765.

8. A. Valentin, P. Ferdinande, ESICM Working Group on Quality Improvement: recommendations on basic requirements for intensive care units – structural and organizational aspects. *Intensive Care Med* 2011; 37: 1575–1587.

9. R. Endacott. The continuing imperative to measure workload in ICU: impact on patient safety and staff well-being. *Intensive Care Med* 2012; 38: 1415–1417.

10. D. Reis Miranda, A. De Rijk, W. Schaufeli. Simplified Therapeutic Intervention Scoring System: the TISS-28 items – results from a multicenter study. *Crit Care Med* 1996; 24: 64–73.

11. D. Reis Miranda, R. Nap, A. de Rijk, *et al.* Nursing activity score. *Crit Care Med* 2003; 31: 374–382.

12. Italian Multicenter Group of ICU research (GIRTI). Time oriented score system (TOSS): a method for direct and quantitative assessment of nursing workload for ICU patients. *Intensive Care Med* 1991; 17: 340–345.

13. T. Campbell, S. Taylor, S. Callaghan, *et al.* Case-mix type as a predictor of nursing workload. *J Nurs Manag* 1997; 5: 237–240.

14. C. Ball, G. Walker, P. Harper, *et al.* Moving on from patient dependency and nursing workload to managing risk in critical care. *Intensive and Critical Care Nursing* 2004; 20: 62–68.

15. D.A. Penoyer. Nurse staffing and patient outcomes in critical care: a concise review. *Crit Care Med* 2010; 38: 1521–1528.

16. A.O.M. Campagner, P.C.R. Garcia, J.P. Piva. Use of scores to calculate the nursing workload in a paediatric intensive care unit. *Revista Brasilera de Terapia Intensiva* 2014; 26: 36–43.

17. D.P. Debergh, D. Myny, I. van Herzeele, *et al.* Measuring the nursing workload per shift in the ICU. *Intensive Care Med* 2011; 38: 1438–1444.

18. D. Reis Miranda, M. Jegers. Monitoring costs in the ICU: a search for a pertinent methodology. *Acta Anaesthesiol Scand* 2012; 56: 1104–1113.

19. P. Hoonakker, P. Carayon, A.P. Gurses, *et al.* Measuring workload of ICU nurses with a questionnaire survey: the NASA task load index (TLX). *IIE Trans Healthcare Syst Eng* 2011; 1: 131–143.

20. G. Iapichino, D. Radrizzani, A. Pezzi, *et al.* Evaluating daily nursing use and needs in the intensive care unit: a method to assess the rate and appropriateness of ICU resource use. *Health Policy* 2005; 73: 228–234.

21. G. Iapichino, D. Radrizzani, C. Rossi, *et al.* Proposal of a flexible structural-organizing model for intensive care units. *Minerva Anestesiol* 2007; 73: 501–506.

22. C.L. Sprung, M. Danis, Iapichino, *et al.* Triage of intensive care patients: identifying agreement and controversy. *Intensive Care Med* 2013; 39: 1916–1924.

23. R.A. Gooch, J.M. Kahn, ICU bed supply, utilization, and healthcare spending: an example of demand elasticity. *JAMA* 2014; 311, 567–568.

24. J. Needleman, P. Buerhaus, V.S. Pankratz, *et al.* Nurse staffing and inpatient hospital mortality. *NEJM* 2011; 364: 1037–1045.

25. D.C. Angus, M.A. Kelley, R.J. Schmitz, *et al.* The Committee on Manpower for Pulmonary and Critical Care Societies (COMPACCS): current and projected workforce requirements for care of the critically ill and patients with pulmonary disease. *JAMA* 2000; 284: 2762–2770.

26. A. Garland, H.B. Gershengorn. Staffing in ICUs: physicians and alternative staffing models. *Chest* 2013; 143: 214–221.

# Chapter 16

# Severity scoring, improved care?

Rui P. Moreno and Joana Manuel

We will have to learn, before understanding any task, to first ask the question, "What information do I need, and in what form, and when." We should begin thinking about the delivery system for the information only when this is clear.

*Peter Drucker*

## Introduction

Intensive care medicine (ICM) was defined many decades ago as the science and art of preventing, detecting, and managing patients at risk of, or already with, established critical illness in order to achieve the best possible outcomes. The delivery of critical care is often a complex process, carried out on heterogeneous patient populations influenced by variables that include patients' and healthcare religious and cultural beliefs, different structures and organizations of healthcare systems within countries (and sometimes even within regions of the same country) and with major differences in the baseline characteristics of the populations [1].

ICM is also a very expensive activity, consuming, at least in the more developed world, a significant portion of the healthcare budget, and is considered to be one of the most expensive hospital assets [2]. At a time of financial constraints, and in the absence of clear and intuitive data about the quality and the adequacy of many ICM practices, it is vital that we can assess performance of individual units to ensure that our resources are wisely spent. This requires a marker of quality (or performance) that can be used both within and between hospitals in an objective and trusted fashion, especially at a time when the initial estimates from the Institute of Medicine that about 98,000 patients died every year due to medical error (based on data from a New York Study from 1984) [3] are now being challenged, and it seems that our lack of active and positive action [4] increased this number to at least 210,000 deaths each year (and more probably 400,000 deaths) just in the USA (not even to mention the burden for the patients, their families, and society of 10–20-fold additional patients with severe injuries) [5].

Finally, it seems there are major variations in the provision of ICM among Western countries [6] or even within different regions of the same country [7] and it is not obvious that these differences (that reach more than seven-fold) correlate with outcomes (at least in surgical patients) [8,9].

---

*Quality Management in Intensive Care*, ed. Bertrand Guidet, Andreas Valentin and Hans Flaatten. Published by Cambridge University Press. © Cambridge University Press 2016.

# From quality evaluation to the quantification of severity of illness

Since possibly the most robust and objective marker of quality and performance is patient all-causes mortality (despite the existence of many others), objective methods to allow the quantification of the severity of illness (and consequently of the predicted mortality of a patient admitted to the intensive care unit [ICU]) have been around since the mid 1980s and are today viewed as a mandatory component of the recently defined indicators to improve the safety and quality of care for critically ill patients proposed by the Task Force on Safety and Quality of the European Society of Intensive Care Medicine (ESICM) by allowing the comparison among ICUs (or within the same ICU over time) of the ratio between the observed mortality at hospital discharge and the hospital mortality predicted by the severity scores – the so-called *standardized mortality ratio* or *SMR* [10].

It was clear many years ago that for mortality to be used as a major component of quality assessment, it must be adjusted for the major determinants of prognosis, from which age, co-morbid diseases, acute reason for ICU admission, and presence and degree of physiological derangement are the most important. As a direct consequence of this need for risk adjustment in the ICU, a series of models have been published trying to take into account this variability in the patient population characteristics. In other words, there is a need to standardize different groups of patients regarding outcome. These risk-adjustment methods then allow us to take into account all of the characteristics of patients known to affect their outcome, irrespective of the treatment received.

As it is impossible to set a-priori mortality targets or to aim at a specific mortality rate – given the difficulty to forecast all the characteristics of the patients that will be admitted in the future, the evaluation of the performance of an ICU in the strictest sense (the level to which the predefined objectives of each ICU are met) has been replaced in real life by the relative evaluation of ICU performance, in which the population of each ICU is compared (after the application of some method for risk adjustment) to a reference database. This process, known as benchmarking, is based on the comparison of the risk-adjusted mortality of each ICU to – as defined in the New Oxford American Dictionary – a standard or point of reference against which things may be compared or assessed. Traditionally based on mortality, this process is now being applied to other outcomes, most if not all related to costs [11]. Despite the increasing use of process-related performance measures [12], the evaluation of ICU throughput has been based until recently almost exclusively on severity-adjusted hospital mortality, on the severity-adjusted length of stay (in the ICU or in the hospital) or on the effectiveness in the use of resources.

Unfortunately, given the probabilistic nature of the instruments used for risk adjustment and the fact that all of them are calibrated with the assumption that the patient will be admitted and cared for in an ICU, it is – by definition – impossible to apply these instruments to individual patients or to know what would be the outcome for any given patient if they were not admitted to the ICU. Also, all these instruments have been calibrated in a certain ICU population used to develop the model and are prone to differences in the population baseline characteristics or in the improvement of outcome in major diseases [13–16].

# The quantification of severity of illness

The evaluation of severity of illness in a critically ill patient is made through the use of general severity scores and general outcome prognosis models:

* Severity scores are instruments that aim to stratify patients according to their severity, assigning to each patient an increasing number of points (or score) as their severity of illness increases.

- Prognostic models, apart from their ability to stratify patients according to their severity of illness, aim to predict a certain outcome – usually the vital status at hospital discharge – based on a given set of prognostic variables and a specific modeling equation. Other outcomes, both for the short and long term can eventually be considered, but most of them are more prone to bias and manipulation or are of little interest to patients, their families and the healthcare providers [1].

Nowadays, almost all instruments used to predict mortality in patients admitted to an ICU are still based on the original concepts developed by Douglas Wagner, William Knaus and co-workers in the acute physiology and chronic health evaluation (APACHE II) system [17], and by Jean-Roger Le Gall and co-workers on the new simplified acute physiological score (SAPS II) [18]. Both use a score, used to measure the severity of illness, and a modeling equation (using just the score or the score plus additional variables) that predicts the outcome at hospital discharge.

Although the methods for selecting the predictive variables vary, all of them use standard logistic regression to develop the equation relating the predictive variables to the probability of the outcome of interest. They allow the user to adjust for the underlying characteristics of the admitted population (case-mix) and to perform indirect standardization of the outcome of different groups of patients, irrespective of the treatment received in the ICU. Since they have been designed to be applied only to heterogeneous groups of patients, their predictions should be used to forecast the aggregated mortality at hospital discharge of all patients from a certain ICU, as if they were treated in a virtual ICU that was used to develop the model. Many other systems have been developed and proposed, but have not gained the widespread use of these two original models. The most recent generations of these instruments have been extensively reviewed and discussed [19]: the APACHE models [20], the SAPS models [21], the Mortality Probability Models [22] and the Intensive Care National Audit & Research Centre (ICNARC) model [23].

An important debate exists about the ideal characteristics of the reference population. This pertains to whether the reference population should be local, with the score adjusted to a certain region or group of ICUs, or if it should include heterogeneity to improve the chances to learn with variation [24]. At the moment, the consensual view seems to be that for benchmarking purposes it is better to sacrifice the greater potential of large, heterogeneous databases to focus on the more homogeneous, actualized, high-quality systems, which introduces the need regularly to reinvent the wheel. This need to change is driven by two main reasons [19]:

1. To ensure that the databases in which the models are developed reflect the underlying characteristics of patients and healthcare delivery systems.
2. To ensure that the relationship between patient underlying characteristics and outcome is still well described by the model.

This allows us to maximize our capability to collect reliable data that are more likely to be adjusted for known, and unknown, confounders, many of them potentially context-dependent [25], and also enables the dataset to be constantly updated, preventing the degrading of the model due to progress and changes over time.

No matter which system is chosen, it is vitally important that all the data needed for computation of the model can be collected in a standard and reliable fashion. This includes such issues as handling of the data before analysis, which must be performed according to the original description of the model; the inclusion of the majority of admissions to the ICU; the model accounting for all the major variables with prognostic significance; and finally, that the dimension of the sample under analysis is large enough to yield the power for detecting significant differences [26,27]. The time frequency of data collection also impacts on the reliability for the calibration of the model. For instance, most systems have been designed in a time when data collection was performed in a manual fashion. Nowadays many units have patient data management systems (PDMS). These can more reliably collect the data, but at a much-increased frequency compared to the older, manual mechanism. This will decrease the calibration of the models due to the high sampling rates, introducing important systematic deviations in the severity scores. Higher sampling rates are associated with higher probabilities of detecting deviations from normality and consequently give higher severity scores (and lower observed to adjusted mortality ratios) [28,29]. This problem is significantly greater for models that use a long observation period – for example, the first 24 hours after ICU admission – and should be small in systems based on admission data only [30,31]. A complete understanding of the methodology (including the methodological problems and limitations) of the severity scores and outcome prediction models is crucial to understanding their use as the basis for risk-adjusted evaluation of mortality [15,16].

# From the quantification of the severity of illness to the computation of predicted hospital mortality

Overall, the process can be described in a sequence of steps:

1. A general outcome prediction model (GOPM) is developed from a suitable database or selected from the existing ones.
2. The model is applied to all patients in the ICU during a certain period of time.
3. The quotient between the observed mortality at hospital discharge and the expected mortality at hospital discharge (based on the risk-adjustment provided by the GOPM selected) is computed, together with the respective confidence intervals, the so-called O/E ratio or standardized mortality ratio (SRM).
4. This one-point estimate is then used to compare the (risk-adjusted) performance of the ICU: if it is significantly lower than 1, the interpretation is that the ICU presents a performance better than the cohort in which the GOPM was derived; if it is significantly higher than 1, the performance of the ICU is judged to be worse than the cohort in which the GOPM was derived. The results can be presented as classical SMR charts (with each ICU plotted by their point estimate and their 95% confidence intervals) (Figure 16.1) or by the more modern funnel plots, where the sample dimension and the confidence intervals are viewed more intuitively (Figure 16.2).

# The multidimensional nature of benchmarking

In a complex activity such as the provision of intensive care, we must keep in mind that benchmarking needs always to be a multidimensional process, in which the assessment of resource use and outcomes must be viewed as being complementary to each other. Other indicators are certainly important, such as communication with the families [32] and respect for their spiritual needs and values [33,34], end-of-life practices [35–37], or relative consumption of resources [11,38].

This issue has been recently addressed using the SAPS 3 database [11]. This group was able to demonstrate a very large variation between different ICUs, encompassing a broad range of structures and processes, within and between geographical regions, based on standardized data collection. Unfortunately, despite these efforts, only a few factors of ICU structure and process were associated with efficient use of the ICU (e.g., multiprofessional rounds,

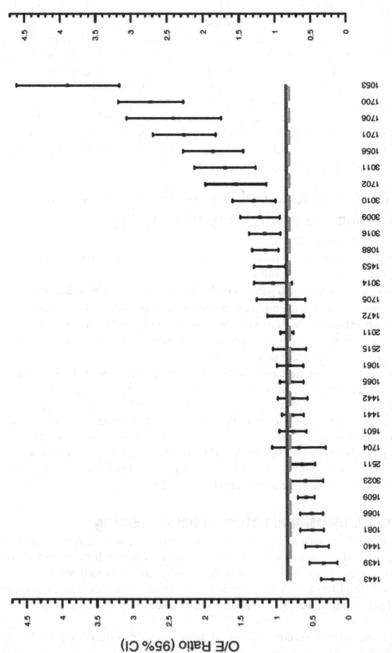

**Figure 16.1** Classical standardized mortality data plot. On the y-axis you can see the SMR (with 1 being the reference and vertical bars representing the 95% confidence intervals) and on the x-axis the identification of a certain ICU.

Data from the Austrian Center for Documentation and Quality Assurance in Intensive Care report for participating ICUs.

## Risk-adjusted mortality vs. number of admissions

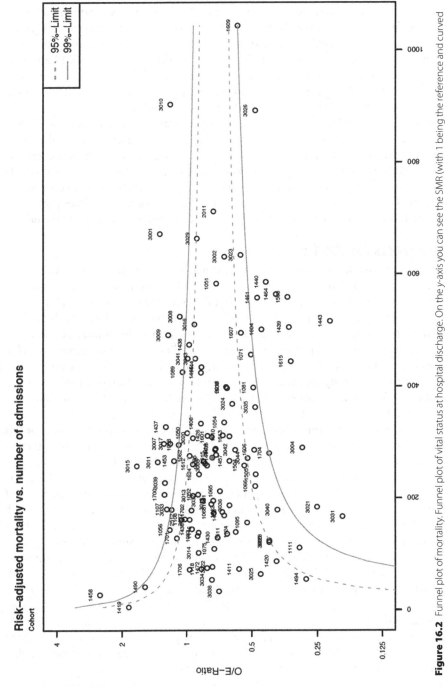

**Figure 16.2** Funnel plot of mortality. Funnel plot of vital status at hospital discharge. On the y-axis you can see the SMR (with 1 being the reference and curved lines representing the 95% confidence intervals) and on the x-axis the identification of a certain ICU.

Data from the Austrian Center for Documentation and Quality Assurance in Intensive Care report for participating ICUs.

presence of an emergency department in the hospital), which suggests that many other confounding factors may play an important role in this variation. The proposed measures in this model were for outcome, the standardized mortality ratio based on the SAPS 3 model (SMR), and for resource use, the standardized resource use (SRU), based on the length of stay in the ICU, adjusted for severity of acute illness (as measured by the SAPS 3 model). The cross-tabulation of these two values allow the authors to split the ICUs into four groups, based on the median SMR and median SRU: "most efficient" included all units whose SMR and SRU were below the median SMR and SRU, respectively; "least efficient" included units in which SMR and SRU were both above the median; "overachieving" or relatively wasteful: low SMR but high SRU; and "underachieving" with a high SMR but low SRU.

This method has never been compared to the method proposed by Rapoport *et al.* in 1994 [39] based on WHD and MPM SMR, the so-called Rapoport–Teres graph, in which the standardized resource use was plotted against the standardized clinical performance use. A new variation of the method was proposed by Nathanson *et al.* [40], using a different way to compute the WHD and the SMR (this time based on the data from project Impact used to develop the MPM III model [31] that is used as the performance indicator. Apart from a Rapoport–Teres plot based on more actual data, the new method did not bring any new concepts to the field.

# New prospects for the future

With a few exceptions, all authors assumed that the performance of an ICU is constant over the whole spectrum of the severity of illness: an ICU with a "good" performance (as demonstrated by an low SMR) is assumed to be uniformly good for both low-risk and high-risk patients; likewise, an ICU with a "bad" performance (as demonstrated by a high SMR) is assumed to be uniformly bad. However, this assumption is most probably not true, since performance might differ over the spectrum of the severity of illness. This assumption, crucial to all the use of O/E ratios for performance assessment, is possibly (probably) not true.

For this reason, our group proposed that we customize the function that predicts hospital mortality at ICU admission for each ICU [41]. The predicted risks of hospital mortality resulting from this function were then compared with the risks that would be obtained using the reference cohort (the one from which the original severity score was developed). For this purpose, we used the original function from the SAPS II publication [18], i.e., the function derived from the SAPS II training sample. By dividing the risk obtained from the ICU-specific function by the risk obtained from the general function, we were able to determine the difference in the risk of dying in the hospital for patients in individual ICUs over the continuum of 5–95% predicted risk. The logistic regression-derived risk ratio was then graphically plotted, together with its confidence intervals. Conventional point-wise 95% confidence intervals for the risk ratios are calculated from the customized logistic models assuming that the expected risk from the original SAPS II risk model in the denominator is a non-random quantity. The result is a risk profile of each ICU over the whole span of the probability of hospital mortality. This method thus allows a direct comparison of individual risk profiles for specific ICUs. Using a simple two-parameter risk model with a form closely related to the model used originally when constructing the SAPS II risk score achieves smoothing of the individual risk profiles with corresponding confidence intervals in moderately small samples. This is different to calculating, e.g., raw ICU-specific risk ratio estimates in risk decile groups with even smaller sample sizes (and potentially wide confidence intervals) [41].

Our results are also concordant with a more rough estimate done during the EURICUS-I study in which three performance variables were computed for each ICU: P20 (performance with low-risk patients, evaluated at the 20th percentile); P50 (performance with medium-risk patients, evaluated at the median); and P80 (performance with high-risk patients, evaluated at the 80th percentile). This method, based on customization of the SAPS II score for each ICU using logistic regression with random effects, allowed the user to compare the performance of an ICU using at least three different points, but not in all of the continuum of severity of illness. Possibly for this reason, and because it implied for each ICU the development of a complex statistical technique, it was almost ignored by the scientific community. Similar results were obtained during the development of SAPS 3, when the relationship between severity of illness and actual mortality was found to differ greatly between different geographical areas, as published in 2005 [42].

## The challenges ahead of us

In this field, as in many others, the challenge to the next years will be:

- to get representative databases (in dimension and in information) about the ICUs participating in a certain benchmarking project; this will need – at least for small countries – the creation of international, scientifically independent, ICU benchmarking centers;
- to incorporate in our plots other dimensions of quality, and not just the relative risk-adjusted mortality;
- to explain to the other professionals and to the population the meaning and interpretation of the plots, in particular about their limitations and their limited (if at all) value for individual patients.

## References

1. Moreno RP, Jardim AL, Godinho de Matos R, Metnitz PGH. Principles of risk-adjustment in the critically ill patient. In: Kuhlen R, Moreno R, Ranieri M, Rhodes A, eds. *25 Years of Progress and Innovation in Intensive Care Medicine.* Berlin: Medizinisch Wissenschaftliche Verlagsgesellschaft, 2007:409–17.

2. Halpern NA, Pastores SM. Critical care medicine in the United States 2000–2005: an analysis of bed numbers, occupancy rates, payer mix, and costs. *Crit Care Med* 2010;38:65–71.

3. Committee on Quality of Healthcare in America IoM. *Crossing the Quality Chasm: A New Health System for the 21st Century.* Washington, DC: National Academy Press, 2001.

4. Howard RJ. Missed opportunities: The Institute of Medicine report – organ donation. opportunities for action. *Am J Transplant* 2006;6:1–3.

5. James JT. A new, evidence-based estimate of patient harms associated with hospital care. *J Patient Saf* 2013;9:122–128.

6. Rhodes A, Ferdinande P, Flaatten H, Guidet B, Metnitz PG, Moreno RP. The variability of critical care bed numbers in Europe. *Intensive Care Med* 2012;38: 1647–1653.

7. Rhodes A, Moreno RP. Intensive care provision: a global problem. *Braz J Intensive Care* 2012;24:322–325.

8. Pearse RM, Moreno RP, Bauer P, *et al.* Mortality after surgery in Europe: a 7 day cohort study. *Lancet* 2012;380:1059–1065.

9. Rhodes A, Cecconi M. Can surgical outcomes be prevented by postoperative admission to critical care? *Crit Care* 2013;17:110.

10. Rhodes A, Moreno RP, Azoulay E, *et al.* Prospectively defined indicators to improve the safety and quality of care for critically ill patients: a report from the Task Force on Safety and Quality of the European Society of Intensive Care Medicine (ESICM). *Intensive Care Med* 2012;38:598–605.

11. Rothen HU, Stricker K, Einfalt J, *et al.* Variability in outcome and resource use

in intensive care units. *Intensive Care Med* 2007;33:1329–1336.

12. Randall Curtis J, Cook DJ, Wall RJ, *et al.* Intensive care unit quality improvement: a "how-to" guide for the interdisciplinary team. *Crit Care Med* 2006;34:211–218.

13. Breslow MJ, Badawi O. Severity scoring in the critically ill: part 1 – interpretation and accuracy of outcome prediction scoring systems. *Chest* 2012;141:245–252.

14. Breslow MJ, Badawi O. Severity scoring in the critically ill: part 2 – maximizing value from outcome prediction scoring systems. *Chest* 2012;141:518–527.

15. Poole D, Bertolini G. Outcome-based benchmarking in the ICU part I: statistical tools for the creation and validation of severity scores. In: Chice J-D, Moreno R, Putensen C, Rhodes A, eds. *Patient Safety and Quality of Care in Intensive Care Medicine*. Berlin: Medizinisch Wissenschaftiche Verlagsgesellschaft, 2009: 141–150.

16. Poole D, Bertolini G. Outcome-based benchmarking in the ICU Part II: Use and limitations of severity scores in critical care. In: Chiche J-D, Moreno R, Putensen C, Rhodes A, eds. *Patient Safety and Quality of Care in Intensive Care Medicine*. Berlin: Medizinisch Wissenschaftiche Verlagsgesellschaft, 2009:151–160.

17. Knaus WA, Draper EA, Wagner DP, Zimmerman JE. APACHE II: a severity of disease classification system. *Crit Care Med* 1985;13:818–829.

18. Le Gall JR, Lemeshow S, Saulnier F. A new simplified acute physiology score (SAPS II) based on a European/North American multicenter study. *JAMA* 1993;270: 2957–2963.

19. Moreno RP. Outcome prediction in intensive care: why we need to reinvent the wheel. *Curr Op Crit Care* 2008;14:483–484.

20. Zimmerman JE, Kramer AA. Outcome prediction in critical care: the Acute Physiology and Chronic Health Evaluation models. *Curr Op Crit Care* 2008;14: 491–497.

21. Capuzzo M, Moreno RP, Le Gall J-R. Outcome prediction in critical care: the Simplified Acute Physiology Score models. *Curr Op Crit Care* 2008;14:485–490.

22. Higgins TL, Teres D, Nathanson B. Outcome prediction in critical care: the Mortality Probability Models. *Curr Op Crit Care* 2008;14:498–505.

23. Harrison DA, Rowan KM. Outcome prediction in critical care: the ICNARC model. *Curr Op Crit Care* 2008;14:506–512.

24. Moreno RP, Afonso S. Building and using outcome prediction models: should we be lumpers or splitters? In: Kuhlen R, Moreno R, Ranieri M, Rhodes A, eds. *Controversies in Intensive Care Medicine*. Berlin: Medizinisch Wissenschaftiche Verlagsgesellschaft, 2008:415–419.

25. Poole D, Rossi C, Anghileri A, *et al.* External validation of the Simplified Acute Physiology Score (SAPS) 3 in a cohort of 28,357 patients from 147 Italian intensive care units. *Intensive Care Medicine* 2009;35:1916–1924.

26. Rowan K. The reliability of case mix measurements in intensive care. *Curr Op Crit Care* 1996;2:209–213.

27. Black NA, Jenkinson C, Hayes JA, *et al.* Review of outcome measures used in adult critical care. *Crit Care Med* 2001;29: 2119–2124.

28. Bosman RJ, Oudemane van Straaten HM, Zandstra DF. The use of intensive care information systems alters outcome prediction. *Intensive Care Med* 1998;24:953–958.

29. Suistomaa M, Kari A, Ruokonen E, Takala J. Sampling rate causes bias in APACHE II and SAPS II scores. *Intensive Care Med* 2000;26:1773–1778.

30. Moreno RP, Metnitz PG, Almeida E, *et al.* SAPS 3 Investigators: SAPS 3 – from evaluation of the patient to evaluation of the intensive care unit. Part 2: development of a prognostic model for hospital mortality at ICU admission. *Intensive Care Med* 2005;31:1345–1355.

31. Higgins TL, Teres D, Copes WS, Nathanson BH, Stark M, Kramer AA. Assessing contemporary intensive care unit outcome: an updated Mortality Probability Admission Model (MPM0-III). *Critical Care Med* 2007;35:827–835.

32. Levy M. Including families in quality measurement in critical care. *Critical Care Med* 2007;35:324–325.

33. Wall RJ, Engelberg RA, Gries CJ, Glavan B, Randall Curtis J. Spiritual care of families in the intensive care unit. *Critical Care Med* 2007;35: 1084–1090.

34. Sprung CL, Maia P, Bulow H-H, *et al.*, The importance of religious affiliation and culture on end-of-life decisions in European intensive care units. *Intensive Care Med* 2007;33:1732–1739.

35. Bertolini G, Boffelli, S Malacarne P, *et al.* End-of-life decision-making and quality of ICU performance: an observational study in 84 Italian units. *Intensive Care Med* 2010;36:1495–1504.

36. Azoulay E, Metnitz B, Sprung C-L, *et al.* End-of-life practices in 282 intensive care units: data from the SAPS 3 database. *Intensive Care Med* 2009;35: 623–630.

37. Randall Curtis J. End-of-life care for patients in the intensive care unit. In: Kuhlen R, Moreno R, Ranieri M, Rhodes A, eds. *25 Years of Progress and Innovation in Intensive Care Medicine.* Berlin: Medizinisch Wissenschaftliche Verlagsgesellschaft, 2007: 469–479.

38. Zimmerman JE, Kramer AA, McNair DS, Malila FM, Shaffer VL. Intensive care unit length of stay: benchmarking based on Acute Physiology and Chronic Health Evaluation (APACHE) IV. *Critical Care Med* 2006;34:2517–2529.

39. Rapoport J, Teres D, Lemeshow S, Gehlbach S. A method for assessing the clinical performance and cost-effectiveness of intensive care units: a multicenter inception cohort study. *Critical Care Med* 1994;22:1385–1391.

40. Nathanson BH, Higgins TL, Teres D, Copes WS, Kramer A, Stark M. A revised method to assess intensive care unit clinical performance and resource utilization. *Critical Care Med* 2007;35:1853–1862.

41. Moreno RP, Hochrieser H, Metnitz B, Bauer P, Metnitz PGH. Characterizing the risk profiles of intensive care units. *Intensive Care Med* 2010;36:1207–1212.

42. Metnitz PG, Moreno RP, Almeida E, *et al.*, SAPS 3 Investigators: SAPS 3 – from evaluation of the patient to evaluation of the intensive care unit. Part 1: objectives, methods and cohort description. *Intensive Care Med* 2005;31:1336–1344.

# Implementation of evidence-based practice

Jeffrey M. Singh and Damon C. Scales

## Introduction

Evidence-based practice involves the thoughtful use of current best evidence in medical decision-making for individual patients or decisions regarding the delivery of health services [1]. Implementing evidence-based practice in the intensive care unit (ICU) is important to provide the best care to an extremely sick and vulnerable population of patients and because the costs of care (in terms of financial and human resources) are extremely high.

Organized and strategic implementation of evidence-based care is important to ensure that the evidence-based practices are actually applied to the patient population of interest. Contemporary literature usually reports the comparative efficacy or benefit of individual therapies or protocols, such as a randomized controlled clinical trial of a specific intervention or protocol. Unfortunately, the efficacy of such treatments, as demonstrated by clinical trials, may be tempered by a variety of patient-, practitioner-, and system-level factors that may reduce their real-world impact or effectiveness. Consequently, the systematic and sequential management of these detracting factors may be required to achieve comparable therapeutic effectiveness, as demonstrated from clinical trials. We propose that implementation of evidence-based practice is best viewed as an exercise in quality improvement, where uptake of evidence-based practice is seen as the quality improvement intervention and its implementation and impact are methodically and iteratively evaluated.

This chapter will provide a framework for the implementation of evidence-based clinical practice and will highlight the importance of pre-specifying the quality goals that will be targeted, evaluating barriers, and facilitators to their uptake, and evaluation of the overall effectiveness of the quality intervention.

## What is evidence-based practice?

Put simply, evidence-based practice is the incorporation of the best available scientific evidence into clinical practice [1]. Practitioners of evidence-based practice seek to the use the highest quality empiric evidence to overcome incorrect decision-making. Usually – but not always – the highest quality and most rigorous evidence comes from large randomized controlled trials. The strength of the evidence base is considered to be greater if multiple well-designed trials have reached similar conclusions about a given therapy.

*Quality Management in Intensive Care*, ed. Bertrand Guidet, Andreas Valentin and Hans Flaatten. Published by Cambridge University Press. © Cambridge University Press 2016.

When clinicians rely solely on clinical judgment and experience, they may reach incorrect conclusions about a treatment's efficacy. For example, clinicians frequently make decisions that are heavily influenced by their recent experiences with similar situations, instead of considering the larger experience of the medical community. Alternatively, clinicians frequently overestimate risks while ignoring small but certain gains that are associated with a treatment. Such errors in judgment can lead to avoidance of potentially helpful therapies, or delivery of treatments that are unlikely to lead to improvements in patients' outcomes. Evidence-based practice does not replace clinical expertise, but it seeks to overcome these heuristics and biases by providing a framework for evaluating the effectiveness of therapies. The overall goals of evidence-based practice are to ensure that proven therapies are appropriately and safely delivered and to eliminate the use of ineffective or harmful treatments.

# Framework for introducing evidence-based practice

Implementation of evidence-based practice in the ICU can be extremely challenging. Evidence-based critical practice can include straightforward decisions regarding specific treatments for eligible patients to highly complex issues related to the delivery of health services within a complex system. However, even simple therapies and treatments can be challenging to implement in the ICU due to the complex and multidisciplinary nature of care. In such an environment, implementing a new practice or changing existing behaviors may require engagement and cooperation with a large number of healthcare providers and stakeholders, each of whom may have their unique facilitators and barriers to behavioral change. For example, although the benefit of lung protective ventilation in patients with acute respiratory distress syndrome (ARDS) is clear [2], there may be multiple barriers and challenges to the consistent, timely, and sustained implementation of this therapy to appropriate patients: the ascertainment of ARDS, setting of the mechanical ventilator, and subsequent management of patient analgesia, sedation, and ventilator synchrony may involve physicians, respiratory therapists, nurses, and pharmacists [3,4]. These challenges are in addition to the other common barriers to change (lack of knowledge, personal motivators, attitudes, available resources, and the physical environment) [5,6]. Implementation of new evidence-based practice initiatives in the ICU requires an organized (and often iterative) framework to address these challenges, and to ensure that the desired practices are applied properly to the patient population of interest.

Many individual therapies or protocols are supported by published studies demonstrating benefits, such as randomized controlled clinical trials. Unfortunately, the efficacy of such treatments outside of the context of a carefully conducted research study may be reduced by a variety of patient-level, practitioner-level and system-level factors. Furthermore, the interdependence of many interventions in the ICU makes it likely that a given practice may be inadvertently affected (positively or negatively) by implementation or change of a different, seemingly unrelated, practice. One example of this could be the impact of implementing a quality improvement intervention to improve adoption of lung protective ventilation on another intervention that aims to reduce the use of sedation medications; if the lung protective ventilation intervention promotes increasing use of sedatives to treat patient–ventilator dysynchrony, it will interfere with the intervention that seeks to decrease sedative use.

We propose that implementation of evidence-based practice is best viewed as an exercise in quality improvement, where evidence-based practice is seen as a quality improvement goal and its implementation and impact are methodically and iteratively evaluated. Hospitals and healthcare teams may employ different conceptual frameworks and models to guide quality improvement activities – for example, Lean, Six Sigma, or the Plan–Do–Study–Act model [7–9]. These frameworks can be useful for providing an organized framework for understanding and organizing the major steps of quality improvement activities. Although the nosology may vary across frameworks, in their most general terms they comprise the following: (1) understanding the desired goal, either a desired care process or clinical outcome; (2) creating an action plan to modify existing process and care practices to reach the desired goal; (3) studying the change in performance, outcomes, and dissemination of these metrics; and (4) planning additional measures to address the quality goal if it has not been achieved. Regardless of the framework used or the nosology, successful completion of these major steps is required for the implementation to be deemed successful.

## Planning a new evidence-based practice intervention

### Identifying the goal

The first major task for the implementation of evidence-based practice is to develop a clear understanding of the desired goal, ideally focusing on processes rather than on downstream clinical outcomes. For example, an appropriate focus could be on correctly implementing lung protective ventilation for patients with ARDS, rather than establishing the efficacy of this treatment approach for reducing mortality rates. The goal of the intervention needs to be explicitly stated so it can be communicated to the various stakeholders in the healthcare team, and clearly understood by all clinicians involved in identifying and implementing targeted care processes.

Targets for implementation of evidence-based practice are typically generated in one of two ways: (1) new high-quality evidence about the efficacy of an intervention becomes available, and this intervention must be introduced into practice (or an existing and widely used intervention is discovered to be unhelpful or harmful and must be removed from practice); and (2) a performance gap or patient safety problem is identified at a local or institutional level and there is a desire to improve practice based on the existing evidence base. It is imperative that the need for a change in current practice is substantiated by observed data that help quantify the existing deviation from the desired goal, since other approaches, including surveys, can be misleading and overestimate or underestimate true practice gaps [10]. These observed data can take the form of performance indicators or data from a critical event, a root cause analysis, or other safety data. The implementation of a new process or a change to an existing process requires a detailed understanding of the current situation, so that the extent and targets for change can be identified, all stakeholders involved can be identified, and that potential consequences of change on other processes and outcomes can be anticipated.

### Communicating the goal

Leaders should take note of the frequently identified barriers to implementation of new research findings into evidence-based clinical practice: lack of knowledge, lack of time, perceived lack of organizational or institutional support, and organizational culture not supportive of change [11,12]. Consequently, these issues should be addressed explicitly in communications with front-line staff members. Given the complexity and membership of healthcare teams in hospitals, clinics, and medical practices, it is also important that leaders ensure that all stakeholders are identified and engaged, and receive these regular communications [13]. Finally, if the proposed goal is just one part of a larger multistep project, it is often helpful that an overview be described in a manner that allows individuals to understand the larger context, and how the component interventions fit together to ultimately achieve the desired quality goal. For example, in implementing a combined bundle of sedation steward-ship, spontaneous breathing trials, delirium screening, and early mobility, team members might be more engaged in sedation stewardship if they also understood the impact of imple-menting improved sedation practices on the other components of the bundle – for example, in reducing delirium and facilitating early mobility initiatives [14].

# Implementing a new evidence-based intervention

## Determining what processes can be modified to improve outcomes

Following the identification of a major target for improvement (e.g., instituting lung pro-tective ventilation for all patients with ARDS; Table 17.1), the next step is to systematically break down the *processes* that surround this target in order to identify items that are required to change (e.g., creation of new lung protective ventilation protocols) as well as items that are required to support implementation of the new practice (e.g., how will ARDS be identi-fied and lung protective ventilation applied?). It is important to recognize that even simple interventions in critical care are often embedded in complex processes. For example, prompt administration of antibiotics to a patient with sepsis seems to be a simple intervention, but is in fact very complicated. Although the medication administration is simple, there are many steps that need to be completed by a variety of healthcare providers in different settings prior to the antibiotics being administered, including but not limited to prompt diagnosis, choice of appropriate antibiotics, preparation and timely medication administration at regular inter-vals, and monitoring for therapeutic effectiveness and safety.

Some quality improvement frameworks such as LEAN or Six Sigma include methods such as "value stream mapping," which help define the current state of a process, identify targets for process improvement, and allow mapping of an improved future process. Such exercises can be helpful at breaking down complex patient care systems into smaller processes and identifying potential targets for intervention. These exercises may also help clarify what the desired process looks like, including identifying obstacles to the desired process and areas where effort must be made to change current practice. Healthcare providers from a clinical background are sometimes challenged by the terms "value" and "waste," which are typically

**Table 17.1** Example of process of breaking down the steps in the provision of lung protective ARDS ventilation

| Goal | Steps required for successful implementation | Potential interventions or action steps |
|---|---|---|
| Provision of lung protective mechanical ventilation to all patients with acute respiratory distress syndrome | 1. Regular screening of PaO$_2$:FiO$_2$ ratios | • Protocolized daily screening by a respiratory therapist |
| | 2. Chest radiograph (completion and interpretation) | • Development of medical directives for chest radiograph in all patients eligible PaO$_2$:FiO$_2$ ratio |
| | 3. Review and ascertainment of ARDS | • Checklist to remind team to review on ICU rounds |
| | 4. Application of standardized ventilator protocol | • Development of an evidence-based ventilation protocol or medical directives |
| | 5. Prescription of adjuncts (additional sedation, analgesia) as necessary | • Implementation of a validated sedation scale in the ICU<br>• Development of standardized sedation protocols |

derived from the manufacturing industries, and have difficulty adapting this to the clinical realm of healthcare. In our experience, however, these methodologies can be helpful tools in identifying areas where processes need to be improved or changed to support implementation of new evidence-based care practices.

It is noteworthy that some evidence-based practices involve the withholding of ineffective or non-beneficial tests or treatments [15]. The implementation of these practices should be approached in the same methodical way: the demonstration of a performance gap followed by a detailed examination of the processes driving this undesirable practice, followed by implementation and evaluation of effectiveness of the quality intervention. Indeed, a thorough mapping of such processes is often even more relevant in this context because a detailed understanding of the external factors or cultural norms that drive provider behavior is necessary to develop effective strategies to change practice.

## Tailoring the intervention to the target population

The factor that has the greatest impact on the success or failure of the introduction of a new evidence-based practice is the extent to which the intervention is planned and tailored to the specific people, context, and environment. Although great emphasis is often placed on the choice of conceptual framework, communication tools, or use of information technology, the most important predictor of success is whether the intervention can successfully engage bedside clinicians and avoid barriers which preclude uptake and behavior change [5,13]. In order to improve success, leaders should keep in mind the common barriers to implementing new practices during development: a lack of knowledge, lack of time, perceived lack of organizational support, and an unsupportive organizational culture [11,12].

During the planning phase, care must be taken in identifying all front-line stakeholders who will be involved in the implementation of the new process. The engagement of the local leadership is particularly important, whether the leaders be explicit (appointed, such as a division head or chief) or implicit (followed voluntarily due to respect or seniority, such as a senior physician), as the support of these leaders is essential for fostering change across the healthcare team. All stakeholders must understand the goal of the proposed new evidence-based process: this includes both *what* is to be implemented, as well as the rationale and *why* the proposed care is superior to the existing care provided. It is helpful when new information is communicated by a trusted source: for example a local expert or recognized leader in the field, even when there is high-quality published evidence supporting the practice. For example, we have found that the presentation of local, high-quality guideline statements tends to generate much less enthusiasm for behavior change than having a local champion discuss the current status of care and the proposed changes based on the guidelines. Front-line healthcare workers, especially physicians, are much more likely to recognize the need for change and exhibit a change in behavior with the latter.

Local barriers and facilitators to implementation should be considered during the development of interventions to implement evidence-based practice. After mapping of the current process, it is useful to explore the determinants of current behavior and what factors reinforce this process. Uptake of new practices are unlikely to be successful unless these factors are addressed, as adoption of new behaviors or processes will be slowed by the persistence of old behaviors. One approach to explore these factors is to evaluate each process step for the likelihood of process adoption using a framework of ability (which includes physical facility, human resource availability, and staff training) and staff disposition or willingness (which encompasses the various motivations and disincentives that govern an individual's willingness to adopt a new process). For example, an individual may not be able to complete the step required because of a lack of training or knowledge, or they may be reluctant to adopt this new practice because of the perceived or real increase in workload or effort, or the cost in time, money, or opportunity, depending on the professional and task involved.

In large interprofessional teams such as the ICU, a thorough understanding of local medical and team culture can be very useful to help identify potential barriers and facilitators to implementation. This includes both the professional culture (e.g., nursing and physician autonomy) and the culture of medical practice (e.g., habitual treatment preferences and patterns). Knowledge of professional culture can be extremely useful in helping target interventions to change behaviors. For example, in a highly hierarchical culture in which physicians hold disproportionate autonomy and power, interventions are unlikely to be effective if the physicians are not engaged and compliant, regardless of the degree of engagement of the other healthcare providers. This knowledge should lead to an educational and communication strategy that puts special emphasis on this group and ensures their collaboration.

Accepting that providers are often very comfortable in their historical clinical practice, understanding the local clinical culture is also helpful. It is important to communicate the reasons why a change in process or new treatment is desired, and acknowledge how it may impact existing care practices. We find that direct comparison of historical and new practices is rarely helpful, but linking the new practice to the benefit or desired outcome is more productive. For example, local beliefs and preferences with regard to administration of analgesia and sedation can have major effects on the success of attempts to implement daily interruptions of sedative infusions. A strong culture of active early patient mobilization (which requires patients to be awake) can reinforce such initiatives, and initiatives should highlight the positive impact of the new initiative on these other, well-established practices in the ICU.

Initiatives should also be supported with adequate human resources, clinical capacity, and time. One important issue is to ensure coordination of various initiatives to ensure: (1) that they are not contradictory or working at cross-purposes; (2) to reduce the number of initiatives competing for the limited time and resources available; and (3) to align common initiatives to reduce duplication of work, overall workload, and prevent fatigue and burn-out.

## Bundling of interdependent processes

Often interconnected or interdependent processes must be addressed in concert to successfully implement a new practice. One example of such is the institution of an ICU early mobility program, which is also highly dependent on the patient's level of consciousness and the presence of delirium, and may be highly impacted by the presence of mechanical ventilation. Consequently, successful programs implementing an early mobility program have done so in concert with concurrent quality improvement initiatives in sedation stewardship, delirium screening, and liberation from the mechanical ventilator [14]. Although the roll-out of interventions designed to address all of these processes does not have to occur simultaneously, it is critically important to identify all potential enablers and obstacles to the successful implementation of a new evidence-based practice so that they can be monitored over time and addressed if they are preventing the planned intervention from being effective.

## Measurement of performance and outcomes

### How will we know that a change is an improvement?

The availability of directly measured data plays a key role in the successful implementation of any evidence-based intervention. Collecting, analyzing, interpreting, and disseminating data are vital to measuring the effectiveness of interventions on uptake of new processes, communicating results to front-line clinicians and other stakeholders, and assessing impacts on downstream outcomes, and any unintended consequences that may result from the initiative. Data collection and feedback are also essential components of the Plan–Do–Study–Act approach to quality improvement.

To motivate front-line clinicians, it is preferable that measured outcomes are both process-oriented and outcome-oriented. Measuring outcomes that actually reflect the targeted care process is key to tracking the success of the intervention. Where possible, measuring outcomes can help highlight the direct impact the intervention has on patients. However, when a quality improvement intervention only involves a single ICU or hospital, the relatively small sample size may make it impractical to actually detect differences in patient outcomes for some care practices. In these instances, we suggest highlighting the established evidence-base supporting the targeted care practice, and emphasizing adherence improvements to the targeted process outcome. Data measurement can quickly become the most labor-intensive aspect of an evidence-based practice intervention. It is important that only data that are used to ensure accountability and that support the process change be collected. There is often an administrative tendency to collect a large number of outcome data that are not directly related to the process being adopted or immediate downstream clinical outcomes. It is imperative that these data be culled to prevent the data collection and management process from becoming overwhelming or stealing energy and resources from implementation activities.

## Challenges to evidence-based practice implementation

One of the greatest challenges to using evidence-based practice is ensuring that it remains current and up-to-date. Unfortunately, much more is known about the challenges of implementing new evidence-based interventions than is known about the challenges of removing from practice treatments that are newly shown to be unhelpful or even harmful. The critical care community has witnessed several seemingly beneficial therapies subsequently proven to be unhelpful in recent years; for example, the use of activated protein C for sepsis, or use of intensive insulin therapy to maintain normoglycemia [16,17]. As the evidence base evolves, the goals of an earlier ICU quality improvement intervention may subsequently become out of date with the publication of additional and larger randomized controlled trials. Practitioners of evidence-based practice must strive to remain current – and also be willing to de-adopt treatments that may have been the focus of previous quality improvement initiatives [18].

Another challenge occurs when there is insufficient or lacking evidence to inform practice. The absence of high-quality evidence about a particular treatment or situation does not necessarily imply an absence of efficacy for that treatment. However, clinicians should be wary of adopting treatments that have not been rigorously evaluated, and which may cause unanticipated harm. Similarly, there may be situations where the existing evidence-base seems contradictory. In these situations, clinicians will need to exercise their judgment, and also to recognize when the existing evidence base cannot be generalized to their own patient.

## Conclusion

Implementing evidence-based healthcare in the ICU is important to provide the best care to an extremely sick and vulnerable population of patients and because the costs of treatment (in terms of financial and human resources) are extremely high. Evidence-based practice helps patients by introducing new treatment approaches where appropriate, by questioning the continued use of ineffective or harmful treatments, and by improving the safety of necessary treatments. Implementing a new evidence-based intervention into the ICU is a complex and challenging process, but can be successful using a quality-improvement framework that includes clear communication of relevant goals, engagement of leadership and front-line staff, tailoring of the intervention to the target population and local culture, and careful and systematic measurement of performance indicators.

# References

1. Cochrane AL. Effectiveness and efficiency. In *Random Reflections on Health Services*. London: Taylor and Francis, 1999.

2. The Acute Respiratory Distress Syndrome Network. Ventilation with lower tidal volumes as compared with traditional tidal volumes for acute lung injury and the acute respiratory distress syndrome. *NEJM*. 2000;342(18):1301–1308.

3. Rubenfeld GD, Cooper C, Carter G, Thompson BT, Hudson LD. Barriers to providing lung-protective ventilation to patients with acute lung injury. *Crit Care Med*. 2004;32(6):1289–1293.

4. Umoh NJ, Fan E, Mendez-Tellez PA, *et al.* Patient and intensive care unit organizational factors associated with low tidal volume ventilation in acute lung injury. *Crit Care Med*. 2008;36(5):1463–1468.

5. Sinuff T, Cook D, Giacomini M, Heyland D, Dodek P. Facilitating clinician adherence to guidelines in the intensive care unit: a multicenter, qualitative study. *Crit Care Med*. 2007;35(9):2083–2089.

6. Sinuff T, Muscedere J, Adhikari NK, *et al.* Knowledge translation interventions for critically ill patients: a systematic review. *Crit Care Med*. 2013;41(11):2627–2640.

7. D'Andreamatteo A, Ianni L, Lega F, Sargiacomo M. Lean in healthcare: a comprehensive review. *Health Policy*. 2015. doi: 10.1016/j.healthpol.2015.02.002.

8. de Koning H, Verver JP, van den Heuvel J, Bisgaard S, Does RJ. Lean Six Sigma in healthcare. *J Healthc Qual*. 2006;28(2):4–11.

9. Nicolay CR, Purkayastha S, Greenhalgh A, *et al.* Systematic review of the application of quality improvement methodologies from the manufacturing industry to surgical healthcare. *Brit J Surg*. 2012;99(3):324–335.

10. Scales DC, Dainty K, Hales B, *et al.* A multifaceted intervention for quality improvement in a network of intensive care units: a cluster randomized trial. *JAMA*. 2011;305(4):363–372.

11. Wallis L. Barriers to implementing evidence-based practice remain high for U.S. nurses: getting past "we've always done it this way" is crucial. *Am J Nurs*. 2012;112(12):15.

12. Grant HS, Stuhlmacher A, Bonte-Eley S. Overcoming barriers to research utilization and evidence-based practice among staff nurses. *JNSD*. 2012;28(4):163–165.

13. Dainty KN, Scales DC, Sinuff T, Zwarenstein M. Competition in collaborative clothing: a qualitative case study of influences on collaborative quality improvement in the ICU. *BMJ Qual Saf*. 2013;22(4):317–323.

14. Services VCfH. ICU delirium and Cognitive Impairment Study Group www.icudelirium.org 2013 (accessed 1 March 2015).

15. Halpern SD, Becker D, Curtis JR, *et al.* An official American Thoracic Society/ American Association of Critical-Care Nurses/American College of Chest Physicians/Society of Critical Care Medicine policy statement: the Choosing Wisely(R) Top 5 list in Critical Care Medicine. *Am J Respir Crit Care Med*. 2014;190(7):818–826.

16. Ranieri VM, Thompson BT, Barie PS, *et al.* Drotrecogin alfa (activated) in adults with septic shock. *NEJM*. 2012;366(22): 2055–2064.

17. Finfer S, Chittock DR, Su SY, *et al.* Intensive versus conventional glucose control in critically ill patients. *NEJM*. 2009;360(13):1283–1297.

18. Niven DJ, Rubenfeld GD, Kramer AA, Stelfox HT. Effect of published scientific evidence on glycemic control in adult intensive care units. *JAMA*. 2015;175:801–809.

# Chapter 18

# Addressing barriers for change in clinical practice

Paul R. Barach

Change is not made without inconvenience, even from worse to better.

*Richard Hooker, 1554–1600*

Changing established behaviour of any kind is difficult. It is particularly challenging in complex critical healthcare settings because of the varied relationships between a wide range of organisations, professionals, patients, and carers. Barriers to change can take a long time to overcome when discussing guidance for implementation in clinical practice; a clinical guideline can take up to 3–5 years to be fully implemented. One may need to consider the scale of change that can be achieved realistically when seeking to implement behavioural change in intensive care units (ICUs); even small changes require trust-building measures and can have a positive impact, especially if the change involves an action that is repeated often. Certain trust-building factors may help to foster an environment that is conducive to behaviour change. An organisation where there is strong leadership, authentic communication, and transparent governance has a much greater chance for success. No matter how necessary change seems to upper management, the barriers must be authentically acknowledged and not swept under the carpet if a strategic change is to be implemented successfully. The key to successful change is in the planning, messaging, and implementation. However, barriers to changing established practice may prevent or impede progress in all organisations, whatever the culture. The three greatest barriers to organisational change are most often the following:

- inadequate culture-shift planning,
- lack of employee involvement,
- flawed communication and leadership strategies.

Organisations also need a clear system in place to support ongoing measurement, implementation, and assessment, and effective ways to address the normalised deviance. This chapter aims to provide practical advice to intensive care providers and administrators on how to encourage and support healthcare professionals and managers to change their clinical practices.

## Complications in critical care

Patient safety and patient-centred care are emerging as key drivers in healthcare reform. Things have changed but often as a by-product of financial reform. Belatedly, safety and quality benchmarks are being integrated into all healthcare organisations' strategic goals. There is

*Quality Management in Intensive Care*, ed. Bertrand Guidet, Andreas Valentin and Hans Flaatten. Published by Cambridge University Press. © Cambridge University Press 2016.

more focus on patient-centred care, but these are early days. Patients still experience needless harm and often struggle to have their voices heard when evidence-based changes are slow to implement and resistance to change causes turmoil.

The critical care setting is one of the most complex environments in a healthcare facility. Critical care units must manage the intersecting challenges of maintaining a high-tech environment and ensuring staff competency in operating the equipment, providing high-quality care to the facility's sickest patients, and tending to the needs of staff members working in stressful environments [1]. While other hospital units may need to manage one or two challenges at a time, critical care settings must manage them all simultaneously, while remaining focused on the delivery of safe patient care.

Before building initiatives to enhance safety, healthcare managers must understand the extent of patient injuries and events in ICUs. Critically ill patients are at high risk for complications due to the severity of their medical conditions, the complex and invasive nature of critical care treatments and procedures, and the use of potent drugs and technologies that carry risks as well as benefits.

The ICU is an ideal laboratory and target-rich environment to study change and implementation. In addition to complications of care, adverse events and errors – many of which are serious – are major risks in ICUs. The 2005 Critical Care Safety Study, found that adverse events in ICUs occur at a rate of 81 per 1000 patient-days and that serious errors occur at a rate of 150 per 1000 patient-days, supporting the findings of an earlier study indicating that nearly all ICU patients suffer potentially harmful events [2]. The study found that the incidence of adverse events (AEs) was 20.2% (13 led to deaths with 55% of these preventable) and there were 223 serious medical errors in a tertiary ICU. The most common serious AE was medication errors, with a cumulative risk of 100% every three days of ICU stay. The Sentinel Evaluation Study found that AEs were associated with patient:nurse ratios, and cost at least $3857 per event and on average led to one extra day in the ICU. Remarkably, nearly half (45%) of the AEs in the safety study were deemed preventable [3]. Common ICU errors are treatment and procedure errors, especially errors in ordering or carrying out medication orders; errors in reporting or communicating clinical information; and failures to take precautions or follow protocols.

# Conceptual framework: a 'whole system' approach

There has been an important re-conceptualisation of clinical risk through emphasising how upstream 'latent factors' enable, condition, or exacerbate the potential for 'active errors' and patient harm. Understanding the characteristics of a safe, resilient, and high-performing system therefore requires research to optimise the relationship between people, tasks, and dynamic environments. The socio-technical approach suggests that adverse incidents can be examined from both an organisational perspective that incorporates the concept of latent conditions and the cascading nature of human error, commencing with management decisions and actions. Some ICU teams are able to recover from errors reliably without leading to patient harm, while others do not learn and repeat the same errors.

This 'systems approach' draws attention to the wider organisation, management, and culture of healthcare. Research reveals, for example, that threats to safety in the ICU are shaped by inter-departmental relationships, attitudinal differences, and cultures that normalise risk. To date, however, this research has tended to focus on single clinical environment or organisational settings, i.e. primary or secondary care, operating theatres, or the emergency department. There is little attention to the threats to patient safety that arise when patients cross these settings – for example, when transferred to a general ward from ICU. Elaborating on this view, it is important to understand the barriers and drivers to patient safety as complex and enmeshed 'constellations' of factors found within and between care processes. This includes regulatory pressures, organisational boundaries, impact of perverse financial incentives, the shifting of professional responsibility, and lack of authentic clinician input and buy-in.

The recent safety checklist study by Urbach *et al.*, demonstrates that the manner in which a checklist is implemented and overseen can contribute to the checklist tool's uptake and compliance by clinicians [4]. Genuine engagement by physicians is critical to the adoption of new care models. Ineffective top-down engagement and inauthentic partnering with clinicians can inhibit positive behaviour change and encourages normalised deviance. Introducing a clinical intervention in an environment characterised by a lack of trust may cause clinicians to feel jeopardised professionally and personally, and encourages gaming.

Glasby suggests three prominent factors influence the participation and engagement of providers in change agency, and are also consistent with the 'whole systems' and 'systems thinking' approaches [5]. These include occupational factors related to the particular knowledge, culture, and practice domains of care providers, such as doctors, social workers, and nurses; organisational factors related to routine working patterns, facilities, capacities, and resources of individual agencies; and compatibility and coordinating factors, which relate to how occupational, organisational, and institutional factors align.

These three factors comprise the following:

- *Knowledge*: related to the epistemological differences between groups, e.g., how they make sense of discharge; understand the role of other professionals; and how meanings are articulated.
- *Culture*: related to the shared meanings, attitudes, and values that shape communication, e.g. when knowledge should be shared and with whom; how norms, identities, and trust reinforce boundaries and knowledge hoarding.
- *Organisation*: related to the influence of departmental, regulatory, and institutional factors that shape knowledge sharing, such as socio-legal rules, professional jurisdictions, organisational priorities, and resource constraints.

## Organisational culture

The most important factor to consider when initiating change relate to the organisational culture, or how providers 'do things here,' and is increasingly appreciated in understanding why persistent variation in practices continues. We define organisational culture as: the socio-organisational phenomena, in terms of behaviour or attitudes, that emerge from a common way of sense-making, based on shared values, beliefs, assumptions, and norms [6]. Evidence suggests that organisational culture may be relevant for successful and sustained improvement efforts.

The cultural barriers are often hidden in the underlying, (invisible) social constructions and attitudes and therefore difficult to identify and assess. A deeper understanding of the relationship between ICU norms and their underlying cultural barriers may contribute to the development and implementation of effective and sustainable interventions to attenuate adverse care events.

## The role of the clinical microsystem

Critical care teams exist within the context of a system. A system is a set of interacting, inter-related, or independent elements that work together in a particular environment to perform the functions that are required to achieve a specific aim. An ICU clinical microsystem is a group of clinicians, nursing staff, and others working together with a shared clinical purpose to provide care for a population of patients [7]. The clinical purpose and its setting define the essential components of the microsystem, which include clinicians, patients, and support staff; information and technology; and specific care processes and behaviours that are required to provide care. The best microsystems evolve over time, as they respond to the needs of their patients and providers, as well as to the external pressures such as regulatory require-ments. They often coexist with other microsystems within a larger (macro) organisation, such as a hospital.

The conceptual theory of the clinical microsystem is based on ideas developed by Deming and others. Deming applied systems thinking to organisational development, leadership, and improvement. The seminal idea for the clinical microsystem stems from the work of James Quinn [8]. Quinn's work is based on analysing the world's best-of-the-best service organisa-tions, such as FedEx, Mary Kay Cosmetics, McDonald's, and Nordstrom. Quinn focused on determining what these extraordinary organisations were doing to achieve consistent, high-quality, explosive growth, high margins, and robust consumer loyalty. He found that these leading service organisations organised around, and continually engineered, the front-line relationships that connected the needs of customers with the organisation's core competency. Quinn called this front-line activity that embedded the service delivery process the *smallest replicable unit* or the *minimum replicable unit*. This smallest replicable unit, or the microsys-tem, is the key to implementing a reliable, effective strategy to provide safe and consistent outcomes.

Nelson and his colleagues have described the essential elements of a microsystem as (1) a core team of healthcare professionals; (2) a defined population they care for; (3) an information environment to support the work of caregivers and patients; and (4) support staff, equipment, and work environment [9]. Linking performance and outcome data to the microsystem model provides a helpful way to identify potential areas for improvement that does not focus on the individual, but instead highlights the system that is producing the processes and outcomes of care.

High-performing clinical microsystems research revealed 43 clinical units that were identified using a sampling methodology. Semi-structured interviews were conducted with leaders from each of the microsystems. Additional research built on the Donaldson and Mohr study in which 20 case studies of high-performing microsystems were collected and included on-site interviews with every member of the microsystem and analysis of individual microsystem performance data. The analysis of the interviews suggested that ten dimensions, shown in Table 18.1, were associated with effective and successful microsystems.

## Organisational environment

In complex organisational environments, teams do not exist in isolation. The performance of individual teams, as well as the team's attitudes towards patient safety, is a function of the milieu, or the culture, in which the team works. Thus, the effectiveness of any particular team cannot be properly assessed without considering the larger system within which the team functions. In a hospital environment, small teams, such as operating teams, coordi-nate with other teams within the perioperative microsystem environment that are involved

**Table 18.1** Ten dimensions of effective clinical microsystems [1,9]

1. Leadership
2. Organisational support of clinicians
3. Staff focus
4. Education and training
5. Interdependence of team members
6. Patient focus
7. Community and market focus
8. Performance results
9. Process improvement
10. Information and information technology

in patient care, and these teams are embedded within larger teams that are directly and indirectly involved in patient care. When looking at the effectiveness of teamwork training for patient safety, one must know how training is supported and reinforced by the organisation in which it occurs.

### Factors that need to be addressed [10]

- Organisational climate: Does the organisational culture support striving for patient safety? Does it allow for non-punitive reporting of problems and near misses?
- Organisational support: Is time for training provided whereby trainees are temporarily relieved of their regular duties? Is training viewed as more than just a necessary checkmark? Is teamwork training widespread and rewarded across the organisation?
- Extent of training: Does the organisation only train isolated teams? Does the training of trauma teams incorporate the 'wider' team members (e.g., including for example, blood bank, radiology, transport, step-down medical, and surgical wards)?

## Tackling change in the ICU

Facilitating change in clinical practice requires an appreciation of barriers at the individual level that may hinder the adoption and implementation of innovation. We have divided the barriers to change in the ICU setting into four sections [11]:

1. understanding barriers to change;
2. identifying barriers to change;
3. overcoming barriers to change;
4. mapping barriers to methods.

## Understanding barriers to change

Recognising the barriers to change of clinical practices requires appreciating the heterogeneity and complexity of interventions implicit in improvement science, including rapid-cycle improvement methods, such as Plan–Do–Study–Act (PDSA) cycles that involve iterative cycles of planning, design, evaluation, and refinement of improvement strategies [12].

The Avedis Donabedian structure–process–outcome model provides the fundamental conceptual framework for evaluating the culture, innovation in the delivery, and organisation of healthcare, and is encapsulated in the well-described PDSA cycle of quality improvement [13].

It is widely understood today that the first step towards improving the safety and quality of care is addressing the varying mental models held by care providers and state agencies.

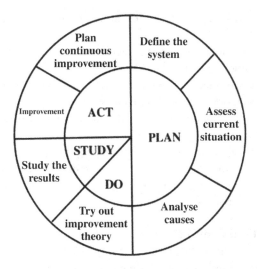

**Figure 18.1** The PDSA cycle.
Adapted from [20].

The implementation and evaluation of changes in structure and process are bound together in a recursive learning cycle of continuous quality improvement. As shown in Figure 18.1 the PDSA model builds on the Donabedian framework and provides clinicians with a structured theory–praxis methodology for routinely evaluating performance and answering the following questions:

- What are we trying to accomplish?
- Are we achieving what we claim and how effective and efficient are we?
- From where we are now, what changes can we make that will result in improvement?
- How will we know that we have achieved the change and that it is an improvement?

The PDSA continuous quality improvement cycle is founded on a thorough understanding of the process being evaluated, gained by detailed mapping of the process of interest, selection of appropriate measurement tools, and identification of an acceptable range of variance.

The PDSA consists of a four-stage process:

1. Plan: What is to be changed, in what way, and how is subsequent performance to be measured and recorded?
2. Do: Implement the plan and collect measurement data on process and outcome.
3. Study: Analyse the data and amend the plan to address the results of the analysis. Rework the process map to identify new nodes, connections, and issues.
4. Act: Implement the amended plan and collect the measurements – again.

## Building trust for organisational resilience

These approaches generate evidence regarding barriers to improvement and help identify solutions and assess their effectiveness using quick turnaround in time and resources. An improvement-science approach recognises the need for customised, site-specific and context-sensitive solutions based on careful study of current practices and local mental models and careful surfacing and recognition of barriers to improvement.

One must start by assessing which barriers and facilitators of change are present at the individual level, including:

1. lack of awareness and knowledge among practitioners and staff of how current ways of working need to change to align with evidence;
2. motivators, both external and internal, such as financial incentives and personal goals and priorities, respectively, or lack of motivators;
3. personal beliefs, attitudes, and perceptions of change, and the associated risks and benefits of the change;
4. individual skills and capacities to carry out the change in practice;
5. practical barriers, including lack of resources, equipment, or staffing; and
6. the external environment, which can influence the individual's ability to adopt a new intervention, such as financial structuring.

## Identifying barriers to change

Conduct a baseline assessment to identify the gap between recommended practice and current ways of working. This baseline assessment of barriers permits tailoring implementation of the innovation. The qualitative data collection methods used to conduct an assessment of barriers include the following:

1. Learn from key individuals with knowledge, authority, and skills to speak to implementation of the innovation.
2. Observe individuals in practice, especially for routine behaviours.
3. Use a questionnaire to explore individuals' knowledge, beliefs, attitudes, and behaviour.
4. Brainstorm informally in small groups to explore solutions to a problem.
5. Conduct a focus group to evaluate current practice and explore new ways of working.

## Overcoming barriers to change

This section examines different strategies for overcoming barriers to implementing change in ICU practice. We outline when specific strategies are used, and briefly discuss evidence of their effectiveness.

The strategies include the following:

1. Educational materials (booklets, CD-ROMs, DVDs, etc.) can raise awareness of a new way of working and are effective in changing behaviour when combined with other strategies. Inadequate education regarding evidence-based interventions such as tight glucose control, handwashing, and central line placement in the ICU is another barrier to achieving reliable ICU quality. Education regarding interventions proven to improve quality of care and patient outcomes is vital in the ICU setting. Multidisciplinary education regarding quality management in the ICU setting is vital to achieving glucose control in critically ill patients. Real innovation in practice led by change in clinician behaviour is best achieved by a combination of interactive education and utilisation of locally developed guidelines or protocols, in addition to continuous quality assessment and feedback [14]. Development of integrated education strategies to improve quality control may be more effective when performed collaboratively in an interdisciplinary manner than within disciplines.
2. Informational meetings (conferences, training courses, lectures, etc.) can increase awareness of change. However, informational meetings with interactive participation, like workshops, are more likely to result in behaviour change.

3.  Educational outreach visits (or academic detailing) involve trained individuals visiting other individuals in their organisation to offer information and support in adopting new ways of working [14]. Outreach visits are effective in changing certain kinds of behaviour, such as the delivery of preventive services or prescribing behaviour.
4.  Opinion leaders can influence their colleagues to adopt an innovation. The use of opinion leaders is an effective way of disseminating information.
5.  Audit and feedback, where information is given back to individuals or teams about their practice as a way to monitor and improve practice, is an effective method for changing behaviour [15]. Audit and feedback are particularly effective when staff buy-in and are involved in the process, when feedback is timely, and when combined with financial incentives.
6.  Reminder systems and decision-support systems are effective in changing behaviour, especially at the point of decision-making. Decision-support systems are effective for specific decisions, such as delivery of preventative services, and less so for complex decision-making [16].
7.  Patient-mediated strategies, which provide information to the general public, are effective in changing the behaviour of practitioners. Such strategies include mass media campaigns, which increase awareness of an innovation among the public and practitioners.

## Mapping implementation barriers to methods

It is essential to choose the methods to map and evaluate the barriers to implementation carefully. Appreciating what others have done and using a series of carefully guided questions to assist in conducting a baseline assessment of barriers can greatly help in overcoming those barriers to assist with implementation change [17].

## Overcoming unseen barriers

Most serious adverse events or industrial disasters do not arise from single point errors, but from many people committing multiple seemingly innocuous errors over time that breach reasonable practice standards. Vaughan describes allowing such process and decision errors to go unattended as 'normalised deviance' [18]. By deviance, we mean organisational behaviours that deviate from normative standards or professional expectations. Outside people see the situation as deviant, whereas inside people get accustomed to it, seeing it as 'routine, rational, and entirely acceptable'. Low handwashing compliance before patient contact, minimal attending oversight of ICU care on weekends, suppressing information about poor care, and the poor handoff communication between ICUs and wards are classic examples of normalised deviance.

Discussion of this sensitive matter using terms such as 'normalised deviance' frequently leads to defensive reactions that halt conversation and require deeper reflection and examination. Ashforth and Anand have described organisational normalised deviance as arising from three mutually reinforcing processes: institutionalisation, rationalisation, and socialisation [19]. During the institutionalisation phase, repetitive practices are enacted without significant thought about the nature of the behaviour. The cause of the behaviour is often external to any one person; instead it emerges from group interaction and socialisation.

A few of these barriers and potential solutions are listed in Table 18.2, which is based on input gathered from healthcare practitioners.

Any of these factors may hold back an organisation, but strong leadership cannot be overemphasised as one of the critical elements for effectively driving change initiatives in

**Table 18.2** Barriers to intensive care change and potential solutions

| Factors inhibiting change | Potential solutions |
| --- | --- |
| Lack of leadership support | Facilitate contact with peers successful in deploying the methodologies. |
| Resistance or scepticism from staff | Develop stakeholder analysis and use a team-based problem-solving approach. |
| Hesitancy to invest time and money | Create a business case supported by sound data (i.e. if the project is to focus on reducing infections, document the costs associated with such occurrences including length of stay, supplies, and added labour). |
| Shortage of internal resources to lead change initiatives | Enlist outside help to drive initial projects or receive training and mentoring in conjunction with projects that produce immediate results. |
| Waning commitment or flavour-of-the-month syndrome | Implement a solid communication plan that reaches all levels of the organisation, and build momentum through early, visible wins. |
| Uncertain roles and/or lack of accountability | Adopt management systems and structures that clearly link projects and performance with overall strategies. |
| This is how we do things here | Addressing actions or care practices that deviate from normative standards or professional society guidelines in a non-accusatory and constructive manner. |

intensive care. To increase efficiency and close the chasm between optimal patient care and that which actually exists, leaders must abandon adherence to obsolete management models.

# Conclusions

Successful change in intensive care practices will be a function of a willingness to adopt new changes, and challenge dogma and the widespread normalised deviance. Dissatisfaction with the present, a shared vision of the future, and mastery of a core set of process improvement tools are needed. Each of these elements is key and needs to be fully leveraged to bring about change. Change leadership is about tirelessly working on each of these elements. Change leadership is also about ensuring all the people in the ICU and those that oversee the ICU in the organisation understand the changes, believe in its personal and organisational impact; and have the capabilities and confidence to flourish in the necessarily changing intensive care environment.

There are, however, a number of barriers to successful change – both in terms of implementation and equally, if not more importantly, in sustaining it. Why are both kinds of change not more successful? Often, the failures can be traced to a few missing ingredients:

1. A fundamental acceptance or realignment in thinking.
2. Appropriate guidance or knowledge.
3. Clear strategies and tactics for maintaining long-term results.

The upside to past failures is that they usually provide some valuable lessons for the future. For instance, ICUs currently contemplating CLABSI or handwashing initiatives as one aspect of transformation can learn from the experiences of other units, both inside and outside their hospital or healthcare system. While avoiding a 'cookie cutter' approach to change initiatives, such examination can provide useful insights into what worked well, and what gaps may have been overlooked. Successful intensive care improvement initiatives can yield a wide range of benefits that are both qualitative and quantitative, including:

- fewer medical errors;
- increased revenue and improved reimbursement;
- better use of advanced technologies (and faster return on investment);
- better accessibility and capacity for patient flow;

- improved organisational communication;
- better nursing and physician satisfaction;
- better patient satisfaction;
- shorter patient wait times;
- investment in staff expertise.

# References

1. Sanchez J, Barach P. High reliability organizations and surgical microsystems: re-engineering surgical care. *Surgical Clinics of North America*, 2012; DOI: 10.1016/j.suc.2011.12.005.

2. Rothschild JM, Landrigan CP, Cronin JW, *et al.* The Critical Care Safety Study: the incidence and nature of adverse events and serious medical errors in intensive care. *Crit Care Med.* 2005;33(8):1694–1700.

3. Valentin A, Capuzzo M, Guidet B, *et al.* Patient safety in intensive care: results from the multinational Sentinel Events Evaluation (SEE) study. *Intensive Care Med.* 2006;32(10):1591–1598.

4. Urbach DR, Govindarajan A, Saskin R, *et al.* Introduction of surgical safety checklists in Ontario, Canada. *NEJM.* 2014;370:1029–1038.

5. Glasby J. *Hospital Discharge: Integrating Health and Social Care.* Oxford: Radcliffe Publishing, 2003.

6. Hesselink G, Vernooij-Dassen M, Barach P, *et al.* Organizational culture: an important context for addressing and improving hospital to community patient discharge. *Medical Care*, 2012; doi: 10.1097/MLR. 0b013e31827632ec.

7. Mohr J, Batalden P, Barach P. Integrating patient safety into the clinical microsystem. *Qual Saf Healthc.* 2004;13:34–38.

8. Quinn JB. *Intelligent Enterprise: A Knowledge and Service Based Paradigm for Industry.* New York: Free Press, 1992.

9. Nelson E, Batalden P, Huber T, *et al.* Microsystems in health care: part 1. Learning from high-performing front-line clinical units. *Jt Comm J Qual Improv.* 2002;28:472–493.

10. Eccles M, Grimshaw J, Walker A, *et al.* Changing the behaviour of healthcare professionals: the use of theory in promoting the uptake of research findings. *J Clin Epidem* 2005;58(2):107–112.

11. National Institute of Health and Clinical Excellence. *Behaviour Change at Population, Community and Individual Levels.* London: National Institute of Health and Clinical Excellence, 2007. www.nice.org.uk/PH006 (accessed 29 May 2015).

12. Donabedian A. Evaluating the quality of medical care. *Milbank Q.* 1966;44:166–203.

13. Lilford R, Chilton PJ, Hemming K, Brown C, Girling A, Barach P. Evaluating policy and service interventions: framework to guide selection and interpretation of study end points. *BMJ* 2010;341:c4413.

14. Greenhalgh T, Robert G, Bate P, *et al. Diffusion of Innovations in Health Service Organisations: A Systematic Literature Review.* Oxford: Blackwell BMJ Books, 2005.

15. Grol R, Wensing M, Eccles M, eds. *Improving Patient Care: The Implementation of Change in Clinical Practice.* Oxford: Elsevier, 2004.

16. van Bokhoven MA, Kok G, van der Weijden T. Designing a quality improvement intervention: a systematic approach. *Qual Saf Healthc.* 2003;12:215–220.

17. Hesselink G, Zegers M, Vernooij-Dassen M, *et al.* Improving patient discharge and reducing hospital readmissions by using Intervention Mapping. *BMC Health Serv Res.* 2014;14:389.

18. Vaughan D. The dark side of organizations: mistake, misconduct and disaster. *Annu Rev Sociol* 1999;25:271–305.

19. Ashforth DE, Anand V. The normalization of corruption in organizations. *Res Organ Behav.* 2003;25:1–52.

20. Langley G, Nolan T, Provost L, eds. *The Improvement Guide*, second edition. San Francisco, CA: Jossey-Bass, 2009.

# Chapter 19

# Teambuilding

Tanja Manser

## Introduction

Intensive care units (ICUs) present a dynamic work environment where patients are critically ill and demands on staff are high. Working in an ICU is cognitively, physically, and emotionally challenging. It requires the collaboration of healthcare professionals from a variety of disciplinary and professional backgrounds in teams. The defining characteristics of a team are that it consists of multiple people with specialised work roles who share resources such as information to achieve a shared goal in a coordinated manner. The shared goal is the key to the work-related interdependencies of team members and the development of and orientation towards shared values. In summary, a team can be defined as an identifiable work unit consisting of two or more people with several characteristics including dynamic social interactions, with meaningful interdependencies, valued and shared goals, a particular lifespan, distributed expertise, and clearly assigned roles and responsibilities [1]. In everyday working life, however, many clinicians seem to perceive only staff from their own discipline or professional group that happen to be working in physical proximity as members of their team. This is often due to the dynamic composition of teams, especially in acute care settings.

However, compared to many other acute care settings, interprofessional ICU teams are rather stable; especially when focusing on the ICU nurses and physicians. Even collaborations with staff from other groups such as pharmacists, physiotherapists, or dietitians occur within rather well-established networks of professionals. Thus, there are real opportunities for teambuilding,[1] that is for developing ways of working together as a team that help to maintain patient safety and clinician health – which in turn is a prerequisite for providing safe care.

This chapter provides an overview of central teamwork concepts and their relevance to critical care. It gives examples for interventions to improve teamwork and discusses the requirements that need to be met for these interventions to be of maximum effect.

---

[1] The term teambuilding is used in different ways. Here it is used in the sense of systematic interventions to support the team in developing effective ways of teamwork and not in the sense of Tuckman's stages of group development [2].

*Quality Management in Intensive Care*, ed. Bertrand Guidet, Andreas Valentin and Hans Flaatten. Published by Cambridge University Press. © Cambridge University Press 2016.

**Table 19.1** Aspects of teamwork relevant to quality and patient safety in acute care settings

| Aspects of teamwork | Examples of safety-relevant characteristics |
| --- | --- |
| Quality of collaboration | Mutual respect (within and across professions and disciplines) <br> Trust <br> Psychological safety |
| Shared understanding | Strength of shared goals <br> Shared situation awareness <br> Shared mental model of team structure, team task, team roles, etc. <br> Transactive memory |
| Adaptive coordination | Dynamic task allocation when new members join the team <br> Shift between explicit and implicit forms of coordination <br> Increased information exchange and planning in critical situations |
| Communication | Openness of communication <br> Quality of communication (e.g. shared frames of reference) <br> Specific communication practices (e.g. team briefing, handover) |
| Leadership | Leadership style (value contributions from staff, encourage participation in decision-making, speaking-up, etc.) <br> Adaptive leadership behaviour (e.g. increased explicit leadership behaviour in critical situations) |

(Adapted from [6])

# Emphasis on teamwork

In recent years it has been widely recognised that effective teamwork is crucial to ensure the quality and safety of patient care and that many of the factors contributing to adverse events in healthcare originate from flawed teamwork rather than from a lack of clinical competence. Especially in acute care settings such as the operating theatre and ICU, the impact of teamwork on clinical outcomes has been well documented. For example, ICUs with high levels of interprofessional collaboration have improved patient mortality rates and reduced average patient length of stay [3]. Another study found that the quality of team functioning perceived by ICU staff (e.g. team members were seen as less dependent and more trusting) was more positive on units with mortality rates that were lower than predicted [4]. Furthermore, ineffective team behaviours such as poor communication during daily rounds and handovers are frequently cited as a main contributory factor to adverse events [5]. These findings are consistent with research from other domains, highlighting the central role of various aspects of teamwork for quality and safety of patient care (see Table 19.1).

# Central teamwork concepts

Team researchers attempting to understand the ways in which factors such as attitudes and behaviours of team members shape team performance often refer to an 'input–process–output' framework [7]. In this context, *input* typically refers to the characteristics team members bring to the team, such as, for example, qualifications, status, professional experience, and personality and demographic attributes. These inputs are often summarised as team characteristics. Other inputs are the characteristics of the task (e.g. routine vs. non-routine) or the level of interdependency. *Process* refers to the work-related interactions of team members that transform inputs into outputs (e.g. sharing of information, distribution of tasks, decision-making). *Output* finally refers to the product of the team's work. This includes outcomes in terms of a product or successful treatment of a patient, but also outcomes in the team members such as work satisfaction or attitudes towards other team members. Over the years this basic framework has been refined, but it is still a very commonly used heuristic to structure our thinking about teamwork (see Figure 19.1).

In the following, selected concepts from this framework will be discussed based on their documented relevance in team research in ICU settings. The study of teamwork in critical care has concentrated either on aspects of team climate or on effective team behaviour during specific work or clinical situations such as daily rounds, shift handover, or resuscitation. The interrelations of these two levels of analysis have rarely been investigated. However, based on conceptual frameworks of team performance (see Figure 19.1) it can be assumed that team climate on the one hand provides the foundation on which the specific teamwork behaviours are enacted, and on the other hand is influenced by the experience of team members during specific work episodes.

## Aspects of team climate

Team climate is a component of organisational culture that has been defined as a team's shared perceptions of organisational policies, practices, and procedures [9]. Two psychological concepts that address specific aspects of these perceptions are psychological safety and the quality of interprofessional collaboration. Both concepts have been applied in research on teamwork in healthcare settings. Some studies have investigated the impact of psychological safety and interprofessional collaboration on patient outcomes, while another line of research has tried to link specific interventions to improvements in either of these team climate aspects.

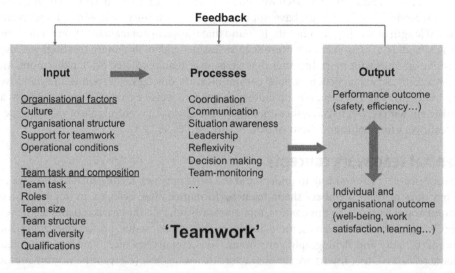

**Figure 19.1** Team performance framework.

Adapted from [8].

## Psychological safety

Psychological safety refers to the degree to which individuals perceive their work environment as supportive of interpersonally risky behaviour, such as seeking help, pointing out mistakes, voicing concerns, or offering suggestions [10,11]. Studies have shown that patients treated in healthcare settings in which staff feel psychologically unsafe often experience adverse events. For example, one study showed that hospitals in which staff reported greater fear of shame and blame performed significantly worse on some patient safety indicators [12]. In the ICU setting, studies found that the perceived communication openness among team members predicted the degree to which individual clinicians reported to understand patient care goals that in turn can be associated with improved care [13].

## Interprofessional collaboration

Interprofessional collaboration (i.e. the quality of collaboration and communication between team members from different professional backgrounds) is one of the major factors for the perceived quality of daily work and is seen as crucial to patient safety [6,14]. At the same time, the interprofessional dimension of teamwork is one for which most studies identified marked differences between the perceptions of professional groups [6]. For example, in a North American study nurses' ratings of the quality of collaboration and communication with physicians (33% positive ratings) were compared with physicians' ratings of the quality of collaboration and communication with nurses (73% positive ratings) [15]. Interprofessional collaboration, or the perception thereof, can be positively influenced by introducing new models of care and by providing teams with opportunities for interprofessional reflection and learning [16]. In the ICU daily rounds and handover situations offer great potential for such reflection and learning that goes beyond the necessary coordination of care.

# Teamwork behaviours during specific work episodes

One of the central team processes mentioned in Figure 19.1 is leadership. Team leader behaviour is a well-documented contributor to team effectiveness via shaping team climate and encouraging positive team behaviour. Apart from facilitating collaboration among the interprofessional team and with other disciplines, team leaders act as role models during daily work. This becomes particularly apparent during rounds and handovers. These two critical communication and decision-making episodes have been studied extensively, leading to a body of knowledge not only regarding effective leadership but also regarding the behaviour of other team members.

## Daily rounds

Interdisciplinary rounds are a foundation of critical care. However, they serve multiple purposes such as decision-making, coordination of care, and education, and have to integrate the priorities and perspectives of multiple professions, disciplines, and hierarchical levels, which sometimes makes it difficult to understand the best possible way to conduct them. The shared goals and thus the need for teamwork can be obscured at times. Research into rounding has highlighted the central role of the leader to structure the communication, to elicit team member contributions, and to establish a climate in which team members feel comfortable to ask questions and raise concerns. A tool that can help the team to summarise the bedside discussion and clarify roles and responsibilities are sheets capturing daily care goals. However, as with many tools, they will not serve their purpose unless the underlying team process, with all its sub-processes (see Figure 19.1), sufficiently supports the development of a shared understanding of the patient and its care.

## Handover

Continuity of care is essential to the quality and safety of patient care in a complex setting such as the ICU. However, the exchange of care-related information at handover points such as end of shift or admission to and discharge from the ICU has been shown to be flawed. This may in part be due to the fact that handover is seen as a mere information transition exercise and not as a critical teamwork episode in which responsibility is handed over along with the tacit knowledge about the patient and her/his needs that may be reflected only incompletely in the patient record and the handover protocols that are increasingly common tools to support patient handover. Handover conversations need to be supported by teamwork behaviours facilitating shared situation awareness as well as trust in other team members and their commitment to the shared goal of providing safe and effective care [17].

# Improvement approaches

Over the past 20 years research on teamwork in the ICU has provided substantial insight into the preconditions and processes of safe performance, and teamwork has become a key component of many education standards for health professions and system-based interventions to improve patient safety. Evidence on the effectiveness and sustainability of team-based interventions is, however, still scarce. This is not necessarily related to a lack of improvement efforts. However, improving teamwork requires a complex set of interventions that combine training elements with work design to facilitate collaboration (e.g. overlapping shift schedules or synchronisation of work schedules across departments to allow for participation of all relevant staff in rounds) and leadership support to allow for successful transfer of teamwork practices into daily work.

However, there are some notable examples for successful interventions focusing on either team climate or teamwork behaviour, or a combination of the two. The majority of interventions aim to improve information exchange as a key to effective teamwork. The introduction of daily care goal sheets and handover protocols are common tools to facilitate this process [6,13]. But the tools themselves are not sufficient to improve the quality of teamwork. The organisation of work, as well as team-oriented leadership behaviour, are needed to support team members in engaging in teamwork, using all available resources to create a shared understanding of patient needs and priorities for treatment, to make care decisions and carry them out in a well-coordinated manner. Concerning the organisational preconditions of teamwork, it is essential to build in the time needed for meaningful reflection as an interprofessional, interdisciplinary team. This is not limited to case conferences or debriefing of resuscitations, but should form an integral part of everyday work and, thus, needs to be planned for when defining rotas and shift schedules.

Teams in the ICU need support in this reflection process. But they also need to be involved in the relevant teambuilding activities and have access to tools that support their reflection and learning. One example of such a tool or technique is the use of video reflection [18]. In the ICU setting this technique has been applied to specific care situations such as handovers [19]. In other settings such as shock trauma it has been used for reflection and debriefing of the interprofessional, interdisciplinary teamwork during actual trauma care. One of the characteristics of this technique that sets it apart from most other teambuilding interventions is that the team itself is in charge of leading this process. The team can decide which care episodes to record, the recordings can be viewed individually or as a team, and with or without the support of an experienced moderator to facilitate reflection. The experience with this technique shows that ICU teams, while first frequently hesitant, appreciate the opportunity to discuss the way they work together as a team and learn how to improve their teamwork by understanding the diverse perspectives of the various professional and disciplinary perspectives on their way of working.

Another study on a multidisciplinary teambuilding intervention in four neonatal ICUs further underlines the importance of a participatory approach to teambuilding [20]. It also highlights the multifaceted nature of such teambuilding, requiring the implementation of a set of intertwined teamwork practices. Further, this study points out the critical importance of leadership commitment and involvement in any component of such an intervention.

The main barriers for implementation of such team development interventions are related to the management commitment necessary to ensure the resources involved in managing comprehensive team training programmes involving staff from multiple disciplines and professions.

## Conclusion

The relevance of effective teamwork to the quality and safety of critical care makes it an ethical imperative to invest in improvements. What implementation science has also made clear within the past decade is that for an intervention to yield improvements in teamwork, whether in the area of team climate or teamwork behaviour, the intervention needs to target the specific team processes relevant to achieving these goals. For example, there is no theoretical foundation for the assumption that a bundle intervention to reduce catheter-related infections should directly influence teamwork. It is more likely for the team process necessary for successful implementation of such rather clinically focused interventions (e.g. agreeing on shared goals, monitoring and discussing changes in infection rates, speaking up to make suggestions for refinement, or questioning aspects of the implementation that do not seem to work) are the ones that contribute to changes in teamwork. This also explains why the same intervention does not necessarily achieve similar improvement in different healthcare organisations.

## Team reflexivity is key

The central role of reflection as a characteristic of true and effective teamwork has been shown across industries [11]. The fact that many teams actually do not have sufficient opportunity for reflection has led to the distinction between authentic and pseudo teams [21]. It has been shown for healthcare that while about 90% of staff report to work in teams, only around 40% indicate that their team has all three defining characteristics of authentic teams: having clear shared goals, working closely and interdependently, and reflecting on effectiveness on a regular basis. Especially the third characteristic was lacking in many healthcare teams, pointing to a high level of pseudo teams. These teams will never be able to fully exploit the potential of teamwork and thus will fall short of the promise of improving the quality and safety of care.

## Holistic view of teamwork gains

This chapter has focused mainly on the effects of teamwork on the quality and safety of care. However, the quality of teamwork also has significant effects on clinicians' psychological health. Burn-out is a core component of reduced work-related psychological health and represents a severe, chronic strain response of the individual to enduring stress at work. It is highly prevalent in healthcare, with a rather alarming increase in recent years; particularly in acute care settings. It has also been shown that high levels of burn-out are not just a problem for the individual clinician, but for the entire team as burn-out might carry over from one team member to another.

From a patient safety perspective, clinician health is critical because burnt-out clinicians lack the necessary resources to perform at the levels necessary in critical care (i.e. reduced vigilance, fatigue, cognitive impairment, emotional distancing or negative attitude towards patients). Thus, errors are more likely to happen and less likely to be detected; especially if other team members are unable to spend additional resources to compensate.

Therefore, preventing or reducing clinician burn-out through work design that supports team-based work and through effective teambuilding might actually have two positive effects: mitigating well-known individual effects such as depression or intention to leave the profession, and helping to maintain patient safety. In turn, improved patient safety has the potential to increase clinicians' feeling of efficacy and potentially buffer negative effects on their health. Considering both outcomes when implementing teamwork improvements is likely to increase not only clinician involvement but also management commitment.

# References

1. Salas E., Rosen M.A., King H. Managing teams managing crises: principles of teamwork to improve patient safety in the Emergency Room and beyond. *Theor Issues Ergonomics Sci.* 2007;8(5):381–394.

2. Tuckman B.W. Developmental sequence in small groups. *Psychol Bull.* 1965;63: 384–399.

3. Baggs J.G., Ryan S.A., Phelps C.E., Richeson J.F., Johnson J.E. The association between interdisciplinary collaboration and patient outcomes in a medical intensive care unit. *Heart Lung.* 1992;21(1):18–24.

4. Wheelan S.A., Burchill C.N., Tilin F. The link between teamwork and patients' outcomes in intensive care units. *Am J Crit Care.* 2003;12(6):527–534.

5. Schmutz J., Manser T. Do team processes really have an effect on clinical performance? A systematic literature review. *Brit J Anaesth.* 2013;110:529–544.

6. Manser T. Teamwork and patient safety in dynamic domains of healthcare: a review of the literature. *Acta Anaesthesiologica Scandinavica.* 2009;53(2):143–151.

7. Guzzo R.A., Shea G.P. Group performance and intergroup relations in organizations. In *Handbook of Industrial and Organizational Psychology.* 3. Palo Alto, CA: Consulting Psychologists Press, 1992: 269–313.

8. Helmreich R.L., Foushee H.C. Why crew resource management? Empirical and theoretical bases of human factors training in aviation. In: Weiner E.L., Kanki B.G., Helmreich R.L., eds. *Cockpit Resource Management.* San Diego, CA: Academic Press; 1993: 3–46.

9. Anderson N.R., West M.A. Measuring climate for work group innovation: development and validation of the team climate inventory. *Journal of Organizational Behavior.* 1998;19(3): 235–258.

10. Kolbe M., Burtscher M.J., Wacker J., et al. Speaking up is related to better team performance in simulated anesthesia inductions: an observational study. *Anesth Analg.* 2012;115(5):1099–1108.

11. Edmondson A.C. Speaking up in the operating room: how team leaders promote learning in interdisciplinary action teams. *J Manage Stud.* 2003;40(6):1419–1452.

12. Singer S., Lin S., Falwell A., Gaba D., Baker L. Relationship of safety climate and safety performance in hospitals. *Health Serv Res.* 2009;44(2 Pt 1):399–421.

13. Reader T.W., Flin R., Mearns K., Cuthbertson B.H. Interdisciplinary communication in the intensive care unit. *Brit J Anaesth.* 2007;98(3):347–352.

14. Zwarenstein M., Bryant W. Interventions to promote collaboration between nurses and doctors. *Cochrane Database of Systematic Reviews.* 2000(2):CD000072.

15. Thomas E.J., Sexton J.B., Helmreich R.L. Discrepant attitudes about teamwork

among critical care nurses and physicians. *Crit Care Med.* 2003;31(3):956–959.

16. Martin J.S., Ummenhofer W., Manser T., Spirig R. Interprofessional collaboration among nurses and physicians: making a difference in patient outcome. *Swiss Med Wkly.* 2010;140:w13062.

17. Manser T., Foster S. Effective handover communication: an overview of research and improvement efforts. *Best Prac Res Clin Anaesthesiol.* 2011;25(2):181–191.

18. Iedema R. Creating safety by strengthening clinicians' capacity for reflexivity. *BMJ Quality Saf.* 2011;20(Suppl 1):i83–i86.

19. Broekhuis M., Veldkamp C. The usefulness and feasibility of a reflexivity method to improve clinical handover. *J Eval Clin Prac.* 2007;13(1):109–115.

20. Brown M.S., Ohlinger J., Rusk C., Delmore P., Ittmann P. Implementing potentially better practices for multidisciplinary team building: creating a neonatal intensive care unit culture of collaboration. *Pediatrics.* 2003;111(4):7.

21. West M., Lyubovnikova J.R. Real teams or pseudo teams? The changing landscape needs a better map. *Ind Organ Psychol.* 2012;5(1):25–28.

# Chapter 20

# Conflict management in the intensive care unit

Katerina Rusinova and Elie Azoulay

## Introduction

Communication tensions and conflicts are normal parts of human communication, a "natural remedy" for stressful situations that are common in the intensive care unit (ICU) setting. The current understanding of conflicts labels them as potentially having both negative and positive consequences [1]. For instance, little conflict leads to less creativity and team-building strategies. Such teams experience little change or motivation. An optimal amount of conflict can generate creativity, strong team spirit, and motivation. Conversely, too much conflict is burdensome for the entire ICU team. They result in a huge loss of energy, decreasing productivity, increasing stress, and, finally, disintegration.

The area of healthcare, especially the ICU, is susceptible to conflict emergence and escalation due to the highly complex medical decision-making involved in life-threatening situations and the emotionally charged life stories of patients. In recent years special attention has been paid to understanding conflicts in the critical care settings. Conflicts are common in the ICU, and are often accompanied by intense experiences. Recent quantitative and qualitative studies have helped understand that ICU conflicts are a dynamic process that needs to be understood via a careful and comprehensive listening and analysis of all stakeholders. Also, the number of reported ICU conflicts has increased following the use of an operational definition of ICU conflicts established by the ethics section of the European Society of Critical Care (ESICM). Conflicts are then defined as "dispute, disagreement, incompatibility, opposition, or difference of opinion involving more than one individual". This could be related to patient management (including admission, discharge, care, nursing, treatment decisions, respect of a patient's preferences and values), or to interpersonal conflict. Conflicts can be measured by nurses, physicians, patients, or family members. They can be assessed during an interview or by a questionnaire survey, during the ICU stay or after patient's discharge.

This review has the main objective to provide critical care clinicians with the knowledge that conflicts can be both measured as any ICU acquired event, but also can be used as an outcome variable. Readers using these data may be able to recognize situations at risk for conflict within different ICU stakeholders.

*Quality Management in Intensive Care*, ed. Bertrand Guidet, Andreas Valentin and Hans Flaatten. Published by Cambridge University Press. © Cambridge University Press 2016.

# Experiencing conflicts in the ICU

## Definition

The question of conflict is primarily addressed and largely explored by the social sciences, mainly psychology. The term "conflict" from a psychological perspective is usually defined as a process that begins when one party perceives their interests, norms, values, opinions, or viewpoints as being opposed, insulted, or resisted by another [1].

The interest in studying conflicts, associated with specific intensive care environments, has grown over the past two decades, mostly in relation to end-of-life issues and withholding/withdrawing life-sustaining treatment at the end of life [2]. The ethics section of the ESICM suggested, in 2007, the following definition reflecting expert opinion: "conflict refers to a dispute, disagreement, or difference of opinion, related to the management of a patient in the ICU involving more than one individual and requiring some decision or action."

## Epidemiology

Based on a modified definition of conflict by Studdert *et al.* [3], a detailed epidemiology of conflict in the ICU was reported in the Conflicus study, which was the largest explorative international one-day cross-sectional study. The study provided prevalence data on perceived conflicts, risk factors, and resolution modalities of intra-team conflicts [4].

In the study, conflicts were perceived by 5268 (71.6%) respondents from 323 ICUs in 24 countries. Considerable variation across countries (from 26% to 100%) was reported. Data from previous studies, in specific patient cohorts, supported these findings [5–7].

## Conflict characteristics

### Parties involved in ICU conflicts

Individuals, groups, or organizations can be involved in conflicts, i.e., the ICU and referring teams (inter-team conflict), members of the ICU team (intra-team conflict), and conflicts between the ICU team and patients' family/substitute decision-maker (SDM). Figure 20.1 describes the people involved in ICU conflicts as they are usually characterized in clinical studies.

Most of the conflicts occur either between families and ICU staff members [7] or within the ICU team [8]. Intra-family conflicts or conflicts with patients are less frequent. When the ICU stay is prolonged, nearly one-third (31.8%) of patients experience conflicts associated with their care, as shown in a study by Studdert and colleagues [3], where nurses reported all types of conflict more frequently than physicians, especially intra-team conflicts.

### Sources of conflict

Many sources of conflict have been identified in ICUs. In the Conflicus study [4], half of the intra-team conflicts were related to end-of-life issues. Poor communication (in quality and in quantity) [9] and general and interpersonal behavior (Figure 20.2) are the most frequent and critical problems creating conflicts. Family needs, in term of communication, in the context of shifting from curative to palliative care, includes the need for timely information, the need for honesty, the need for clinicians to be clear, and the need for clinicians to listen [2]. When these needs are unmet, they frequently contribute to a conflict emergence and may

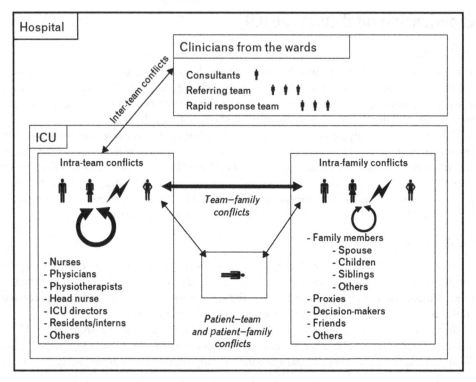

**Figure 20.1** People involved in ICU conflicts. The thickness of the arrows reflects the estimated prevalence of conflicts. Intra-team and team–family conflicts are more frequent than intra-family conflicts or conflicts with patients.

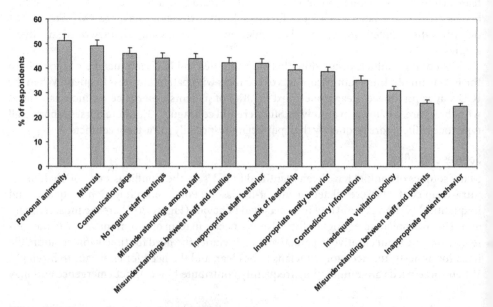

**Figure 20.2** Sources of behavior-related conflicts.

contribute to the frustration of nurses with overly authoritarian intensivists [10]. A study by Danjoux *et al.* found that every disagreement over treatment goals was potentially a major source of conflict [10].

### Conflict severity and impact
In the Conflicus study [4], conflicts were perceived as severe in more than half of cases (53%). Conflicts were not resolved, at the time of the study, in about 40% of cases and respondents frequently reported that the same type of conflict was anticipated to reoccur. About 25% of them indicated that the reported conflict was related to a previous conflict.

Conflicts are usually perceived as draining energy, reducing focus, and causing discomfort and hostility. In the critical care setting, this impact can be harmful not only for the healthcare team (conflicts have been consistently shown to be strongly associated with burn-out syndrome in nurses and physicians [11–13]), but may also possibly affect patient safety and the quality of care [14,15].

# Managing conflicts
## Theoretical perspectives
Most of the understanding regarding conflict function, role, and management is derived from non-intensive care literature [1] and is poorly studied in ICU settings [16–18]. Further qualitative and interdisciplinary research is needed to better understand the typology of ICU-specific conflicts, classification of their severity and impact in terms of both usefulness and harmfulness [19].

Recently, a promising simulation experiment method was introduced to evaluate and study important communication skills of ICU clinicians [20]. Using best-practice guidelines and an iterative, multidisciplinary approach, a simulation involving a critically ill patient was developed and refined. This model proved to be feasible, acceptable, and realistic. Its use offers an opportunity and method for pursuing an in-depth understanding of ICU conflicts.

## Results of interventional studies
Interventional research in the area of ICU conflicts prevention and management requires a thorough interdisciplinary approach with fundamental input of social science theories [1].

So far, only a limited number of studies have tested interventions aimed specifically at conflict reduction. Burns *et al.* [21] evaluated the intervention of social workers in the ICU, who intervened as facilitators of family–ICU staff communication and gave feedback to the clinical team. This intervention, however, failed to demonstrate any change with regard to satisfaction of care, information sharing/content, or involvement in the decision-making process.

Although there is, as yet, no known effective intervention for reducing ICU conflicts (based on clinical research), the field of ICU communication (whose description is beyond the scope of this chapter) is well studied and there is available evidence-based recommendations regarding structured communication and family conferences [22].

# How to turn conflict into an opportunity for improvement
After reviewing current evidence on conflicts in the ICUs, the following part of the paper briefly reports on some of the general practical aspects for approaching and handling conflict situations, many of which are unavoidable in daily ICU routines: e.g., conflict phases and

styles, the process of negotiation, and the role of emotional communication and social skills in managing conflicts.

## Understanding conflict phases and styles

Recognizing the five basic conflict phases may offer better insight into the process of conflict [16]:

1. latent conflict (opposing forces or ideas exist)
2. conflict emergence (explicit voicing of the conflict)
3. conflict escalation (standpoints are firmly taken and expressed)
4. conflict de-escalation (characterized by an openness to a possible settlement of the conflict)
5. post-conflict peace-building phase (creates a potential for a conflict to become an opportunity for improvement).

### Conflict style

The results of the conflict and the relationship with the other party are the two variables that define the style of a conflict.

For example, urgent situations in the ICU can justify the use of an assertive style: one cannot engage in lengthy discussions in urgent situations, even at a cost of possible (temporary) loss of a good relationship with the family/team [16].

On the other hand, the assertive (so-called win–lose) style is probably harmful in other situations, e.g., while discussing goals of care and unfavorable prognosis with patients and families. In this context refined and nuanced communication aimed at building a trusting relationship with the family has been shown to be effective in preventing family/staff conflicts and may also help families better process a poor prognosis emotionally, as emphasized by Anderson *et al.* in a recent study [23].

## Negotiation

Conflicts can be resolved by the process – some say "art" – of negotiation. Therefore, interpersonal communication skills rank highly among the most important personal attributes. A conscious approach to techniques of negotiations include several well-described strategies [24]: (1) staying in control under pressure, (2) defusing anger and hostility, (3) finding out what the other side really wants, (4) using power/persuasion to bring the other side back to the table, and (5) reaching agreements that satisfy the needs of both sides.

For example, discussing treatment alternatives relative to an unfavorable prognosis or end of life is a situation known to be associated with increased risk of conflict [4] and hence requires empathetic communication and careful negotiation. It has been demonstrated that not only knowledge (about advance directive laws, training on how to deliver bad news, etc.), but also what can be called perceived self-efficacy plays a major role in the ability to attend to the emotional needs of patients and surrogates and succeed in this negotiation process [25]. This finding, so far unmentioned in the available qualitative research in the field of ICU conflicts, clearly illustrates how complex it is to get deeper insight into the problem of negotiation in the context of critical illness, and highlights the importance of multimodal research design in this area.

## Conclusion

Although a thorough exploration of conflicts in the ICU environment has been developed only recently, we have gained important insight through both quantitative and qualitative research. However, current knowledge is still incomplete and further research is needed, especially in refining a reliable definition of conflicts in the ICU and in the typology of conflicts related to critical care. Management of conflicts relies mainly on principles taken from the social sciences and has not yet been sufficiently explored in the ICU setting. So far only a limited number of educational interventions aimed at improving the ability of intensivists to handle conflicts have been tested. The problem of conflicts in the ICU is a complex issue involving specific social skills and requiring knowledge and practice of specific communication strategies. This suggests that while better insight through continuing high-quality research is necessary, it will be crucial to develop targeted medical education in order to improve conflict management.

## Acknowledgment

Zuzana Čepelíková for insightful comments.

## References

1.  Dreu CKW de, Gelfand MJ, eds. *The Psychology of Conflict and Conflict Management in Organizations*. New York: Lawrence Erlbaum Associates, 2008.

2.  Norton SA, Tilden VP, Tolle SW, Nelson CA, Eggman ST. Life support withdrawal: communication and conflict. *Am J Crit Care Off Publ Am Assoc Crit-Care Nurses*. 2003;12(6):548–555.

3.  Studdert DM, Mello MM, Burns JP, *et al.* Conflict in the care of patients with prolonged stay in the ICU: types, sources, and predictors. *Intensive Care Med.* 2003;29(9):1489–1497.

4.  Azoulay E, Timsit J-F, Sprung CL, *et al.* Prevalence and factors of intensive care unit conflicts: the Conflicus study. *Am J Respir Crit Care Med.* 2009;180(9):853–860.

5.  Breen CM, Abernethy AP, Abbott KH, Tulsky JA. Conflict associated with decisions to limit life-sustaining treatment in intensive care units. *J Gen Intern Med.* 2001;16(5):283–289.

6.  Way J, Back AL, Curtis JR. Withdrawing life support and resolution of conflict with families. *BMJ.* 2002;325(7376):1342–1345.

7.  Abbott KH, Sago JG, Breen CM, Abernethy AP, Tulsky JA. Families looking back: one year after discussion of withdrawal or withholding of life-sustaining support. *Crit Care Med.* 2001;29(1):197–201.

8.  Ferrand E, Lemaire F, Regnier B, *et al.* Discrepancies between perceptions by physicians and nursing staff of intensive care unit end-of-life decisions. *Am J Respir Crit Care Med.* 2003;167(10):1310–1315.

9.  Rusinova K, Kukal J, Simek J, Cerny V. Limited family members/staff communication in intensive care units in the Czech and Slovak Republics considerably increases anxiety in patients' relatives. *BMC Psychiatry.* 2014;14:21.

10. Danjoux Meth N, Lawless B, Hawryluck L. Conflicts in the ICU: perspectives of administrators and clinicians. *Intensive Care Med.* 2009;35(12):2068–2077.

11. Aiken LH, Clarke SP, Sloane DM, Sochalski J, Silber JH. Hospital nurse staffing and patient mortality, nurse burnout, and job dissatisfaction. *JAMA.* 2002;288(16):1987–1993.

12. Poghosyan L, Clarke SP, Finlayson M, Aiken LH. Nurse burnout and quality of care: cross-national investigation in six countries. *Res Nurs Health.* 2010;33(4): 288–298.

13. Embriaco N, Azoulay E, Barrau K, *et al.* High level of burnout in intensivists: prevalence and associated factors. *Am J Respir Crit Care Med.* 2007;175(7): 686–692.

14. Tarnow-Mordi WO, Hau C, Warden A, Shearer AJ. Hospital mortality in relation to staff workload: a 4-year study in an adult intensive-care unit. *Lancet.* 2000;356(9225):185–189.

15. Manser T. Teamwork and patient safety in dynamic domains of healthcare: a review of the literature. *Acta Anaesthesiol Scand.* 2009;53(2):143–151.

16. Strack van Schijndel RJM, Burchardi H. Bench-to-bedside review: leadership and conflict management in the intensive care unit. *Crit Care Lond Engl.* 2007;11(6):234.

17. Hawryluck LA, Espin SL, Garwood KC, Evans CA, Lingard LA. Pulling together and pushing apart: tides of tension in the ICU team. *Acad Med J Assoc Am Med Coll.* 2002;77(10 Suppl):S73–76.

18. Lingard L, Espin S, Evans C, Hawryluck L. The rules of the game: interprofessional collaboration on the intensive care unit team. *Crit Care Lond Engl.* 2004;8(6): R403–408.

19. Fassier T, Azoulay E. Conflicts and communication gaps in the intensive care unit. *Curr Opin Crit Care.* 2010;16(6): 654–665.

20. Chiarchiaro J, Schuster RA, Ernecoff NC, Barnato AE, Arnold RM, White DB.

Developing a simulation to study conflict in ICUs. *Ann Am Thorac Soc.* 2015;12(4):526–532.

21. Burns JP, Mello MM, Studdert DM, Puopolo AL, Truog RD, Brennan TA. Results of a clinical trial on care improvement for the critically ill. *Crit Care Med.* 2003;31(8):2107–2117.

22. Curtis JR, White DB. Practical guidance for evidence-based ICU family conferences. *Chest.* 2008;134(4):835–843.

23. Anderson WG, Cimino JW, Ernecoff NC, *et al.* A multicenter study of key stakeholders' perspectives on communicating with surrogates about prognosis in intensive care units. *Ann Am Thorac Soc.* 2015;12(2):142–152.

24. Ury W. *Getting Past No: Negotiating With Difficult People.* New York: Bantam Books, 1991.

25. Sulmasy DP, Sood JR, Ury WA. Physicians' confidence in discussing do not resuscitate orders with patients and surrogates. *J Med Ethics.* 2008;34(2):96–101.

# From polio to hospital-wide care

## The evolution of intensive care

Ken Hillman, Michael Parr, and Anders Aneman

The specialty of intensive care has made remarkable progress in a relatively short time. The birth of the specialty was in the early 1950s when the anaesthetist Bjørn Ibsen intubated (by tracheostomy) and ventilated patients who were unable to breathe effectively because of poliomyelitis. He was able to maintain life until the patients recovered sufficiently to breathe spontaneously again. By moving the patients into dedicated ward areas with adequate equipment and staffing, the mortality of patients with acute poliomyelitis was reduced from 80% to 40% [1]. Intensive care has moved a long way from treating young patients with acute but reversible single-organ failure to managing aged patients with chronic and severely restricted physiological reserves in multiple-organ systems. Yet the models of care, and expectations to defy mortality, have not changed to a similar extent. The organisation of hospitals has furthermore remained largely unchanged, meaning that many generic principles regarding attending to patients on wards are the same today as half a century ago. However, the population of patients and their level of complexity have changed considerably.

Like all novel and iconoclastic advances in medicine, it took time for the specialty of intensive care to be universally accepted. Before the specialty of intensive care became recognised, the admitting team caring for the patient would also manage the patients when they became seriously ill, whether they were appropriately trained or not (Figure 21.1). Needless to say, the outcome of many patients was extremely poor [2]. Up to 40% of admissions to intensive care units (ICUs) were found to be potentially avoidable because of sub-optimal care, lack of knowledge, lack of organisation, and failure to seek advice [3]. The admitting team caring for patients on the wards often did not recognise patients were at risk of serious deterioration. Studies showed that the majority of cardiac arrests, potentially avoidable deaths, and admissions to an ICU were not sudden and unexpected but preceded by slow deterioration which was not responded to appropriately [2]. More recent data published in 2014 suggest that such shortcomings on a system level remain [4].

## Rapid response systems

Intensivists could not help but notice that many of the patients admitted to an ICU from the general wards could have been diagnosed and resuscitated at a much earlier stage in their illness. A hospital-wide system to recognise and respond to seriously ill patients was established using a set of criteria based on abnormalities in vital signs and other observations.

*Quality Management in Intensive Care*, ed. Bertrand Guidet, Andreas Valentin and Hans Flaatten. Published by Cambridge University Press. © Cambridge University Press 2016.

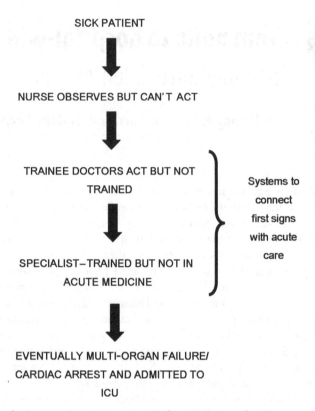

**Figure 21.1** System for detecting deteriorating patients before introduction of rapid response teams.

This allowed ward staff to call clinicians who had appropriate skills, knowledge, and experience to deal with seriously ill patients on the ward [5]. As a result, a large number of cardiac arrests, unexpected ICU admissions, and deaths could be avoided. The system was known as the medical emergency team (MET) and is now known by many other names under the generic label of rapid response systems (RRSs). It was a natural transition for intensivists to not delay until the patient was seriously ill or near death before intervening in an appropriate way. The challenges in establishing RRSs were the same challenges as those faced by the pioneers who established the specialty of intensive care. Originally they had to convince colleagues that the specialty of intensive care required dedicated training supported by its own textbooks, journals, conferences, and other sources of continuing education. Intensivists then had to convince colleagues that patients can be seriously ill both within an ICU and in the general wards of a hospital. In fact, the level of illness and mortality rates of patients subject to MET calls is much the same as patients in the ICU [6].

Rapid response systems have now been introduced in one form or another in the majority of hospitals in Australasia, North America, and the United Kingdom [2]. They are also being introduced in many European, Asian, and South American hospitals [2]. Moreover, there continues to be active research around the world in RRSs (Figure 21.2).

The core aim of intensive care is to manage seriously ill patients. Both ICUs and RRSs are systems designed around the needs of patients. Both have limited evidence that they achieve their goals. Both interventions are based on the intuitively appealing premise that it

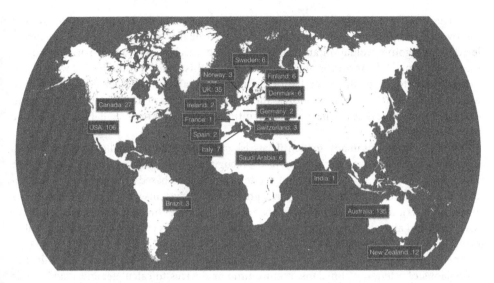

**Figure 21.2** The world of RRS research.

is necessary to provide timely care to the seriously ill using staff who have appropriate skills, knowledge, and experience.

In the largest meta-analysis, paediatric hospitals with a RRS have reduced their mortality and death rates by about one-third [7]. Approximately the same reduction is seen in cardiac arrest and death rates in adult hospitals [7–9].

While this is an achievement, the failure to recognise the seriously ill on the general floors in acute hospitals remains the most common cause of potentially preventable mortality [4]. Patients rarely suffer unexpected deaths or cardiac arrests in monitored environments such as operating rooms or ICUs [2]. We then have to ask ourselves why most of the unexpected deaths and serious adverse events occur in the general wards of hospitals. Part of the reason is the population of hospitalised patients is now more prone to serious illness and deterioration on the general floors of hospitals. Despite this, they are monitored in much the same way as they have been for over 100 years [10]. Interestingly, there has been little research on how patients are monitored on the general wards, despite it being the most commonly performed intervention in acute hospitals. There are few, if any, evidence-based guidelines on issues such as the ideal intervals for measurement; the variability of measurement for different patients; and what actions and outcomes were associated with abnormal values. In one of the few studies in the area there was marked variation in the accuracy and frequency with which vital signs are documented [11].

In the largest study conducted on the effectiveness of RRSs, over 50% of patients who died, had a cardiac arrest, or were admitted to an ICU had no vital signs measured within eight hours of the event [12].

Thus, even if the most appropriate clinician, with the most appropriate skills, could be urgently summoned to a deteriorating patient, the weak link, and the difference between patients in ICUs and the general floors, is that they are not continuously and accurately monitored. If patients on the general floors are becoming more at risk, then monitoring vital signs irregularly and inaccurately is probably not acceptable. Great variations in the clinical state can occur within the eight hours between vital sign recording. It is not surprising, therefore, that early attempts are being made to improve the monitoring of patients on general floors.

Intensive care physicians will no doubt be closely involved in the research and in ways to improve the recognition of deteriorating patients. While it is early days, some of the newer devices undergoing evaluation are patient-worn and wireless, with multi-parameter real-time monitoring [13]. As the systems become more sophisticated it could be that we move to universal monitoring on the general wards, where the signals become algorithms for different degrees of alert. This may help to address the current weakness of RRSs, in that while urgent and appropriate expertise can be provided, it ultimately depends on irregular and inaccurate manual monitoring.

As well as variations in how to identify at-risk patients on the general floors, there are also many variations in the way at-risk patients are recognised and a response triggered. They can be divided into either single abnormality systems or triggers based on a score [2]. Both systems rely on similar abnormalities in vital signs. However, systems which use a single serious abnormality as a trigger for urgent assistance also include life-threatening observations such as seizures and airway obstruction. Moreover, scoring systems can be inaccurate, as well as introducing significant intra- and inter-rater reliability errors [2].

The major concern with using scores for triggers is that they ignore the skills and impressions of attending clinicians, require time or devices to calculate, and may impede an experienced clinician escalating the care of a patient who 'just does not look right'. Score-based systems may not allow for this 'concern' factor when attempting to identify seriously ill patients [2].

No monitoring system, regardless of its level of sophistication, can ever change clinical outcomes unless coupled with appropriate therapeutic interventions. All RRSs attempt to urgently provide a clinician with appropriate skills, knowledge, and experience at any time of the day. This is why many systems employ staff from the ICU. There are many minor variations on the way RRSs are implemented, including more involvement by the admitting team with a two tiered system [2]. Outreach systems provide specialised nursing staff to educate staff on general floors and act as a consultant for patients who may deteriorate [14].

## Other intensive care initiatives operating outside ICUs

### High dependency units

Another intervention to make hospitalised patients safer and to reduce the gap between the care given in ICUs and the general floors is the development of high dependency units (HDUs) [15]. They take many different forms, sometimes staffed by fully trained intensivists and other times by specialists, such as in respiratory medicine, general medicine, or surgery. There is probably greater nursing expertise and a higher nurse:patient ratio in HDUs. Despite the widespread implementation of HDUs, there are few robust data on their overall performance and cost-effectiveness.

### End of life

Intensivists have become increasingly involved with the appropriate management of patients at the end of life (EOL). Many of the patients in the ICU have been admitted by well-meaning colleagues who are programmed to provide active management in the hope that patients will be 'cured' [16]. The difficult discussions about how to explain to patients and their carers are then left to intensivists.

Similarly, with rapid response calls, over one-third of all calls are for matters related to EOL care [17]. This highlights a matter of great importance for healthcare generally. Specialist doctors in acute hospitals often do not recognise patients at the EOL and it is only when the patient is extremely ill and the subject of a rapid response call that further active management may be seen as being futile.

The management of patients at the EOL is a core business of the specialty of intensive care medicine [17]. Over 90% of all deaths in the ICU are as a result of actively withdrawing and withholding treatment.

Whether it is an ideal situation or not, intensivists have become important when diagnosing patients at the EoL. While many of us are not comfortable with this role, it may be related to the way modern medicine has developed. Up until the 1950s, the diagnosis of dying was usually made by the family practitioner. As technology developed, acute hospitals acquired diagnostic and therapeutic interventions that meant seriously ill patients were admitted to acute hospitals under specialist physicians and surgeons. They became the ones who diagnosed dying when further treatment was deemed to be futile.

As the specialty of intensive care developed, our specialist colleagues would often refer patients to the ICU when they had exhausted other options. Thus, the intensivist was increasingly the person who would make the decision that further treatment would be futile. Thus the diagnosis of dying has gradually become an important role for intensivists, not only within the ICU but also as a critical role for patients subject to a rapid response call. An RRS has, in many cases, performed a surrogate EOL function [18]. While not necessarily anticipated or planned that way, it is important that intensivists be involved in improving the way patients are managed at the EOL and that dying becomes a major quality issue for hospitalised patients. Intensivists are increasingly becoming the gatekeepers for admissions to ICU. This can put great pressure on them as both the community and our medical colleagues often have unrealistic expectations of what modern medicine can deliver. In the face of uncertainty it is therefore common that intensivists succumb to that pressure and, as a result, there are increasing numbers of frail, elderly patients where continued treatment is often futile. Intensivists will probably be increasingly involved in this delicate issue outside the ICU as part of RRSs or ward consultations.

## Post-ICU discharge

Intensivists are also becoming increasingly aware of the impact that admission to an ICU has on patients when they are discharged from the ICU. They are becoming more involved in clinical follow-up and research in this area.

There is an increasing incidence of critical illness poly-neuropathy (CIP) and/or myopathy (CIM) in seriously ill patients with multi-organ failure [19]. Many of these patients after discharge from the ICU are severely de-conditioned and debilitated and remain so, even many years after hospital discharge [20].

Other problems that are encountered after hospital discharge can be roughly divided into physical issues, such as organ dysfunction and negative impact on activities of daily life; and non-physical issues such as mental and emotional problems and quality of life [19]. Symptoms include anxiety and depression, which can manifest in many ways from insomnia to severe post-traumatic stress disorders (PTSD). Cognitive dysfunction can occur, especially in the short term after hospital discharge, but tends to improve over time.

We are just beginning to learn about the long-term impact on patients after an ICU admission. Intensivists in some units are establishing follow-up clinics as well as ways of explaining to patients and their carers that following discharge from the ICU and hospital, they may have long-term physical and non-physical impairment [20]. It will become increasingly important for intensivists to become familiar with their own follow-up data in order to educate and prepare patients and their carers for the issues that many may face in the post-hospital period.

Perhaps if we knew more about the post-ICU state of our patients we could share that information with our community, to be used in their decision-making about whether they indeed wanted to embark on such complex interventions.

## Other involvement outside the ICU

Intensivists are involved in many other activities outside the four walls of intensive care, including research and teaching. They also play important roles in professional organisations and the publication of journals and books.

They may be involved in healthcare administration at many levels. This is not surprising as hospitalisation is the largest component of healthcare costs and the majority of this expenditure is in the last year of life. Critical care contributes considerably to these costs. Patients do not necessarily want to spend the last few days or weeks of their lives in an ICU. Moreover, there is a general impression in society that the daily reported medical miracles in all forms of media mean that even the most parlous clinical conditions can be addressed and reversed.

Individual intensivists and the profession of intensive care collectively have a duty to begin a dialogue with our society explaining that while the specialty of intensive care has contributed greatly to the prolongation of life, ageing and dying are natural processes and medical miracles cannot postpone them indefinitely. This is probably the most important challenge for intensivists outside the four walls of our ICUs.

## References

1. H.C.A. Lassen. A preliminary report on the 1952 epidemic of poliomyelitis in Copenhagen: with special reference to the treatment of acute respiratory insufficiency. *Lancet* 1953; 1(6749): 37–41.

2. K. Hillman, D. Jones, J. Chen. Rapid response systems. *Med J Aust* 2014; 201: 519–521.

3. D.R. Goldhil, A. Sumner. Outcome of intensive care patients in a group of British intensive care units. *Crit Care Med* 1998; 26: 1337–1343.

4. L.J. Donaldson, S. S. Panesar, A. Darzi. Patient-safety-related hospital deaths in England: thematic analysis of incidents reported to a national database, 2010–2012. *PLoS Med* 2014; 11: e10016667.

5. A. Lee, G. Bishop, K. M. Hillman, K. Daffurn. The medical emergency team. *Anaesth Intensive Care* 1995; 23: 183–186.

6. M. Buist, S. Bernard, T. V. Nguyen, et al. Association between clinically abnormal observations and subsequent in-hospital mortality: a prospective study. *Resuscitation* 2004; 62: 137–141.

7. P.S. Chan, R. Jain, B.K. Nallmothu, R.A. Berg, C. Sasson. Rapid response teams: a systematic review and meta-analysis. *Arch Intern Med* 2010; 170: 18–26.

8. J. Chen, R. Bellomo, A. Flabouris, et al. The relationship between early emergency team calls and serious adverse events. *Crit Care Med* 2009; 37: 148–153.

9. J. Chen, L. Ou, K.M. Hillman, et al. Cardiopulmonary arrest and mortality trends and their association with rapid response system expansion. *Med J Aust* 2014; 201: 167–170.

10. R. Bellomo, K. Hillman, A. Flabouris, et al. Triggers for emergency team activation: a multicenter assessment. *J Crit Care* 2010; 25: e1–7.

11. J. Chen, K. Hillman, Bellomo, et al. The impact of introducing medical emergency team system on the documentation of vital signs. *Resuscitation* 2009; 80: 35–43.

12. K. Hillman, J. Chen, M. Cretikos, et al. Introduction of the medical emergency team (MET) system: a cluster-randomised controlled trial. *Lancet* 2005; 365: 2091–2097.

13. P. Pawar P.V. Jones, B.-J.F. van Beijnum, H. Hermens. A framework for the comparison of mobile patient monitoring systems. *J Biomed Inform* 2012 45: 544–556.

14. L. Esmonde, A. McDonnell, C. Ball, *et al.* Investigating the effectiveness of critical care outreach services: a systematic review. *Intensive Care Med* 2006; 32: 1713–1721.

15. D.R. Gerber. Structural models for intermediate care areas: one size does not fit all. *Crit Care Med* 1999; 27: 2321–2322.

16. D.C. Angus, A.E. Barnato, W.T. Linde-Zwirble, *et al.* Use of intensive care at the end of life in the United States: an epidemiologic study. *Crit Care Med* 2004; 32: 638–643.

17. D. Jones, S.M. Bagshaw, J. Barrett, *et al.* The role of the medical emergency team in end-of-life care: a multicentre prospective observational study. *Crit Care Med* 2012; 40: 98–103.

18. M.J.A. Parr, J.H. Hadfield, A. Flabouris, G. Bishop, K. Hillman. The Medical Emergency Team: 12 month analysis of reasons for activation, immediate outcome and not-for-resuscitation orders. *Resuscitation* 2001; 50: 39–44.

19. H. Flaatten. Mental and physical disorders after ICU discharge. *Curr Opin Crit Care* 2010; 16: 510–551.

20. M.S. Herridge, J. Batt, C. Dos Santos. ICU-acquired weakness, morbidity and death. *Am J Resp Crit Care* 2014; 190 360–361.

| Chapter **22** | # Patient and family satisfaction |
| --- | --- |

Ruth Endacott

## Context
### Why is it important?
Satisfaction with healthcare has become an important marker of quality and is increasingly likely to be linked to funding [1]. In the UK, satisfaction has been subsumed to a certain extent by loyalty, with patients and visitors asked 'would you recommend us to your family and friends?'. While ICU patients and family members in most countries have little choice about where they receive care during a period of critical illness, the importance of patient and family satisfaction as quality markers has increased.

### Satisfaction and needs
Satisfaction is described as multidimensional and an abstract concept, but is helpfully defined by Rothen *et al.* as: 'the amount of fulfilment of perceived or real, implicit or explicit needs and expectations of an individual or a group of persons' [2, p624]. Hence, at a simplistic level, satisfaction and needs can be viewed as two sides of the same coin: when perceived needs are met, satisfaction is likely to be higher [2]. However, Heyland and colleagues [3] caution that this over-simplifies the relationship: unmet needs do not necessarily result in dissatisfaction, or vice versa. While patient and family satisfaction with care in ICU has come to prominence over the past 15 years, family needs have been the subject of research studies for almost four decades [4]. The most commonly used instrument – the Critical Care Family Needs Inventory (CCFNI) – has 30 statements grouped into five domains (information, proximity, assurance, support, and comfort) and respondents rate (1) the importance of each need statement and (2) the extent to which it has been met [4]. The most commonly used family satisfaction instrument [2] is the Family Satisfaction-ICU (FS-ICU). The FS-ICU has two subscales: satisfaction with care and satisfaction with decision-making. Many of the FS-ICU items are similar to the CCFNI statements but FS-ICU requires the family member to rate satisfaction with care provided to the patient, rather than simply unmet family member needs.

Not surprisingly, greater attention has been paid to family satisfaction in the field of paediatric intensive care, with a number of surveys exploring parents' satisfaction with care [5].

---

*Quality Management in Intensive Care*, ed. Bertrand Guidet, Andreas Valentin and Hans Flaatten. Published by Cambridge University Press. © Cambridge University Press 2016.

While paediatric ICU satisfaction instruments are not addressed in this chapter, reviews in paediatric and adult ICU reveal similar domains used in satisfaction questionnaires [5,2]:

- clinical care
- information, communication, and decision-making
- hospital infrastructure.

## Factors linked to satisfaction

Communication with clinicians is the most common cause of dissatisfaction [6] and the information needs of family members are a common focus in research studies. However, findings can be distinctly different: a recent review [7] revealed that information needs were the most frequently *unmet* need in studies conducted in Belgium and Jordan, and the most frequently *met* need in studies conducted in China and the United States.

A systematic review of studies exploring family satisfaction with end-of-life care in the ICU found that a number of characteristics, such as good-quality communication, were associated with high satisfaction, but few interventions actually increased satisfaction [8]. Authors of a systematic review of randomised controlled trials designed to test communication interventions in ICUs reported that 12 of the 21 included studies used family and/or patient satisfaction as an outcome measure [9]. Ten of these studies reported negative or neutral impact on satisfaction; however, several studies had low response rates. The authors suggest that satisfaction alone is not a sufficient measure of intensive care outcome.

Studies have identified a number of patient characteristics linked with higher family satisfaction in ICU, including higher severity of illness [10] and the need for mechanical ventilation [11], with family of non-survivors also more likely to report higher satisfaction scores [12], although another study did not identify survivorship as a predictor for satisfaction [13]. These indicators significantly associated with higher family satisfaction indicate that the amount of physician and nurse time that the patient and family receive might be important, although this has not been explored in empirical work. One study measuring satisfaction across four units in one hospital reported high but significantly different satisfaction levels, not explained by patient characteristics, indicating that ICU-level factors are important.

## Measuring satisfaction

As identified above, satisfaction has been measured largely using quantitative survey instruments, although the psychometric properties of instruments vary considerably. Some researchers have used instruments with no evidence of validity [14,15].

The most commonly used family satisfaction instrument [2], the FS-ICU, was developed by the Canadian researchers at End of Life Network (CARENET) [3,12], has gained international acceptance, and is used in countries such as Germany [13], Switzerland [10], the Netherlands [16], the USA [11], and the United Kingdom [20]. It has been translated into ten languages (www.thecarenet.ca).

The FS-ICU originally contained 34 items, and has been reduced to a 24-item instrument, a common feature in scale development. Items were removed during development of the smaller FS-ICU-24 version primarily because they threatened scale integrity. Hence the authors recommend use of FS-ICU-24 for research studies but, as some of the 'dropped' items may be useful for quality improvement, the full set of items (FS-ICU-34) remains on the website (see full explanation at http://thecarenet.ca/docs/fss/FS_Reduction.pdf).

The FS-ICU includes three free-text questions, although few published studies report these findings. Schwarzkopf and colleagues [13] report integrated qualitative and quantitative findings from their use of FS-ICU with 215 family members of patients admitted to four ICUs in a single centre. One hundred and eleven family members provided qualitative comments; respondents who were highly satisfied were more likely to provide positive comments. The five themes arising from the qualitative analysis were: care; communication; respect and compassion shown to family; family participation; and ICU environment.

A team in Australia measured family satisfaction using a locally developed ten-item questionnaire incorporating visual analogue scales ($n = 84$ family members) [15]. Overall family satisfaction was high, with highest scores recorded for communication with nursing staff, while lowest scores were for frequency of doctors' communication. There was no difference in the reported satisfaction of families of patients who died compared to those who survived, but the study may be underpowered to detect such a difference. Sample size was calculated based on a ratio of 70:30 non-survivors:survivors whereas the sample was not recruited to maintain this ratio and comprised 15:85 ($n = 13$ non-survivors). Families were more likely to report satisfaction with care if there was a documented meeting with medical staff or social worker in the case notes (relative risk 0.14; confidence interval 0.03–0.59; $p = 0.08$; relative risk 0.23; confidence interval 0.07–0.81; $p = 0.02$). No validity or reliability testing is reported by the authors, and respondents who completed the survey over the phone gave poorer scores than those who completed the mailed version.

Boev [14] used a previously unpublished 26-item patient satisfaction instrument to measure relationship between patient satisfaction and nurses' work environment. While the study results reveal a significant association between patient satisfaction and nurses' perceptions of nurse leadership, the study had a number of limitations: (1) no evidence of validity testing was provided for the patient satisfaction survey; (2) the patient or family member completed the survey, with no distinction between responses; (3) the study design relied on secondary data analysis.

## Patient or family satisfaction?

### Which do we use?

Intensive care patients commonly have a compromised mental state due to injury, delirium, or sedation. In the absence of the patient voice, it has been common practice to measure family needs and family satisfaction as a form of proxy. As with any proxy measure, the main challenge is the extent to which these are legitimate proxies, with evidence that caregivers or relatives may overestimate a patient's anxiety or distress.

The FS-ICU has been adapted by research teams in the Netherlands [16] and Switzerland [17] to capture patient satisfaction. It is not clear what items were included in the version by Stricker and colleagues [17], hence comparison between the two studies is not feasible. Results from this study, conducted in Switzerland with family members ($n=996$) and patients ($n = 235$) [17], revealed no significant differences between paired next of kin and patient satisfaction ratings. Agreement was highest (measured using Cohen's kappa) when the proxy was the spouse or partner, rather than a non-partner/spouse family member. Of note, patients were least satisfied with the management of agitation and restlessness, highlighting the importance of attempting to capture patient satisfaction prospectively to inform day-to-day management of the patient in ICU. The study conducted in the Netherlands [16] was conducted primarily to examine the effect of ICU environment on patients' ($n = 274$) and families' ($n = 323$) satisfaction, using a pre–post design, and the researchers did not intend to

**Table 22.1** Timing of satisfaction survey data collection

| Authors and country | Instrument and sample | Survey distribution |
|---|---|---|
| Stricker et al. [17] Switzerland | FS-ICU (n = 996)<br>Patient Satisfaction (n = 235) | 2 days after patient admission to ICU<br>At ward round on day of ICU discharge |
| Jongerdan et al. [16] Netherlands | FS-ICU (n = 323)<br>PS-ICU (n = 274) | 10 weeks after ICU discharge<br>10 weeks after ICU discharge |
| Osborn et al. [18] United States | FS-ICU & QODD-1 (n = 1290) | 4–6 weeks after patient's death |
| Sundararajan et al. [15] Australia | Unvalidated Family Satisfaction (n = 84) | 4–6 weeks after ICU discharge |
| Hunziker et al. [11] United States | FS-ICU (n = 449) | 3 days after ICU discharge; 7 weeks after death for non-survivors |
| Schwarzkopf et al. [13] Germany | FS-ICU (n = 215) | During ICU stay |
| Boev [14] | Unvalidated Patient Satisfaction (n = 1532) | Not stated |
| Heyland et al. [3] Canada | FS-ICU (n = 624) | At ICU discharge; 3–4 weeks after death for non-survivors |

match family and patient satisfaction. Mean satisfaction scores for both phases were higher for family members than for patients (69.5 [SD 16.6] vs 63.6 [SD 18.3] pre and 74.1 [SD 15.2] vs 69.6 [SD 18.3] post), indicating the importance of capturing the patient's ICU experience. The increasing emphasis on patient-reported outcome measures and changes in the sedative regimen suggest that more efforts should be made to capture patient satisfaction.

## When to measure

Regardless of the instrument used to measure satisfaction, the timing of data collection is variable, making comparison across studies of limited value (see Table 22.1). Few authors provided a rationale for the timing of survey distribution. By contrast, Stricker and colleagues [17] administered the FS-ICU to family members two days after the patient was admitted to ICU and the PS-ICU to the patient at the ward round on the day of ICU discharge. This approach was taken to minimise the likelihood that patients and family members would collude.

## Can we influence satisfaction?

Communication is a common cause of dissatisfaction. In the single-centre, four-ICU study undertaken by Schwarzkopf and colleagues [13], 'clarity and completeness of information' and 'compassion towards families' were identified as areas for improvement. In the single-centre, nine-ICU study undertaken by Hunziker and colleagues [11], incomplete information was strongly associated with low satisfaction [OR: 4.4 95% CI: 2.4–8.1] and disagreement within the family about care on admission is a predictor for lower satisfaction with the ICU. Stricker and colleagues [10] found that understandable, clear, complete information had a high impact on satisfaction, but families overall had low satisfaction with information they were given.

As highlighted previously, communication interventions intended to improve family satisfaction had a neutral or negative impact in 10 out of 12 studies [9]. One of the successful trials conducted by Azoulay and colleagues achieved significant improvements in patient satisfaction and comprehension of information following introduction of a family information leaflet [6]. Dhillon and colleagues [19] report some promising outcomes from a small study reporting a proactive approach to communication with family members ($n = 139$). They instigated a 'bundled' informed consent using an early family meeting to provide an explanation of common ICU interventions and procedures. They measured FS-ICU using a pre–post, control–intervention design and found that family satisfaction was higher in the intervention group ($95.4 \pm 4$ vs $78.2 \pm 22$; $p < 0.001$) [19]. A similar approach was taken by Higginson and colleagues [20], who developed and implemented the Psychological Assessment and Communication Evaluation (PACE) to improve communication in ICUs. They reported significantly higher satisfaction with symptom control and the honesty and consistency of information from staff for family members of patients who received the PACE [20].

The level of caring and emotional support reported by family members is also linked with satisfaction. Hunziker and colleagues found dissatisfaction with concern and caring by ICU staff was strongly associated with low overall satisfaction [OR: 5.0 95% CI: 1.9–12.6] [11]. Stricker and colleagues also found that emotional support had a high impact on family satisfaction but families reported overall low satisfaction [10].

Several studies have established links between nurses' work environment, burn-out, and job satisfaction [see 14]. Boev [14] explored the relationship between patient satisfaction and nurses' perception of the working environment in four adult ICUs over a five-year period ($n = 1532$ patients). Patients' overall satisfaction was high but with significant differences between ICUs. Multilevel modelling of patient satisfaction revealed a significant association with nurses' perception of nurse leadership (estimate 0.424; CI 0.074–0.775; $p = 0.018$). Regardless of the limitations noted earlier for this study, the findings suggest that the work environment for nurses is likely to be of importance for patient satisfaction.

The impact of physical environment of the ICU on satisfaction (measured using FS-ICU and PS-ICU) was examined in a single-site, pre–post study conducted in the Netherlands [16]. The unit was migrating from an open-plan ward environment to a new setting with single rooms. The researchers found both family members and patients had higher satisfaction scores in the new, single-room ICU. Total family satisfaction scores increased from 69.5 [SD 16.6] to 74.1 [SD 15.2], $p = 0.01$ and total patient satisfaction scores increased from 63.3 [SD18.9] to 69.6 [SD18.3], $p = 0.02$. Scores for the 'satisfaction with decision-making' subscale increased for family members and patients but did not reach significance. As both questionnaires were sent to the family ten weeks after discharge, the extent of collusion between patient and family member was not known.

## Summary

Quantitative measures are useful and provide a picture of some dimensions of satisfaction across a large sample. However, they can only be considered as a key part of a quality improvement approach to ICU care if they are used in conjunction with qualitative measures. These are more challenging to collect but essential if we are to mediate between expectations and experience and capture the sort of data that tells us how it really was for the patient and family. The lack of response to satisfaction surveys, a feature in several studies, indicates that we have some way to go to really capture the patient and family experience. Qualitative data also provide useful feedback, especially important when satisfaction levels are high, which may otherwise lead nurses and physicians to believe that there is little or no room for improvement. The timing of satisfaction data should also be carefully considered. The collection of data some ten weeks after patient discharge [16] runs the risk of becoming an intellectual, or research-driven, exercise rather than an iterative process that informs care for the patient and family in front of you. The key to successful use of satisfaction data is the way in which the outcomes are linked to quality improvement actions.

# References

1. J. Wise. Part of hospitals' funding will depend on patient satisfaction ratings from 2010–11. *BMJ* 2009; 339: b5451.

2. H.U. Rothen, K.H. Stricker, D.K. Heyland. Family satisfaction with critical care: measurements and messages. *Curr Opin Crit Care* 2010; 16: 623–631.

3. D.K. Heyland, G.M. Rocker, P.M. Dodek. Family satisfaction with care in ICU: results of a multi-centre study. *Crit Care Med* 2002; 30: 1413–1418.

4. N.C. Molter. Needs of relatives of critically ill patients: a descriptive study. *Heart Lung* 1979; 8: 332–339.

5. J.M. Latour, A.J. Hazelzet, A.J. van Heijden. Parent satisfaction in paediatric intensive care: a critical appraisal of the literature. *Pediat Crit Care Med* 2005; 6: 578–584.

6. E. Azoulay, S. Chevret, G. Leleu, *et al.* Half the families of intensive care unit patients experience inadequate communication with physicians. *Crit Care Med* 2000; 28:3044–3049.

7. R. Khalaila. Meeting the needs of patients' families in intensive care units. *Nursing Standard* 2014; 28 (43): 37–44.

8. L.J. Hinkle G.T. Bosslet, A.M. Torke. Factors associated with family satisfaction with end of life care in the ICU: a systematic review. *Chest* 2014; doi:10.1378/chest.14-1098.

9. L.P. Scheunemann, M. McDevitt, S.S. Carson, L.C. Hanson. Randomized, controlled trials of interventions to improve communication in intensive care. *Chest* 2011; 139: 543–554.

10. K.H. Stricker, O. Kimberger, K. Schmidlin, M. Zwahken, U Mohr, H.U Rothen. Family satisfaction in the intensive care unit: what makes the difference? *Intens Care Med* 2009; 35: 2051–2059.

11. S. Hunziker, W. McHugh, B. Sarnoff-Lee, S. *et al.* Predictors and correlates of dissatisfaction with intensive care. *Crit Care Med* 2012; 40:1554–1561.

12. R.J. Wall, J.R. Curtis, C.R. Cooke. Family satisfaction in ICU: differences between families of survivors and nonsurvivors. *Chest* 2007; 132:1425–1433.

13. D. Schwarzkopf, S. Behrend, H. Skupkin *et al.* Family satisfaction in the intensive care unit: a quantitative and qualitative analysis. *Intensive Care Med.* 2013; 39: 1671–1679.

14. C. Boev. The relationship between nurses' perception of work environment and patient satisfaction in adult critical care. *J Nurs Sch* 2012; 44: 368–375.

15. K. Sundararajan, T.S. Sullivan, M. Chapman. Determinants of family satisfaction in the intensive care unit. *Anaesth Intensive Care* 2012; 40: 159–165.

16. I.P. Jongerdan, A.J. Slooter, L.M. Peelen, *et al.* Effect of intensive care environment on family and patient satisfaction: a before–after study. *Intens Care Med* 2013; 39: 1626–1634.

17. K.H. Stricker, O. Kimberger, L. Brunner, H.U. Rothen. Patient satisfaction with care in the intensive care unit: can we rely on proxies? *Acta Anaesthesiol Scand* 2011; 55:149–156.

18. T.R. Osborn, J.R. Curtis, E.L. Neilsen A.L. Back, S.E. Shannon, R.A. Engleberg. Identifying elements of ICU care that families report as important but unsatisfactory: decision-making, control and ICU atmosphere. *Chest* 2012; 142: 1185–1192.

19. A. Dhillon, F. Tardini, E. Bittner, U. Schmidt, R. Allain, L. Bigatello. Benefit of using a 'bundled' consent for intensive care unit procedures as part of an early family meeting. *J Crit Care* 2014; 29: 919–922.

20. I.J. Higginson, J. Koffman, P. Hopkins, *et al.* Development and evaluation of the feasibility and effects on staff, patients, and families of a new tool, the Psychosocial Assessment and Communication Evaluation (PACE), to improve communication and palliative care in intensive care and during clinical uncertainty. *BMC Medicine* 2013; 11: 213.

# Chapter 23

# Follow-up after intensive care

Folke Sjöberg and Lotti Orvelius

## Introduction

Almost 50 years ago Donabedian suggested evaluating quality of care on the basis of three different components: structure, process, and outcome. Structure indicators are related to rather fixed resources (e.g., number of rooms and number of ventilators, and also such factors as staffing). Process indicators refer to the activities related to treatment and care (e.g., time to first antibiotic and prevention bundles, such as raising the head, reduce the use of gastric ant- acid treatment and decontaminating the oral cavity to reduce the risk of ventilatory induced pneumonia (VAP)). Outcome is defined as changes in the state of health of a patient that can be attributed to an intervention or to the absence of an intervention, e.g., ICU or hospital mortality or patient reported outcome measures (PROM) such as health-related quality of life (HRQoL). It may also be based on patient-reported experience measures (PREM), as has been increasingly addressed recently. Measuring outcome after critical illness is important for many reasons, particularly mortality has historically been used as a sturdy measure of the effectiveness of the intensive care treatment [1]. ICU outcome has often been investigated and been of interest as such care is highly costly and most often the most resource-demanding process in hospitals.

Outcome measures after critical illness can be viewed from at least three separate perspec- tives: that of the patients and relatives; the clinical staff; and the managers of the healthcare system [2]. Very important in this aspect is, of course, the patient's perspective as the con- sumer of healthcare, and in this chapter we will focus particularly on this perspective. There are many patient-related outcome measures that have been used in the medical setting, and up till recently mortality has been mostly commonly used as mortality is easily assessed and has also been one of the major goals of the critical care process. However, in recent times mor- tality rates have been decreasing and not uncommonly today constitutes a problem for only a minority of the patients, as fewer will face such a risk. The decreasing mortality rate has led to the need for other outcome measures and also increasing interest has further been directed toward the patient perspective, such as HRQoL, and also including important long-term effects depicting, e.g., functional ability/disability, cognitive function, and return to work, which in themselves are important for the HRQoL experience.

Many factors will affect the long-term HRQoL outcome after critical care; this includes, not least, factors from before ICU care, such as socioeconomic status and pre-existing

*Quality Management in Intensive Care*, ed. Bertrand Guidet, Andreas Valentin and Hans Flaatten. Published by Cambridge University Press. © Cambridge University Press 2016.

diseases, as well as ICU-related factors (admission diagnoses; APACHE IV score, length of ventilator or ICU stay, and organ failure), and possible new diseases that have been brought about during the ICU care (i.e., critical illness due to a complication, etc.). All of these may for obvious reasons affect the HRQoL outcome from many perspectives after both ICU and hospital discharge. Interest in outcome measures after critical care has during the last decade been increasingly directed toward also examining patient subjective measures of function for general ICU patients, as well as for specific diagnoses groups (Table 23.1) [2–7].

The incidences of post-traumatic stress disorder (PTSD), anxiety, and depression in ICU survivors are high, but it is unclear what influences emotional outcome. One suggestion is that delirium related to memories could be important, but results are conflicting [2].

In addition, delirium has also been found to be related to long-term cognitive problems [3], and acute psychological reactions during ICU care have been found to be strong risk factors for developing mental illness in the long term following critical illness [4]. Both physical and psychological limitations are common, but vary due to the underlying diagnoses in an often heterogeneous ICU population. A recurring and important factor during ICU care which has been found important for a reduced long-term HRQoL outcome after ICU care has been a pre- or peri-ICU care-related respiratory impairment or failure [5,6].

Further, sexual dysfunction was common 3–8 years after the acute illness in a group of critically ill patients after trauma; it was also associated with a high rate of depression [7].

**Table 23.1** Morbidity after critical care

| Author, (pub. year) | No. of patients | ICU designation | Factor | Follow-up period | Mean age (years) | Instruments used for measurement |
|---|---|---|---|---|---|---|
| Ulvik et al. 2008 [7] | 156 | Trauma | Sexual function | 3–8 years | 46 | British instrument |
| Nouwen et al. 2012 [2] | Review | General | Delirium Memories PTSD Anxiety | ICU stay–5 years | NA | CAM-ICU, ICU-MT PTSS-10, PTSS-14, PDS, HADS, IES-R |
| Van den Boogaard et al. 2012 [3] | 915 | General | Delirium | 18 months | 65 | CAM-ICU |
| Dowdy et al. 2009 [5] | 160 | ALI | Depression | 6 months | 49 | HADS |
| Wade et al. 2012 [4] | 100 | General | Psychological morbidity | 3 months | 57 | Profile of Mood States, ICUSS, BIPQ |
| Herridge et al. 2011 [6] | 64 | ARDS | Functional disability | 3 months–5 years | 44 | Interview, physical examination |

ALI: acute lung injury; ARDS: acute respiratory distress syndrome; BIPQ: brief illness perception questionnaire; CAM-ICU: confusion assessment method – intensive care unit; HADS: hospital anxiety and depression scale; ICU: intensive care unit; ICU-MT: intensive care unit-memory tool; ICUSS: intensive care stress reaction scale; IES-R: impact of events score (revised); NA: not available; PDS: post-traumatic diagnostic scale; PTSD: post-traumatic stress disorder; PTSS-10 and PTSS-14: post-traumatic stress scale version 10 and 14.

# Patient reported outcomes in the Swedish National Quality Registries

Patient-reported outcome measures are important in the healthcare system and can, together with professional/clinical data, provide important information on the patient's condition based on the patient's perception of health and functioning – i.e., the effects of the treatment. In the Swedish healthcare system, 93 of the 108 National Quality Registries include some form of PROM or PREM. The registries are increasingly using the patient-reported data as a basis for quality improvement work such as shared decision-making in clinical encounters, a basis for care plans, clinical decision-aids, and treatment guidelines, to improve the precision of indications for surgery, to monitor complications after the patient has left the hospital, and to improve patient information. One of those registries is the Swedish Intensive Care Registry (SIR). It is a quality registry for all intensive care units (general, burns, thoracic, neurosurgery, and pediatric) in Sweden. The registry uses PROM data to identify risk groups as well as for decision-making in clinical encounters to examine whether improvement of medical treatment and care is indicated, before, during and/or after the intensive care period [8]. In addition, the registry also uses PROM data at an individual level during the follow-up visit for shared decision-making, together with the patient and next of kin. In a European perspective, however, the use of PROM in quality registries unfortunately has not attained the same level of interest.

## Health-related quality of life

Health-related quality of life can be defined as the level of well-being and satisfaction associated with a person's life and how it is affected by disease, accident, and treatment [1]. The most important aspects of HRQoL are physical and mental health, social function, role function, and general well-being, because the goal of healthcare is to maximize the health component of quality of life [9]. For survivors of intensive care the most important outcome variable for assessing the effectiveness of the intensive care treatment has been claimed to be HRQoL [10]. It is well known that HRQoL is reduced up to two years after intensive care compared with that in the general population adjusted for age and sex [11]. However, it is not known how much of this decrease is already present in the period before the intensive care. Present data do not support a large HRQoL effect of intensive care-related factors such as length of stay in the ICU or hospital or time on the ventilator. It is also uncertain when the pre-ICU HRQoL level is reached, although most of the published data suggest that pre-ICU levels seem to be reached approximately at one year after the ICU period.

## Scoring systems for health-related quality in healthcare

Patient-reported outcome measures are often divided into two main types – disease-specific or generic. A disease-specific instrument is adapted for special groups and examines dimensions specific for an illness or treatment for a single disease group of patients or area of function (www.proqolid.org). Generic instruments include health profiles and instruments that generate health utilities that can be applied to any patient groups and is not related to a specific disease. Today, two of the globally most commonly used generic measures of health-related quality of life are the EQ-5D [12] and the SF-36/RAND-36 [13].

EQ-5D was originally intended to be used in health economic evaluations and should therefore essentially be used for that, or in combination with a disease-specific or general instrument. HRQoL questionnaires, such as the SF-36, are made up of a number of items or questions. These items are added up in a number of domains or dimensions. A domain or dimension refers to the area of behavior or experience that the investigator is trying to measure. For some instruments the evaluation exercises are of importance for each item rate in relation to the others. For other instruments items are equally weighted, which assumes that their value is equal. The HRQoL questionnaires can be administered by trained interviewers, self-administered, by computer, or be web-based.

As the intensive care population are heterogeneous, generic instruments are recommended [10] as they are of relevance for all kinds of diseases and health states, can facilitate comparisons across patient groups and populations, as well as comparisons across ICU patients and non-ICU patients.

## Challenges when assessing HRQoL in former intensive care patients

As there is a natural lack of data for HRQoL patient data from the period before the intensive care period, several investigators have tried to ask the patients to report the HRQoL that they experienced before their time in the ICU. This is likely to lead to "recall bias." Retrospective assessment of HRQoL is always influenced by the critical illness and the pre-morbid HRQoL is claimed to be experienced falsely high in that a present poor status may lead to an overrating of the pre-ICU HRQoL [14]. Other investigators, therefore, instead have asked the next of kin to report the patient's HRQoL before the patient was admitted to the ICU. This approach is also beset with methodological difficulties. Relatives are claimed to overestimate the patient's physical dysfunction and at the same time to underestimate the mental limitations relative to the measures presented by patients themselves [15]. From a philosophical point of view, HRQoL is a unique personal perception and therefore the best description of the HRQoL most certainly will have to come from the patient him/herself. Given that it is not possible to assess properly the HRQoL of patients before their stay in the ICU, the approach can be to choose a control group and adjust for differences in age, sex, and comorbidity, and to measure HRQoL over time on several occasions to get an estimate of the effect of the ICU care.

## Factors of importance for HRQoL after intensive care

A considerable number of ICU outcome studies have explored potential determinants for the low HRQoL levels often depicted in former ICU patients, but such predictors of HRQoL are inconsistent. One of these determinants has been claimed to be length of stay in the ICU. As lengths of stay in ICUs are decreasing and nowadays in Sweden are often fewer than three days (mean) (www.icuregswe.org), the impact of length of ICU stay on HRQoL is anticipated to be of reduced importance. In a recent systematic review it is concluded that the previous health state, age, severity of disease (APACHE-II), admission diagnostic category (scheduled surgery, trauma, or medical), and in addition anxiety-, depression-, and PTSD-related factors significantly decreases HRQoL [16]. In our own research with a long follow-up period (three years) we have found that factors that have an impact on the HRQoL after ICU care can be divided into:

1. patient-related factors such as age and sex;
2. patient-acquired factors such as previous health state, socioeconomic factors, sleep patterns, mastery, level of hopelessness, and social network;
3. intensive-care-related factors such as diagnosis on admission, severity of illness (APACHE II), time on ventilator, severity of injury (trauma), or organ dysfunction; and
4. factors related to the time period after the critical care, such as new or remaining sleep disturbances or pain (Figure 23.1).

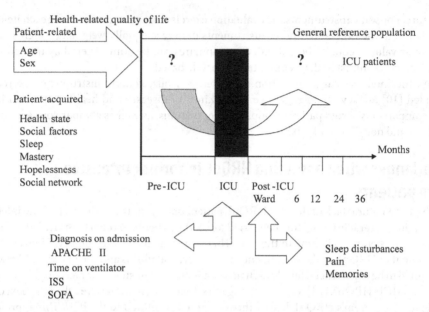

**Figure 23.1** Factors which impact the HRQoL for the ICU patient. HRQoL is reduced up to two years after intensive care compared with that in the general population. It is not known if the decrease is already present in the period before the intensive care, or if it is the result of the circumstances of the intensive care period. It is also unknown when the HRQoL returns to the pre-ICU level. Factors that have been found to have an impact on the HRQoL for the ICU patient are patient related, patient acquired, intensive care related, and factors after the critical care period.

In our model we found that the most important factor for the decrease of HRQoL after intensive care is the level of pre-existing chronic disease [17,18], and approximately 50% of the decrease in self-reported HRQoL can be predicted by this factor. For the remaining decrease the factors of importance are largely unknown, and therefore of special interest for future HRQoL investigations.

## HRQoL changes over time after ICU care

Although we cannot yet describe all factors of importance for HRQoL after intensive care, we do know that improvements in HRQoL after ICU care occur over time. The level of HRQoL are particularly decreased at two months after ICU discharge compared with age-, sex-, and comorbidity-adjusted reference groups, and a clear recovery is seen at six months post-ICU; this seems to level off at the 12-month assessment after ICU care. On a group level no further improvements over time seem to occur [17].

## Physical and psychological recovery

Due to different study designs, patient populations, HRQoL instruments, follow-up times, and response rates, results differ in HRQoL follow-up studies after intensive care. Review articles conclude that mainly the physical dimensions improve over time [16]. For the mental health outcome, acute psychological reactions in the ICU were the strongest risk factor for developing mental illness after intensive care [4]. When adjusting for age, sex, and co-existing conditions we found in a large multicenter study for general intensive care patients that up to 22% of the patients had decreased levels in the mental dimensions as compared with a general control group [17]. This group was characterized by more often being male, single, on sick leave before admission to ICU, and having a short survival time after discharge from the ICU.

## Future directions

From the data presented and the conclusions drawn, it appears important to separate the risk groups presented above that have a low HRQoL and to do interventions that we think may improve their HRQoL. For these patients, follow-up visits may empower the patient and be of help in the physical and psychological rehabilitation process, which may include contact with a counselor, psychologist, physiotherapist, or an outreach clinic.

A remaining paradox in the data presented is the recurring finding that ICU patients who are healthy before the ICU period, and that do not attain a chronic disease during the ICU period, do not reach the same level on HRQoL as that registered in healthy control groups (age and sex adjusted) [17]. This finding needs to be further explored; one hypothesis is that it may be due to new socioeconomic effects, possibly work-related due to having been critically ill.

# References

1. Nouwen MJ, Klijn FA, van den Broek BT, Slooter AJ. Emotional consequences of intensive care unit delirium and delusional memories after intensive care unit admission: a systematic review. *J Crit Care.* 2012;27(2):199–211.

2. Ridley S. Non-mortality outcome measures. In *Outcomes in Critical Care.* Oxford: Butterworth-Heinemann; 2002, 120–138.

3. van den Boogaard M, Schoonhoven L, Evers AW, van der Hoeven JG, van Achterberg T, Pickkers P. Delirium in critically ill patients: impact on long-term health-related quality of life and cognitive functioning. *Crit Care Med.* 2012;40(1):112–118.

4. Wade DM, Howell DC, Weinman JA, *et al.* Investigating risk factors for psychological morbidity three months after intensive care: a prospective cohort study. *Crit Care.* 2012;16(5):R192.

5. Dowdy DW, Bienvenu OJ, Dinglas VD, *et al.* Are intensive care factors associated with depressive symptoms 6 months after acute lung injury? *Crit Care Med.* 2009;37(5):1702–1707.

6. Herridge MS, Tansey CM, Matte A, *et al.* Functional disability 5 years after acute respiratory distress syndrome. *NEJM.* 2011;364(14):1293–1304.

7. Ulvik A, Kvåle R, Wentzel-larsen T, Flaatten H. Sexual function in ICU survivors more than 3 years after major trauma. *Intensive Care Med.* 2008;34:447–453.

8. Berkius J, Engerstrom L, Orwelius L, *et al.* A prospective longitudinal multicentre study of health related quality of life in ICU survivors with COPD. *Crit Care.* 2013;17(5):R211.

9. Bowling A. *Measuring Health: A Review of Quality of Life Measurement Scales.* third edition. Milton Keynes: Open University Press, 2005.

10. Angus DC, Carlet J. Surviving intensive care: a report from the 2002 Brussels Roundtable. *Intensive Care Med.* 2003;29(3):368–377.

11. Niskanen M, Kari A, Halonen P. Five-year survival after intensive care: comparison of 12,180 patients with the general population. Finnish ICU patients. *Crit Care Med.* 1996;24:1962–1967.

12. The EuroQol Group. EuroQol: a new facility for the measurement of health-related quality of life. *Health Policy.* 1990;16:199–208.

13. Ware J, Snow K, Kosinski M, Gandek B. *SF-36 Health Survey: Manual and Interpretation Guide* Boston, MA: The Health Institute, 1993.

14. Wehler M, Geise A, Hadzionerovic D, *et al.* Health-related quality of life of patients with multiple organ dysfunction: individual changes and comparison with normative population. *Crit Care Med.* 2003;31(4):1094–1101.

15. Scales DC, Tansey CM, Matte A, Herridge MS. Difference in reported pre-morbid health-related quality of life between ARDS survivors and their substitute decision makers. *Intensive Care Med.* 2006;32(11):1826–1831.

16. Granja C, Amaro A, Dias C, Costa-Pereira A. Outcome of ICU survivors: a comprehensive review. The role of patient-reported outcome studies. *Acta Anaesthesiol Scand.* 2012;56(9): 1092–1103.

17. Orwelius L, Nordlund A, Nordlund P, *et al.* Pre-existing disease: the most important factor for health related quality of life long-term after critical illness: a prospective, longitudinal, multicentre trial. *Crit Care.* 2010;14:R67.

18. Orwelius L, Willebrand M, Gerdin B, Ekselius L, Fredrikson M, Sjoberg F. Long term health-related quality of life after burns is strongly dependent on pre-existing disease and psychosocial issues and less due to the burn itself. *Burns.* 2013;39(2):229–235.

# *In situ* small-scale simulation

Pascale Gruber and Rebecca Lea-Smith

Simulation-based training (SBT) has become increasingly popular in the past few years, with many intensive care units (ICUs) embracing this approach to deliver team training. SBT facilitates experiential learning, allowing participants to practise both routine and complex infrequent clinical scenarios in a safe and controlled setting. *In situ* SBT has the advantage that training is delivered to teams which normally work together, within their own clinical domain, while using their own equipment, thus closely replicating the complexities of the typical working environment [1–8]. *In situ* SBT enhances the learning experience for participants by adding context and realism to the scenario. In addition, it may also prove to be a useful tool for quality improvement. Patient safety and clinical care can be improved by identifying organisational weaknesses and inefficiencies during *in situ* simulation. Quality markers and measures of efficiency can be assessed, allowing detection of processes that require change, while facilitating focused training tailored to individuals' and teams' needs. In this chapter we discuss the benefits and challenges of running a small-scale *in situ* SBT programme in the ICU, and describe how SBT can be used to support quality improvement.

## *In situ* simulation in healthcare

There has been rapid expansion in the use of simulation as an educational tool in medicine, nursing, and many other clinical groups. This has been driven by a decrease in opportunity for clinical teaching by the bedside, a need to train in new technologies, and an acknowledgement that poor teamwork and communication often contribute to medical error [9]. Simulation provides a 'hands on' experiential educational opportunity, enabling healthcare professionals to repeatedly practise clinical scenarios in a safe and controlled learning environment [1–8]. Studies have shown that simulation training leads to improved knowledge, skills, and clinical competence [10,11]. Skill retention and quality of care have also been demonstrated to improve when simulation is used in addition to traditional medical teaching [10,11]. Furthermore, Cook *et al.* were able to show notable improvements in patient-related outcomes [12].

SBT has been demonstrated to be particularly effective in enhancing non-technical skills (human factors) such as communication, decision-making, leadership, and situation awareness [13]. Poor communication, teamwork, and leadership have repeatedly been shown to contribute to medical errors in the ICU [9]. Non-technical skills training during SBT has been

*Quality Management in Intensive Care*, ed. Bertrand Guidet, Andreas Valentin and Hans Flaatten. Published by Cambridge University Press. © Cambridge University Press 2016.

shown to help improve patient safety and care [13]. However, SBT goes beyond individual and teamwork competencies. The delivery of high-quality and safe patient care is affected by the wider, complex healthcare system [14]. As reported by the Institute of Medicine document, *To Err is Human*, the majority of medical errors result from failure of systems and processes, not individuals [14]. The clinical environment, work processes, local policies, equipment availability, and staffing levels can all influence patient outcome and unit safety [15]. Incorporating the clinical environment into simulation training allows the team to identify organisational and system-based weaknesses that create barriers to optimal care delivery [1,2,15,16]. Latent system errors or flaws may often be identified during scenarios. Each drill should be viewed as an opportunity to improve patient safety and staff effectiveness, through better preparation and a greater understanding of the processes involved in high-quality care delivery [8].

Several published studies have demonstrated the benefits of *in situ* SBT for unit and organisational level learning [1,2,15,16]. For example, Lighthall *et al.* identified a number of significant events that occurred during cardiac arrest simulations, which could have compromised patient care had they been 'real' cardiac arrests [1]. Walker *et al.* were also able to show a number of latent systems errors (e.g. lack of swipe card access, poorly stocked resuscitation trolley) during their unannounced cardiac arrest simulations [2]. Similarly, Patterson *et al.* employed *in situ* simulation training to identify latent errors and reinforce critical safety competencies [16].

The ICU is a challenging environment, but offers a unique opportunity to run small-scale SBT programmes. The high acuity, high-stakes environment, complexity of illnesses, and multidisciplinary nature of the specialty means that ICU teams rarely have the chance to train together. As a result, error is common. *In situ* SBT enables participants to undertake training in their own clinical environment alongside teams they normally work with, at the place where they usually work, using the equipment that is normally available to them. This means targeted training can be delivered directly to the multidisciplinary team in the ICU while minimising time out from clinical duty. Meurling *et al.* were able to show improved perceptions of teamwork, safety, and working conditions in their ICU after implementation of a small-scale *in situ* SBT programme [5].

Nowadays, *in situ* SBT has expanded beyond just multidisciplinary training within confined units (e.g. ICUs, operating theatres, wards). Recent studies have demonstrated the benefit of full hospital simulation across the whole patient pathway [17]. Such macro-simulations take into account the wider hospital organisation that impact on coordination of patient care. Quality improvement may be delivered at every stage of the patient pathway by integrating the varied training needs of expert clinicians, with testing of 'fitness for purpose' of whole hospitals.

## *In situ* simulation as a quality improvement tool

SBT is a useful adjunct to quality improvement. Quality improvement initiatives permeate throughout modern healthcare, with various approaches described [18]. However, no single tool or approach has clearly been shown to be superior to another. The principles that underpin quality improvement processes remain largely the same. These include the use of performance indicators to identify processes with suboptimal outcomes, undertaking an analysis of information obtained, instituting change, and, finally, reassessing performance to determine if the change was successful [19]. Processes, procedures and care pathways can be evaluated during *in situ* simulation scenarios. Further exploration during debrief may identify areas for individual and team development, with a view to enhancing patient safety, efficiency, and care delivery through education, reflection, behavioural change, and repeated supervised practice.

Change plays a key part in any quality improvement process. Embedding change into clinical practice is often difficult. Studies have repeatedly shown that despite good-quality evidence for certain guidelines, some are better adopted into clinical practice than others [19]. Results suggest that change and adoption into clinical practice are closely associated with factors such as better quality of evidence supporting the recommendation, close compatibility of the recommendation with existing unit values, reduction in the complexity of the decision-making, a concrete description of the desired performance, an understanding of the potential obstacles to change, and staff and organisational support for change (i.e. strong leadership, incentives) [19]. A multimodal approach that targets different groups and is tailored to the specific needs of each group is recommended [19]. SBT facilitates change implementation by demonstrating the desired performance in the real clinical environment, enabling it to be 'tested' prior to roll-out, and encouraging staff engagement and feedback during debrief. For example, *in situ* scenarios can be used to pilot the impact of a change process as part of the Plan–Do–Study–Act (PDSA) cycle. Measures of success or failure can be reviewed during the pilot scenario prior to real-life change implementation.

While it is often difficult to predict the shortfalls of an untested environment, mock scenarios can be a useful way to test the local impact of a change process; this may include new patient pathways, policies, equipment, or working environment. Examples include opening of a new ICU, implementation of an electronic medical record system, or automated drug dispensary [4]. Here, *in situ* simulation scenarios can be used to identify latent system threats to patient safety, and to screen for unintended consequences of the proposed change. In one study, running *in situ* SBT identified incorrect defibrillator pads stocked on the resuscitation trolley, thus avoiding a potential adverse event [2]. Engaging individuals and teams during scenarios where change is being tested motivates them to participate in the change process, allowing them to reflect on the potential barriers to change and identify solutions with a greater likelihood of buy-in.

Finally, efficiency measurements of process can be embedded into a simulation drill. For example, in testing the hospital's ability to cope with a major haemorrhage in the ICU, measurement of time from initiating a major haemorrhage protocol to receiving blood products on the ICU could be recorded [8]. This provides quantitative evidence of system strengths and weaknesses, identifying processes that require change and giving a measure of efficiency (Figure 24.1) [8].

## Advantages of using *in situ* SBT in intensive care

A number of advantages of running *in situ* SBT programmes have been described in the literature [1,2,3,5,7,8,15,16]. These are outlined below:

1. *Multidisciplinary team training. In situ* SBT enables delivery of a complete package of training to the entire ICU team (doctors, nurses, laboratory services, allied health professionals). Multidisciplinary team involvement during scenario design, implementation, and debriefing ensures that the training delivered is both realistic and relevant to clinical practice. It pays attention to the educational and developmental needs of all learners, while reinforcing the benefit of interdisciplinary instruction. This models best practice for teamwork and collaborative interactions for the whole ICU team [7]. Collaborative training results in an increased understanding of each profession's complex prioritisation and helps better define each team member's role and responsibilities [8]. While particularly important in crisis situations, these skills may also be helpful in preventing routine situations from rapidly deteriorating into emergency

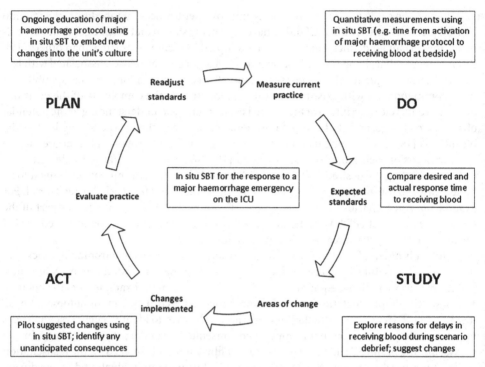

Ongoing education of major haemorrhage protocol using in situ SBT to embed new changes into the unit's culture

Quantitative measurements using in situ SBT (e.g. time from activation of major haemorrhage protocol to receiving blood at bedside)

Readjust standards

Measure current practice

**PLAN**

**DO**

In situ SBT for the response to a major haemorrhage emergency on the ICU

Evaluate practice

Expected standards

Compare desired and actual response time to receiving blood

**ACT**

**STUDY**

Changes implemented

Areas of change

Pilot suggested changes using in situ SBT; identify any unanticipated consequences

Explore reasons for delays in receiving blood during scenario debrief; suggest changes

**Figure 24.1** Use of *in situ* simulation-based training as a tool for quality improvement in response to major haemorrhage in the ICU.

events. A 'simulated mock run' of a procedure can be a useful task to undertake with the team prior to the real procedure. For example, when performing a percutaneous tracheostomy, a 'mock run' will ensure that each individual team member clearly understands the tasks required of their role, how this fits with the duties of the other team members, the sequential steps undertaken during the procedure, and the potential risks at each stage. This results in vigilant team members who are able to recognise and vocalise potential complications should they occur, thus improving collaborative teamwork and patient safety during the procedure. A number of studies have demonstrated better collaborative practice and communication following introduction of multidisciplinary *in situ* SBT in the ICU [3,5].

2. *Time and accessibility.* Duty hour restrictions such as those imposed by the European Working Time Directive, conflicting schedules, and differing shift patterns of ICU team members mean that there is often limited time for dedicated training outside clinical duty. By increasing the opportunity for integration into clinical schedules, *in situ* SBT maximises the accessibility of simulation as an educational tool for the unit.

3. *Relevant and individualised learning.* Learning objectives can be tailored to the needs of the ICU. Learning may be focused around critical incidents, suboptimal processes, and pathways, providing individually tailored scenarios for deliberative practice that are specific and relevant to the ICU and its team. For example, during crisis events in the ICU, complex arrangements of multiple pieces of equipment necessary for patient care may complicate communication, teamwork, and healthcare providers' access to the

patient. Teams can practice, reflect, and provide solutions to barriers to optimal care delivery in their own clinical environment.

4. *Enhanced realism.* Features of effective simulation are immediate feedback, active participation, and fidelity [6]. The equipment, environment, and the participants' psychological state add to the degree of believability. *In situ* SBT enhances fidelity, with the contextual cues, practical difficulties, and distractions of the real-life clinical environment adding to candidates' perception of realism and suspension of disbelief [6]. Increased authentic experiential learning has been shown to improve the transfer of learned skills, and to promote behavioural change through an increased emotional response in the learners [6].

5. *Reduced start-up and maintenance costs.* *In situ* small-scale SBT programmes can provide a cost-effective alternative to SBT delivered in purpose-built simulation centres. A study in a paediatric teaching hospital demonstrated implementation of a mobile simulation cart to be a cost-efficient means of delivering small-scale *in situ* SBT [20].

## Challenges of using *in situ* SBT in intensive care

Despite the numerous advantages to *in situ* SBT, there are some challenges to adopting an *in situ* SBT programme in the ICU. These are outlined below.

1. *Resources.* The concept of *in situ* simulation is attractive, but relies on the availability of resources such as empty ICU bed spaces and available staff. With most ICUs running to full capacity and increasing demands on clinical time, sessions may be difficult to schedule reliably, particularly where more than one discipline is involved.

2. *Minimising disruption to patient care.* The potential for scenarios to disrupt patient care, and for sessions to be interrupted by the need for clinical care, creates a conflict between the educational and clinical needs of the department. This is particularly the case for unplanned or unannounced scenarios. Running planned sessions allows dedicated time out from clinical duty for candidates participating in the scenario. Appropriate prior notification of the staff and an assessment of the unit workload on the allotted day should help to mitigate this risk.

3. *False alarms.* Unplanned or unannounced scenarios have the risk of repeated false alarms, such that staff may not respond promptly in the event of a true emergency. Careful planning and prior staff notification should alleviate this risk.

4. *Patient and family perceptions.* There is a theoretical perception that patients and visitors may be distressed or worried by seeing staff train in nearby clinical areas. A less than perfect mock scenario could potentially undermine patient and family confidence in healthcare providers. Interestingly, a study addressing relatives' perception of *in situ* simulation demonstrated the opposite effect and families 'were glad the health care teams were practicing for high-risk situations', providing they were notified beforehand [3]. Some studies have demonstrated that use of coloured vests or sashes to differentiate simulation group participants from clinical staff was particularly useful in avoiding confusion for patients and visitors [8].

5. *Equipment and medications.* Equipment and drugs used for simulation should be clearly separated, labelled, and stored to ensure that they are not inadvertently used for clinical care. Equipment (e.g. resuscitation trolleys, airway trolleys, practical procedural trays) not specifically designated for simulation and used clinically should be checked after use to ensure that they are not damaged or items are not missing.

6. *Lack of environmental control.* The challenge of an unpredictable environment is particularly pertinent when running unplanned sessions. The simulation team needs to be sensitive to unexpected changes in ICU workflow, a sudden large volume of unanticipated patient admissions, or clinical emergencies during planned sessions. These may impact the number or type of participants. The simulation team needs to exhibit flexibility in order to keep the session running smoothly.

7. *Participant 'buy-in'.* When designing clinical scenarios the simulation team should aim to ensure that the scenario content is context specific and clinically applicable. Scenarios that are overly complex may devalue the educational benefits and can lead to unnecessarily high levels of participant stress [3]. The degree of anxiety experienced during *in situ* simulation may be significant, as poor performance observed by colleagues can be regarded as erroneously reflecting poor clinical performance. A number of preventative measures to alleviate anxiety among participants have been described [6]. These include the use of non-judgemental feedback, carefully constructed debriefing, close consideration to the emotional safety of participants, and pre-scenario clarification regarding the purpose of the session. In some SBT programmes candidates are expected to sign a formal written contract outlining the terms of participation, such as strict confidentiality. Effective participant 'buy-in' is crucial, without which the simulation team can be met with resistance and failure of SBT programme implementation.

## Conclusion

*In situ* SBT has been shown to lead to safer clinical practice, better multidisciplinary team-work, and improved patient care in the ICU. The use of *in situ* SBT as an adjunct for quality improvement is increasingly being recognised. Here, it can be used to evaluate existing or pilot new care process and pathways, as a tool to support change, and to offer quantitative measures of efficiency. There are a number of advantages but also challenges in running an *in situ* SBT programme on a busy ICU. Ultimately, how SBT is used and best delivered is determined by local needs and available resources.

## References

1. Lighthall GK, Poon T, Harrison TK. Using in situ simulation to improve in-hospital cardiopulmonary resuscitation. *Jt Comm J Qual Patient Saf* 2010;36:209–216.

2. Walker ST, Sevdalis N, McKay A, *et al.* Unannounced in situ simulations: integrating training and clinical practice. *BMJ Qual Saf* 2013;22:453–458.

3. Patterson MD, Blike GT, Madkarni VM. In situ simulation: challenges and results. In: Henriksen K, Battles JB, Keyes MA, *et al.* eds. *Advances in Patient Safety: New Directions and Alternative Approaches,* Vol. 3: Performance and Tools). Rockville, MD: Agency for Healthcare Research and Quality (US), 2008. www.ncbi.nlm. nih.gov/books/NBK43682/ (accessed 11 September 2014).

4. Geis GL, Pio B, Pendergrass TL, *et al.* Simulation to assess the safety of new healthcare teams and new facilities. *Simul Healthc* 2011;6:125–133.

5. Meurling L, Hedman L, Sandahl C, *et al.* Systematic simulation-based team training in a Swedish intensive care unit: a diverse response among critical care professions. *BMJ Qual Saf* 2013;22:485–494.

6. Wang EE. Simulation and adult learning. *YMDA* 2011;57(11):664–678.

7. Allan CK, Thiagarajan RR, Beke D, *et al.* Simulation-based training delivered directly to the pediatric cardiac intensive care unit engenders preparedness, comfort, and decreased anxiety among multidisciplinary resuscitation teams. *J Thorac Cardiovasc Surg* 2010;140:646–652.

8. Hansen SS, Arafeh J. Implementing and sustaining in situ drills to improve multidisciplinary health care training. *J Obstet Gynecol Neonatal Nurs* 2012;41:559–571.

9. Reader TW, Flin R, Cuthbertson BH. Communication skills and error in the intensive care unit. *Curr Opin Crit Care* 2007;13:732–736.

10. Wayne D, Didwania A, Feinglass J, *et al.* Simulation-based education improves quality of care during cardiac arrest team responses at an academic teaching hospital. *Chest* 2008;133:56–61.

11. McGaghie WC, Issenberg SB, Cohen MER, *et al.* Does simulation-based medical education with deliberate practice yield better results than traditional clinical education? A meta-analytic comparative review of the evidence. *Acad Med* 2011;86:706.

12. Cook DA, Hatala R, Brydges R, *et al.* Technology-enhanced simulation for health professions education. *JAMA* 2011;306:978–988.

13. Flin R, Maran N. Identifying and training non-technical skills for teams in acute medicine. *Qual Saf Health Care* 2004;13:80–84.

14. Kohn LT, Corrigan JM, Donaldson MS. *To Err is Human: Building a Safer Health System*. Washington, DC: Institute of Medicine, National Academy Press, 1999.

15. Salas E, Paige JT, Rosen MA. Creating new realities in healthcare: the status of simulation based training as a patient safety improvement strategy. *BMJ Qual Saf* 2013;22:449–452.

16. Patterson MD, Geis GL, Falcone RA, *et al.* In situ simulation: detection of safety threats and teamwork training in a high risk emergency department. *BMJ Qual Saf* 2013;22:468–477.

17. Arora S, Cox C, Davies S, *et al.* Towards the next frontier for simulation-based training: full-hospital simulation across the entire patient pathway. *Ann Surg* 2013; 260:252–258.

18. Langley JG, Nolan KM, Nolan TW, *et al.* *The Improvement Guide: A Practical Approach to Enhancing Organizational Performance*. New York: Jossey-Bass, 1996.

19. Grol R. Successes and failures in the implementation of evidence-based guidelines for clinical practice. *Med Care* 2001; 39:46–54.

20. Weinstock PH, Kappus LJ, Garden A, Burns JP. Simulation at the point of care: reduced-cost, in situ training via a mobile cart. *Pediat Crit Care Med* 2009;10: 176–181.

Chapter

# National ICU registries

25

Sten M. Walther and Göran Karlström

In the late 1980s, efforts were being made to collect information in intensive care databases to be used for the purpose of describing and defending intensive care. Information was initially limited to provision of resources or services such as intensive care unit (ICU) bed availability, equipment, staffing, occupancy, and numbers of patients and interventions, with minimal, if any, patient-level data. Registries were typically started within national borders, healthcare systems, or large research projects where shared values and service models facilitated collection and interpretation of data. With time, detailed patient-level data and outcomes were added to the registries.

## Perspectives and goals

The forces driving joint collection of patient data and analysis of outcomes have varied over time and across healthcare systems. Multiple goals have often been expressed, indicating the wide scope and importance ascribed to the use of intensive care databases. Some early examples demonstrated this idea by showing how observing and reporting practice in the "real world" could change practice and delivery of intensive care. In an analysis of the observational SUPPORT study database, which was collected for research purposes during 1989 to 1994, the use of the pulmonary artery catheter was suggested to be harmful [1]. Proper randomized controlled studies followed that led to the gradual abandonment of the, at that time in the USA, quite extensive use of the pulmonary artery catheter. In another analysis of two databases in the UK, discharge from ICU at night was found to be associated with increased mortality. This association, which disappeared after adjusting for perceived premature discharge, put focus on the comparatively low provision of ICU beds in the UK [2]. While perspectives of the main stakeholders in intensive care are tightly connected and overlap, they do not always match and sometimes come into conflict.

## The professional perspective

The initial attempts of joint collection of ICU information reflected a professional need to discuss patient management and share experiences in the treatment of the critically ill. One very early instance of collection of detailed data was presented in 1960 at the World Congress of Anesthesiologists in Toronto when Norlander et al. reported their experience with prolonged

*Quality Management in Intensive Care*, ed. Bertrand Guidet, Andreas Valentin and Hans Flaatten. Published by Cambridge University Press. © Cambridge University Press 2016.

controlled ventilation in a heterogeneous group of critically ill patients treated in six different hospitals [3]. Assembling this report in a young discipline required developing common terminology and definitions, a process central also to current intensive care registries. The principal difference compared to a national registry was the limited scale and duration of data collection.

In the 1980s several professional initiatives to collect and analyze comprehensive sets of information from multiple ICUs emerged, e.g., the EURICUS project from the Foundation for Research on Intensive Care in Europe (FRICE), the Winnipeg ICU database, and the Finnish ICU Study Group [4]. These initiatives were partly driven by the rapidly increasing cost of intensive care and the need for healthcare professionals to respond to arguments about ineffectiveness and poor performance of intensive care. National registries started to grow from some of these large collaborations: National Intensive Care Evaluation (NICE) in the Netherlands; the Intensive Care National Audit & Research Centre (ICNARC) Case Mix Programme Database in England, Wales and Northern Ireland; Intensium in Finland; and the Australian and New Zealand Intensive Care Society (ANZICS) CORE registries, to name but a few [4]. In addition, registries collecting data from large clusters of ICUs appeared, e.g., Project IMPACT from the Society of Critical Care Medicine (SCCM) in the USA; CUB-REA network in Paris, France; and Gruppo Italiano per la Valutazione degli Interventi Terapia Intensiva (GiViTI) in North Italy [4]. Throughout, the main mission of intensive care registries has been to support the medical profession to carry out clinical audit, inform the planning and management of services, and provide clinicians with accurate estimates of the outcome of their care.

## The patient perspective

The growth of patient autonomy in healthcare decision-making and the growing realization that the application of high-technology care must be balanced with the ability to improve quality of life has influenced delivery of intensive care and how ICU registries operate. Although public accountability for outcomes derived from delivered health services has been a growing expectation of consumers, the move to provide patients with data on the performance of individual doctors, teams, and hospitals has accelerated after widely published examples of poor performance and malpractice. However, presenting and interpreting health service information is challenging and, for ICUs, requires an ability to evaluate the incremental benefit of intensive care services on patient outcomes. Public disclosure of performance data is not without its problems. In addition to gathering, interpreting, and building an infrastructure for reporting complex information, mechanisms must be in place to support underperforming ICUs. Although data collected in this way are meant to support decision-making and quality assurance, there is evidence that public reporting of patient outcomes may result in reduced ICU admission of the sickest patients and increased transfer of critically ill patients to other hospitals [5].

The patient perspective has also led to a move away from process targets to a focus on delivering the outcomes that matter most to people. Patient-reported outcome and experience measures are just becoming part of the routine dataset of ICU registries. This trend is in line with a general trend of looking at healthcare services, which has changed toward assessing the value to patients that they create.

## The provider perspective

Concern and attention to costs of healthcare have led to increased scrutiny of ICU performance as this is usually one of the most expensive types of medical service. Purchasers vary from national governments to regional providers of healthcare to companies and private payers, sometimes acting in concert, as in the Cleveland Health Quality Choice (CHQC) program, which already in the 1980s demanded hospitals to submit performance data to the public [6]. In this and other similar initiatives [7], ICU care was selected not only because of cost, but also because of high mortality rate, data showing large variations in performance as measured by risk-adjusted mortality rates, and evidence that interventions could improve outcomes. By collecting and presenting registry data, hospitals and clinicians would have benchmarks to use in setting quality improvement goals. Consumers could incorporate the information into decisions about their choice of caregiver, but only if ICU performance could be assessed accurately using methodology accepted by all parties. For that purpose risk adjustment models were customized and adapted to the local environment [6,7]. Although some of the resulting registries remain, most have been short-lived or lost momentum, partly due to criticism of risk-adjustment models, accusations of "gaming" the system by discharging patients too early, or lack of data to support any improvement in performance over time [5,8].

## Management of registries

Most successful registries were started by initiatives from ICU physicians and nurses, usually with ties to their professional societies. Management and funding developed over time in parallel with growth in coverage and scope. Regardless of organization, boards are still dominated by professionally active physicians and nurses. Financing varies from total membership subscription to total government funding. Although few registries present clearly their sources of income, their management, and their ownership, some examples may illustrate the current state and trends.

## Organization and funding

The registry of the Austrian Center for Documentation and Quality Assurance in Intensive Care (ASDI), created in 1994 and now expanded to include Italian and Portuguese units, is run as a non-governmental organization by an Austrian board of physicians [4]. The German registry (Register Versorgungsforschung Intensivmedizin, REVERSI), under construction since 2012, is run by the German Interdisciplinary Association of Critical Care and Emergency Medicine (DIVI). The same professional setup applies for the registries run by the Spanish Society of Intensive Care, Critical Care and Coronary Units (SEMICYUC), where data collection seems to be split into several diagnosis- and method-specific registries, often in collaboration with other professional bodies. GiViTI, initially a professional northern Italy network starting in 1991, has grown to a large organization with ICUs in most parts of Italy. Funding was from the start by industrial grants but has changed to 54% public Italian, 37% public from outside Italy, and the remainder from sponsors. The ANZICS-CORE registries are primarily funded by the departments of health of Australia and New Zealand and run by the national professional societies. ICNARC (the case-mix program) in the UK, except Scotland, is a charity that depends on membership fees from ICUs and research grants, quite similar to the Dutch NICE-foundation which is financed by membership fees. In Scotland the national ICU database was from its origin in 1995 part of the Scottish Intensive Care Society, but joined in 2006 a division of NHS National Services Scotland. The Swedish Registry was created as a separate national body by a handful of intensivists maintaining tight links with the Swedish Society of Anaesthesia and Intensive Care, but became part of the national health system in 2008 in response to new legislation. The Norwegian registry, with many similarities to the Swedish registry, is entirely financed by the government, with a steering group of elected ICU doctors and nurses from the participating units. The Malaysian Registry of Intensive Care (created in

2003 and reorganized in 2009) and the new Sri Lankan registry are both government funded and have strong professional ties. Intensium in Finland, among the first with a nationwide registry, was created as a private company because of lack of support from national and professional bodies, but with tight ties to the profession. It rapidly gained momentum to become a nationwide registry and software developer, which recently was bought by a software company with presently little information open to the public. The SCCM Project IMPACT database has undergone a similar transition to become a joint venture with industry, focusing on the measurement and improvement of ICU performance.

# Registry design

Registries offer opportunities to carry out comparative audit, to inform about management of services, and provide sources for evaluative research. Proper design and valid and reliable content are all central to meeting these expectations. While pioneering registries provided "snap-shot" data over time or recruited patients for a limited period, most current large-scale registries include consecutive patients continuously. Reliability has improved in mature registries by moving from collecting data that were defined retrospectively and identified in discharged patients' charts, to data defined in advance and entered manually or automatically.

## Definitions

The intensive care episode is one link in a chain of episodes of care, and its boundaries may not always be easily defined. Likewise, the terms "intensive care unit" and "intensive care bed" may not mean the same to its various users, which points to the need for standardization of concepts and language. This need may be true within a given healthcare system or country, and even more obvious when making comparisons across systems and countries [9]. How do lower intensity levels of care which is provided in general ICUs in a hospital differ from intermediate, step-down, and high-dependency units in another hospital? The population for which the results from the data are generalizable must be identified by defining who is included (the clinical scope) and from where (e.g., geography, healthcare system). Whether defined by an administrative arrangement (e.g., admission to a physical ICU or an ICU without walls) or a common circumstance (e.g., severe organ failure), arriving at common definitions is an absolute prerequisite for data collection within a registry.

## Confidentiality

At some stage registries need to hold ICU and patient identifiable information. This information may at a later stage be reversibly or irreversibly anonymized. The need to maintain anonymity of the provider, the ICU, has gradually changed toward a development where the identity of the ICU has become open, at least to other participating ICUs within the registry. This change has been important to quality management by stimulating and facilitating clinical audit and benchmarking.

The need to inform patients and relatives and obtain consent varies according to local regulations and laws. Subjects may not be informed at all, or only collectively through posters and leaflets displayed in the ICU. Alternatively, patients that recover may need to be informed individually and signed consent must be obtained before their data can be transferred to the database. Varying practices may lead to markedly biased inclusion of patients.

Because patient privacy and confidentiality must be secured at all times, individual data are protected to the same extent as during care in the ICU. However, a unique individual local or global "key code" may be included to make possible reversing the anonymity of the data. The "key code" allows tracing patients through more than one episode of care within the registry. This helps identify multiple admissions and the temporal sequence in which events occur. The "key code" makes it also possible to link with external registries and obtain additional information, e.g., vital status after discharge from hospital.

## Data quality

Incomplete coverage and poor accuracy are two main threats to reliability, internal validity, and generalizability of intensive care registries. Black and Payne developed a practical checklist where coverage and accuracy were described in ten items (four for coverage and six for accuracy), with four levels of attainment per item (Table 25.1) [10].

Four items related to coverage were deemed important in this context. First, how representative is the registry of the country or the healthcare system as a whole? Second, to what extent have all eligible patients been included in the registry? Third, does the dataset cover the most important aspects of intensive care? Fourth, is data collection complete? While representativeness, completeness of patient recruitment, and complete collection of data are fairly straightforward items to assess, it may be more difficult to assess whether the included dataset variables are complete. A standard dataset typically includes information on demographics, case-mix variables (in addition to those which are part of the risk adjustment model that is in use), workload, and ICU and hospital outcome. Potential additional variables include descriptors of procedures, therapies, evolution of organ failure, resuscitation code status, and complications in the ICU, as well as outcomes after discharge from ICU, including health-related quality of life. These and additional variables may be used singly or in combination to assess quality of care. However, the usefulness of collecting many of these variables needs to be determined to avoid registration fatigue and overloading the registry with information that may never be used. Six items related to accuracy were described in detail. In which form were quantitative data collected (raw vs. processed)? Were explicit definitions of variables available and used? Were explicit rules for data collection present and was coding reliable? Reliability includes validation of the main outcome variable, which for intensive care usually is survival at the unit or hospital, which is quite clear-cut. It also includes the extent to which data are validated. The relevance of these ten items and the feasibility of the checklist for intensive care have been tested and approved [11].

## Reports and feedback

A functioning system for quality management must not only comprise one or more registers, but also the analyses, feedback reports, and a structure in which ICUs discover and discuss the implications in order to improve treatment and organization. To meet this aim data must be easily available, updated, relevant, and reliable, and allow for necessary comparisons over time and between units.

## Report cycle

The standard audit report cycle varies. Annual reports are probably too infrequent to serve as quality instruments, but they may be used for historical analyses and dissemination to authorities, funders, and other interested parties. Biannual and quarterly reports may be adequate for most quality aspects but some (e.g., presence of bacterial multi-resistance) may need more frequent feedback, particularly given that reports are produced with delay. Best use of the registry is to allow data to be analyzed locally by the ICU, in addition to centralized production of reports. An added advantage of local analysis is that data are often of better quality if those collecting them are involved in using and analyzing them. Transparent access to data from other participants of the registry adds further to the usefulness of the registry.

**Table 25.1** Criteria for assessing the coverage and accuracy of a clinical database [10]

| | Level 1 | Level 2 | Level 3 | Level 4 |
|---|---|---|---|---|
| 1. Extent to which the eligible population is representative of the country. Specify country: | No evidence or unlikely to be representative | Some evidence eligible population is representative | Good evidence eligible population is representative | Total population of country included |
| 2. Completeness of recruitment of eligible population. State when and how completeness was determined: | Few (<80%) or unknown | Some (80–89%) | Most (90–97%) | All or almost all (>97%) |
| 3. Variables included in the database | • identifier<br>• admin info<br>• condition or intervention | • identifier<br>• admin info<br>• condition or intervention<br>• short-term or long-term outcome | • identifier<br>• admin info<br>• condition<br>• intervention<br>• short-term or long-term outcome major known confounders | • identifier<br>• admin info<br>• condition<br>• intervention<br>• short-term outcome<br>• major known confounders<br>• long-term outcome |
| 4. Completeness of data (percentage variables at least 95% complete). State when completeness was last determined: | Few (<50%) or unknown | Some (50–79%) | Most (80–97%) | All or almost all (>97%) |
| 5. Form in which continuous data (excluding dates) are collected (percentage collected as raw data) | Few (<70%) or unknown | Some (70–89%) | Most (90–97%) | All or almost all (<97%) or no continuous data collected |
| 6. Use of explicit definitions for variables | None | Some (<50%) | Most (50–97%) | All or almost all (>97%) |
| 7. Use of explicit rules for deciding how variables are recorded* | None | Some (<50%) | Most (50–97%) | All or almost all (>97%) |
| 8. Reliability of coding of conditions and not tested interventions. State when and how it was most recently tested: | Not tested | Poor | Fair | Good |
| 9. Independence of observations of primary outcome | Outcome not included or independence unknown | Observer neither independent nor blinded to intervention | Independent observer not blinded to intervention | Independent observer blinded to intervention or not necessary as objective outcome (e.g., death or lab test) |
| 10. Extent to which data are validated | No validation | Range or consistency checks | Range and consistency checks | Range and consistency checks plus external validation using alternative source |

*For example, timing of physiological measures or distinguishing primary from secondary diagnoses.

One impediment for timely feedback is the frequency with which data are sent from local ICUs to the central database. This will be a minor concern if data are submitted regularly with short time intervals (weekly or bimonthly) and the central update of the registry is rapid. However, a real-time database, where data are automatically sent to the central database as soon as they are entered into the local system, may be used to analyze day-to-day changes in bed occupancy, and for immediate planning of service delivery and patient transfers within a network of hospitals. Although a real-time registry could be preferable, it may be better with some time lag to allow for completion of each episode of care before merging with the central registry. Alternatively, export of data generated locally can be limited to completed care episodes, although this may bias some aspects of the feedback reports (e.g., assessment of workload over time), particularly in ICUs with patients that have extended care episodes.

## Access to reports

In this context two extremes of reporting may exist, both maintaining patient anonymity. The first is when access to reports is strictly limited to the participating ICU; participants can identify their own information but other units' data are either anonymized or aggregated. The other extreme is when information is identifiable per ICU and open to the public. Maintaining the first extreme is difficult in the long run for a registry if the purpose is to perform comparative audit. It may be a first step while gradually developing a valid dataset and building trust between participants. It must be followed by sharing data if improvement of quality by learning from others is a main purpose.

The other extreme with maximal openness is feasible when trust and willingness to measure and share results, also when suboptimal, are present. Whereas this approach has been considered controversial in some healthcare models [5,8], it may be possible in models where the main means of financing is by taxation, as shown in Sweden where continuously updated data have existed online, open to the public since 2005. There are many variations between these two extremes, some which provide password-protected interactive tools for participants only to access the database and generate results, as in Austria (ASDI), the Netherlands (NICE), and Italy (GiViTI); and others which provide identifiable ICU outcome data on a regular basis to the public, as in Scotland and Malaysia [4]. Regardless of details, public access to data needs to involve a communication strategy that includes readiness to educate media and laymen.

## Future outlook

### Dataset extensions

A significant development of registry datasets would be to include a time-fixed outcome measure, e.g., 30- or 90-day survival. This advance is required when using hospital mortality as a primary outcome variable, to minimize bias due to differing transfer and discharge practices. An outcome variable with some distance to the time of hospital discharge is also better for assessing the true patient value of intensive care, although practical and judicial obstacles are considerable in many countries.

Patient-reported outcome measures (e.g., health-related quality of life) and patient- (or next-of-kin) reported experience measures may also prove important in the near future to assess ICU performance and the value of the care given.

### Automated data capture

Registration fatigue leading to missing and incorrect information is threatening the validity of registries. Integration with patient data management systems used for daily care are operative in some environments [12], but further progress is needed with automatic and semi-automatic transfer of information from laboratory systems and patient files to data repositories for secondary validation.

## From national to international

Several registries have developed from regional to international collaborations: Intensium (recruiting from Finland, Estonia, and Switzerland), ASDI (Austria, Portugal, and Italy), ANZICS-CORE (Australia, New Zealand, and Hong Kong), ICNARC Case Mix Programme (England, Wales, and Northern Ireland), and GiViTI (Italy, Afghanistan, Cyprus, Greece, Israel, Poland, Slovenia, Sudan, and Hungary), to name a few examples [4]. Starting new registries in environments that lack such activity is facilitated by collaborations with mature registries. Also, increasing diversity by sharing information from other intensive care settings may give valuable insights to all participants. In 2000 the European Society of Intensive Care Medicine (ESICM) took the initiative to identify all ICUs in "Greater Europe" and collect at least some common information from each (The European registry of Intensive Care, ERIC [4]). An obvious extension would be to offer external audit and certification of registries by a common body, which was done by ESICM, who in 2010 certified the Austrian benchmarking project [4]. However, this activity and ERIC seems to have lost momentum and there is little current activity and no published reports.

## From ICU performance to patient value

Intensive care is one episode, sometimes unwanted, of many episodes of care in a patient's disease course. Collecting information from the entire course together with the value created by caregivers from the patient's viewpoint (e.g., long-term survival, health-related quality of life) may offer a better understanding of where improvement is needed. This is, admittedly, most easily done in diseases with distinctly identified care processes (e.g., ischemic heart disease, colonic cancer, asthma); it is much more complex for the frail, elderly patient with multiple chronic conditions. The approach, however, will put ICU care in a wider perspective and may give insights into how to identify risk and prepare patients earlier to generate the best value. Delivery and volume of intensive care may change when incentives are structured so that quality, measured by outcomes that matter for patients, and not merely the provision of the least expensive care, is fairly compensated.

## References

1. A.F. Connors Jr, T. Speroff, N.V. Dawson, et al. The effectiveness of right heart catheterization in the initial care of critically ill patients: SUPPORT Investigators. JAMA 1996; 276: 889–897.

2. C. Goldfrad, K. Rowan. Consequences of discharges from intensive care at night. Lancet 2000; 355: 1138–1142.

3. O.P. Norlander, V.O. Bjork, C. Crafoord, et al. Controlled ventilation in medical practice. Anaesthesia 1961; 16: 285–307.

4. Swedish Intensive Care Registry. Intensive care registries. 2015. www.icuregswe.org/registries (accessed 30 September 2015).

5. L.A. Reineck, T.Q. Le, C.W. Seymour, et al. The impact of publicly reporting intensive care unit (ICU) in-hospital mortality on ICU case-mix and outcomes. Ann Am Thorac Soc 2015; 12: 57–63.

6. C.A. Sirio, L.B. Shepardson, A.J. Rotondi, et al. Community-wide assessment of intensive care outcomes using a physiologically based prognostic measure: implications for critical care delivery from Cleveland Health Quality Choice. Chest 1999; 115: 793–801.

7. California Intensive Care Outcomes project (CALICO). 2007. www.oshpd.

ca.gov/HID/Products/PatDischargeData/ICUDataCALICO/CALICO_05-07.pdf (accessed 30 September 2015).

8. D. Neuhauser, D.L. Harper. Too good to last: did Cleveland Health Quality Choice leave a legacy and lessons to be learned? *Qual Saf Health Care* 2002; 11: 202–203.

9. A. Rhodes, P. Ferdinande, H. Flaatten, *et al.* The variability of critical care bed numbers in Europe. *Intensive Care Med* 2012; 38: 1647–1653.

10. N. Black, M. Payne. Directory of clinical databases: improving and promoting their use. *Qual Saf Health Care* 2003; 12: 348–352.

11. D.A. Harrison, A.R. Brady, K. Rowan. Case mix, outcome and length of stay for admissions to adult, general critical care units in England, Wales and Northern Ireland: the Intensive Care National Audit & Research Centre Case Mix Programme Database. *Crit Care* 2004; 8: R99–111.

12. M. Reinikainen, P. Mussalo, S. Hovilehto, *et al.* Association of automated data collection and data completeness with outcomes of intensive care: a new customised model for outcome prediction. *Acta Anaesthesiol Scand* 2012; 56: 1114–1122.

# Chapter 26

# Quality indicators

Peter van der Voort

## Introduction

Professionals are trained to provide care based on the principles of evidence-based medicine [1]. However, many recommendations in guidelines appear to lack sufficient evidence [2]. As a result, part of clinical practice is dependent on local and individual preferences. Consequently, clinical practice and the actually delivered care generally show variability between medical doctors and institutions [3]. Insight into the variability and quality of the delivered care can only be accomplished by collecting data. For several years now, medical professionals have been increasingly interested in measuring the quality of their work. Previously, each doctor had his or her internal quality control by seeing and listening to the patients who returned for a follow-up visit. However, it is now broadly agreed that an active quality improvement programme based on measurements should be present in each hospital department, including the intensive care unit (ICU). The ICU, where complex care is provided and many physiologic signs are measured and recorded, is a logical place to have a quality improvement programme based on the available data. These data can be used to gain insight into the quality of care. Such data are called indicators. Indicators can be used to compare the chosen aspects of the quality of care over time but also to compare with other ICUs (benchmark). Measuring and analysing these indicator data can lead to adjustments in caregiving in order to improve the outcome for the patients.

## What is a quality indicator?

The definition of an indicator is: a measurable feature of healthcare, which gives an indication of the quality of care.

In this definition three words are important. First, an indicator is a measurable aspect of caregiving. Only quantifiable items can be used for comparison and benchmark and thus an indicator should be measurable. Second, an indicator provides information on the quality of care. Quality of care is a broad concept and can be defined in several ways. The six domains of quality as defined the Institute of Medicine are a useful categorization in this respect [4]. Third, an indicator gives an indication and is not an absolute qualification. This implies that the results obtained from the indicator may be flawed for several reasons. For instance, when the indicator data are, at first sight, not as good as expected,

*Quality Management in Intensive Care*, ed. Bertrand Guidet, Andreas Valentin and Hans Flaatten. Published by Cambridge University Press. © Cambridge University Press 2016.

**Table 26.1** Characteristics of a quality indicator

Relevant for clinical decision-making.
Related to an outcome or to a process that is related to an outcome.
Can lead to actions leading to improvement.
Easily measurable.
Quick and available in a timely fashion.
Can be used in different institutions.
Based on evidence or evidence-based guidelines.

a thorough analysis of determinants should be performed before a definite conclusion about the quality of care can be made. The characteristics of indicators determine how well the indicator will perform in describing the quality of care. These are shown in Table 26.1. The first characteristic, the relevancy for clinical decision-making, embraces the frequency of occurrence of the measured item and the associated risk for patients. When an indicator measures something that nearly never happens, it will not be relevant. In addition, the indicator should measure something that is risky or beneficial for patients; otherwise the information will not motivate action.

## Types of indicators

Donabedian made a categorization of indicators around 1970 [5–7]. He made a distinction between structure, process, and outcome indicators. This categorization is easy to use for both policy-makers and professionals [8]. The indicators can be conveniently arranged in this way, which helps to clarify the field of quality improvement. This categorization is therefore widely used. Structure indicators describe the organization, facilities, and personnel. Examples of structure indicators in the ICU are the number of ICU beds, the number and availability of intensivists, and the availability of nurses to provide care. Structure indicators usually describe aspects that can be improved by increasing investment. It may take a lot of time, however, to realize improvement, e.g., to increase the number of ICU beds.

The process indicators describe the process of care between caregiver and patient. The indicator should address processes that are directly related to outcomes. These process indicators are preferentially used because they are relatively easy to measure and it is relatively easy to change aspects of the caregiving processes. Examples of process indicators are the length of stay, glucose regulation, and the adherence to guidelines. Though process indicators have attractive characteristics, it is the outcome that ultimately counts. The outcome is measured by outcome indicators. These give insight into the outcome, preferably at the patient level. A typical outcome indicator in the ICU is the standardized mortality rate (SMR).

Indicators that are used by organizations or professionals themselves to improve care are called internal indicators. These data are not publicly available and cannot lead to league tables in the media. It implies that these internal indicators can be more loosely defined than external indicators because aberrations can be discussed internally and will not immediately lead to publicity with blame and shame. After thorough analysis, these internal indicators may lead to improvements in either the registration of data or the delivery of care. External indicators are meant to provide information to outsiders. The outsiders can be the public, governmental organizations, insurance companies, or health-care inspectorates. These indicators should be robust in registration, interpretation, and conclusion as they may be used for league tables and public debate. External indicators help to provide the transparency of healthcare, which is often asked for. To serve these goals, external indicators must fulfil five criteria (see Box 26.1).

---

**Box 26.1**

Characteristics of external indicators

1. Designed for accounting to external stakeholders.
2. High precision.
3. Reproducible.
4. Univocal interpretation.
5. Low risk for manipulation of data.

---

# How to develop an indicator (set)

Because indicators are measurable features of healthcare, a numerator with a denominator usually defines them. An example is the nurses:patients ratio. In this indicator the numerator is the number of nurses and the denominator is the number of patients. As a result, multiple data need to be collected and put into a formula to determine the value of the indicator. In this example, the number of nurses and the number of patients may be counted each nursing shift for a period of time. For each shift the mean nurses:patients ratio can be calculated, which may lead to a mean for a given period of time. Moreover, one can also look for the percentage of shifts in which the nurses:patients ratio is lower than the minimum set. For each indicator the population should be defined as well. For instance, the nurses:patients ratio can be measured in all ICU patients or in mechanically ventilated patients. This example shows that the collection of the same data can lead to different indicators. Beforehand, it should be clear what one wants to measure and to achieve and the exact definition of the indicator should match with this goal. The development of an indicator or set of indicators should therefore start with a clear description of the goals [9]. The second step is to choose the items that should be measured by the indicators. The indicators themselves should preferably have a high validity. The higher the validity, the more the indicator really measures what it should measure. Several aspects of validity exist, but the most important are face validity and construct validity. Face validity is the opinion of the experts in the field where the indicator will be used. When the experts in the field deem the indicator invalid, it is unwise to implement it, as it will probably lead to insufficient effects. In that case the results will not be seen as relevant and the data will not easily lead to quality improvement. Construct validity determines whether the indicator is related to the quality of care based on scientific rationale. Indicators that are derived from clinical guidelines should have high construct validity as the (evidence-based) guideline has critically appraised the literature on this subject.

Delphi techniques are often used when indicators are being developed. However, other methods can be used as well. In the Delphi method experts discuss and make their choices in several rounds, based on evidence and expert opinion.

In the development phase of indicators, the face validity and construct validity should be carefully determined for each indicator. When indicators are based on recommendations of guidelines, the evidence that is summarized in the guideline usually guarantees the construct validity. A tool to check the validity of indicators is the AIRE instrument [10,11]. Indicators that are used together in a set will usually be chosen for their interrelationship. The set as a whole will give insight into the quality of care in the field where the set has its focus.

## The indicator in a PDCA cycle

Quality improvement can be achieved by using a quality improvement model. The four-phased Plan–Do–Check–Act cycle is the most widely used quality improvement model. Indicators are crucial elements of such a PDCA cycle. The first phase, usually called the plan phase, is characterized by defining the goals of a chosen quality improvement project. In the second, the do phase, the implementation of the intervention takes place. In the next phase, the check phase, it is checked whether the intervention works and improvement is made. In this phase data collection is necessary and this is the moment at which most indicator data are collected. Collecting indicator data at this moment is a crucial step in continuing the PDCA cycle. Based on the analysis of indicator data, one can enter the next step of the PDCA cycle, which is the act-phase. The action should lead to the continuous improvement of the care delivery process and it may lead to re-writing the plan. As such, the cycle is re-entered and a continuous improvement can be achieved. Indicators can only ground this continuous quality improvement cycle when they meet the standards for indicators as summarized in Table 26.1. In addition, the registration must be reliably and carefully executed and the registry must also be complete and enclose all consecutive patients. The implementation of indicators or a set of indicators can be seen as a PDCA cycle by itself, as will be shown later.

## Definition and registration

Indicators measure specific aspects of healthcare in order to compare an ICU over time or to compare an ICU with other ICUs. This implies that the definition and registration of data for a specific indicator should be consequently the same over time and in between different ICUs. It is often seen that the interpretation of the results will lead to questions about the use of the correct definition and whether the registration was performed well. It is hard to compare with previous data or with your benchmark when a definition is unclear. The same is true when definitions are not used correctly at all times. As a consequence, these less reliable data will decrease the trust in the data and this will make users reluctant to make changes that may be necessary to improve. An incomplete registration will lead to biased results, which may or may not be obvious, and invalid conclusions may arise. Thus, the indicator data can lead to discussions about definition or registration and the final step to improvement is therefore not made. To reduce this risk, the people who are responsible for the registration should be well prepared for their job by education and clear instructions. It is advised to use bedside computerized systems for the registration instead of paper-assisted registration [12].

## Interpretation of indicator data

The analysis of indicator data may be hampered by unavailable data on determinants of the indicator. For instance, mortality is often used as an outcome indicator in intensive care. However, mortality has a lot of determinants, of which many are not routinely measured.

This makes it difficult to take appropriate steps in order to reduce mortality when mortality is high. In general, this is more often the case with outcome indicators compared to process and structure indicators [9]. In addition, some indicators are measures within a particular model or reference set which may not be well calibrated for a particular ICU. For instance, mortality can be related to severity of illness by using a reference database. This can be the APACHE or SAPS reference database and its associated prediction model. However, each chosen model will have its own limitations and strengths. In order to perform a thorough analysis of the SMR of a population based on one of these models one should have a clear view on the model's characteristics and the case-mix of the included population. The same models may also be used to predict length of stay in the ICU, but appear to have limitations [13].

## The feedback of analysed indicators

Indicators used for benchmarking are usually collected in a larger (national) database. Most indicators are composed of several items, which are usually uploaded to a central office of a registry where the indicator data are calculated from the items and then entered into the database [14]. These registries usually report to the ICUs on a regular basis. The reports include the indicator data but may also include quality reports of the uploaded data. The reports provide comparisons over time and a benchmark report with other ICUs. The feedback reports can be provided in several ways; the way the feedback is performed has implications for its use, the interpretation of the indicator data, and also for the subsequent steps to quality improvement. The simplest form of feedback of the indicator data is by sending a document with the results. The feedback reports can also be provided in combination with other feedback methods [14,15]. Such multifaceted feedback, in which several methods of feedback are combined, appears to be more effective than the documented report alone [15]. The multifaceted approach may include, for example, in addition to the standard reports, online admission to the database with the possibility to perform individual queries, the combination with expert meetings, the implementation of a quality improvement team or specific analyses based on specific data. In that respect, statistical process control (SPC) can help to get warning signals in time to make appropriate adjustments in structure or process aspects of caregiving [16].

## How to achieve improvement

It has been shown that a multifaceted intervention can lead to quality improvement [17,18]. In addition, the use of indicators can help to improve hospital care [15]. The collection of indicator data is usually the method to identify opportunities for improvement. However, quality improvement appears difficult to achieve even when the indicator results are clear [19,20]. To achieve improvement, additional steps must be taken after the indicator determines a less than optimal result. First, it is necessary to know whether the registration of the data is performed in the right way. At this stage, the construct validity may be checked as well. Often, one gets stuck in these issues and the final steps that should be undertaken for improvement are not made. When outcome indicators are used, it is more difficult to determine which necessary steps should be taken to achieve improvement than for process indicators. This is caused by the fact that multiple determinants are involved in the outcome. To overcome these problems and to achieve improvements it may be helpful to focus the project on a limited area of healthcare and to make someone or a small group of people responsible for the results [9,12]. In addition, it is of utmost importance that the leaders of the ICU actively support the project.

# What indicators are currently used in intensive care medicine?

Pronovost was one of the first to describe indicators that may be used in the critical care setting, followed by others [9,21–23]. Table 26.2 summarizes the mostly reported indicators. European indicators were described by the ESICM in 2012 [24]. In a review in 2012 it was shown that indicators that are used on a national level are highly variable between countries [25]. Sixty-three indicators appeared to be used in eight countries, but none of them was used in all of them. Mortality was used most often, in six out of eight countries, followed by measurements of patient/family satisfaction, presence of an ICU specialist 24/7, and the occurrence

**Table 26.2** Quality indicators as described in the literature

| Structure | Process | Outcome |
|---|---|---|
| Availability of ICU specialists | Re-admission rate | Mortality (standardized) |
| Staffing level | Adherence to VAP protocol | VAP rate |
| Nurse:patient ratio | Analgesia monitoring/protocol | Decubitus incidence rate |
| Number of ICU beds | Early enteral nutrition | Patient/family satisfaction |
| Multidisciplinary rounds | Sedation monitoring/protocol | Blood stream infections |
| Availability of ventilators | Correct antibiotic use | Central line infections |
| Availability of other equipment | Adherence to hygiene protocol | Prevalence of multi-resistant bacteria |
| Rapid response team | Inter-clinical transport | Occurrence of thromboembolism |
| Number of patients/volume | Occupancy rate | Costs |
| Fulfilment of national requirements to provide ICU care | Night discharge | Workload |
| Adverse event reporting system | Delayed ICU admissions or discharge | Long-term survival |
| Availability of a pharmacist | Length of stay | Rate of CPR on the ICU |
| | Duration of mechanical ventilation | Rate of new GI bleeding |
| | Documented meetings with family | Rate of unplanned extubation |
| | End-of-life protocol | Staff turnover and satisfaction |
| | Use of daily goals | Rate of severe adverse events |
| | Therapeutic hypothermia | |
| | Reintubation rate | |
| | Use of stress ulcer prophylaxis | |
| | Adherence to sepsis guidelines | |
| | Inappropriate red blood cell transfusion | |
| | Rate of cancelled surgery | |
| | Rate of ARDS patients with low tidal volume | |
| | Glucose regulation/hypo- and hyperglycaemia | |
| | Rate of adverse drug events | |
| | Adherence to medication protocol | |
| | Use of handovers between shifts and other services | |
| | Continuing medical education | |

GI; gastro-intestinal, ARDS; adult respiratory distress syndrome, VAP; ventilator-associated pneumonia, CPR; cardio-pulmonary resuscitation.

of ventilator-associated pneumonia, all used in five out of eight countries. Complications may also be seen as indicators when they are defined as a ratio with a numerator and denominator. As such, they may be incorporated in national indicator sets as well.

## Implementation of a quality indicator set

The implementation of a set of quality indicators can be seen as a quality improvement project by itself (Figure 26.1). It means that for the implementation of the set of indicators, a PDCA cycle can be used as well. First, a plan should be made in which the relevant items for implementation are described. It comprises how to do the registration, who is responsible for the registration, which software will be used, and how the registered data are aggregated and uploaded to a database. In our experience, in the do-phase the implementation of indicators will more likely succeed when the aforementioned items are clearly defined [12]. In addition, a computerized data registration will more likely succeed than a paper registration [12]. Also, when the registration is embedded in the daily workflow and when the workflow is limited, the implementation of the indicator registration will be more successful. In the next steps one should evaluate whether the indicators are correctly and completely registered. If not, action should be undertaken to improve the implementation of the indicator set. When a correct and continuous data registration is guaranteed, someone needs to be responsible for the overall process of quality improvement based on the indicator data.

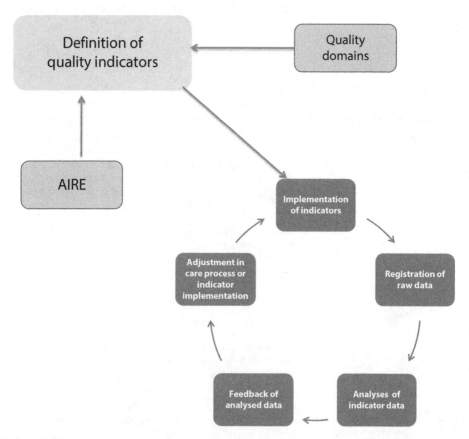

**Figure 26.1** Framework for implementation of quality indicators.

# Limitations in the use of quality indicators

The use of quality indicators is an essential part in quality improvement cycles. However, it is often difficult to see a direct association between indicator results and good outcome [19,20]. Several reasons may cause this paradox. It may be caused by insufficient validity of the indicators themselves or limited changes are made following the analysis of indicator results. In our experience, this last step in the quality improvement cycle is difficult to make. In addition, it may not always be easy to copy quality improvement projects from the literature [26] as they are context dependent and barriers and facilitators differ from one institution to the other.

External indicators are increasingly used for accountability reasons. Especially outcome indicators are used to make league tables and to show new patients how the organization or individual physician performs. Unjustified punishment or rewards may follow when the results of indicators are overinterpreted or the data are incorrect. Gaming behaviour and manipulation may be the effect [27]. In addition, high-risk patients may be deprived of care to achieve optimal results on the institutional level.

# References

1. Greenhalgh T, Howick J, Maskrey N. Evidence based medicine: a movement in crisis? *BMJ* 2014;348:3725.

2. McAlister FA, van Diepen S, Padwal RS, Johnson JA, Majumdar SR. How evidence-based are the recommendations in evidence-based guidelines? *PlosOne* 2007;4:e250.

3. The Dartmouth Atlas of Health Care. www.dartmouthatlas.org (accessed 22 March 2015).

4. Institute of Medicine, Committee on Quality of Health Care in America. *Crossing the Quality Chasm: A New Health System for the 21st Century*. Washington, DC : National Academies Press, 2001.

5. Donabedian A. The quality of medical care. *Science* 1978;200:856–864.

6. Donabedian. *An Introduction to Quality Assurance in Health Care*. Oxford: Oxford University Press, 2003.

7. Donabedian. Evaluating the quality of medical care. *Milbank Q* 2005;83:691–729.

8. Thijs LG. Continuous quality improvement in the ICU: general guidelines. *Intensive Care Med* 1997;23:125–127.

9. Pronovost PJ, Miller MR, Dorman T, Berenholtz SM, Rubin H. Developing and implementing measures of quality of care in the intensive care unit. *Curr Opin Crit Care* 2001;7:297–303.

10. De Koning J. Development and validation of a measurement instrument for appraising indicator quality: appraisal of indicators through research and evaluation (AIRE) instrument. www.egms.de/en/meetings/gmds2007/07gmds798.shtml (accessed 22 March 2015).

11. De Koning JS, Smulders A, Klazinga NS. *Appraisal of Indicators through Research and Evaluation (AIRE)*, second edition. Utrecht: Orde van Medisch Specialisten, 2007.

12. de Vos ML, van der Veer SN, Graafmans WC, *et al.* Implementing quality indicators in intensive care units: barriers to and facilitators of behaviour change. *Implement Sci* 2010;5:52.

13. Verburg IWM, de Keizer NF, de Jonge E, Peek N. Comparison of regression methods for modelling intensive care length of stay. *PlosOne* 2014;9(10):e109684.

14. van der Veer SN, de Keizer NF, Ravelli AC, Tenkink S, Jager KJ. Improving quality of care: a systematic review on how medical registries provide information feedback to health care providers. *Int J Med Informatics* 2010;79:305–323.

15. de Vos M, Graafmans W, Kooistra M, *et al.* Using quality indicators to improve hospital care: a review of the literature. *International Journal for Quality in Health Care* 2009;21:119–129.

16. Carey RG. Measuring health care quality: how do you know your care has improved? *Eval Health Prof.* 2000; 23:43–57.

17. Scales DC, Dainty K, Hales B, *et al.* A multifaceted intervention for quality improvement in a network of intensive care units. *JAMA* 2011;305:363–372.

18. Garrouste-Orgeas M, Soufir L, Tabah A, *et al.* A multifaceted program for improving quality of care in intensive care units: Iatroref study. *Crit Care Med* 2012;40:468–476.

19. van der Veer SN, de Vos ML, van der Voort PH, *et al.* Effect of a multifaceted performance feedback strategy on length of stay compared with benchmark reports alone: a cluster randomized trial in intensive care. *Crit Care Med* 2013;41:1893–1904.

20. Neuman MD, Wirtalla C, Werner RM. Association between skilled nursing facility quality indicators and hospital readmissions. *JAMA* 2014;312:1542–1551.

21. Berenholtz SM, Dorman T, Ngo K, Pronovost PJ. Qualitative review of intensive care unit quality indicators. *J Crit Care* 2002;17:1–12.

22. Pronovost PJ, Berenholtz SM, Ngo K, *et al.* Developing and pilot testing quality indicators in the intensive care unit. *J Crit Care* 2003;18:145–155.

23. De Vos M, Graafmans W, Keesman E, Westert G, van der Voort PHJ. Quality measurement at intensive care units: which indicators should we use? *J Crit Care* 2007;22:267–274.

24. Rhodes A, Moreno RP, Azoulay E, *et al.* Prospectively defined indicators to improve the safety and quality of care for critically ill patients: a report from the Task Force on Safety and Quality of the European Society. *Intensive Care Med* 2012;38:598–605.

25. Flaatten H. The present use of quality indicators in the intensive care unit. *Acta Anesthesiol Scand* 2012; 1078–1083.

26. Fan E, Laupacis A, Pronovost PJ, Guyatt GH, Needham DM. How to use an article about quality improvement. *JAMA* 2010;304:2279–2287.

27. Lilford R, Mohammed MA, Spiegelhalter D, Thomson R. Use and misuse of process and outcome data in managing performance of acute medical care: avoiding institutional stigma. *Lancet* 2004;363(9415):1147–1154.

# Chapter 27

# Benchmarking

## From comparison to performance

Bertrand Guidet and Yên-Lan Nguyen

The problem is that not everything that counts can be counted, and not everything that can be counted counts.

*Albert Einstein*

## Introduction

Since we were children, we have loved to compare ourselves to each other. We are living in modern societies with ever-present selection and competition. The media are fond of comparisons and ranking. In most countries, at the regional or national level, data are provided about hospital activities and patient-centered outcomes. More recently, patients associations want to be part of the process and to gain access to quantitative and qualitative information in order to be able to make their own comparisons. Unfortunately these comparisons are often crude (obtained without adjustments to known confounding factors) and do not allow one to obtain accurate performance information for healthcare structures.

## Definition of benchmarking

### Historical background

Benchmarking has been defined by Camp [1] as "the search for industry best practice that leads to superior performance." The three principles of benchmarking are maintaining quality, customer satisfaction, and continuous improvement [2]. First, benchmarking consists of evaluating processes within an organization in comparison to best practice (diagnosis step). Then, the treatment step allows organizations to set goals and to develop action plans on how to adopt such best practice, with the aim of increasing performance. The final step is to check that the results derived from the new methods meet customers' expectations (monitoring step). This approach was first used by Xerox Corporation in the late 1970s, when the company was under pressure and losing market share. Since then, benchmarking has gained popularity among all major companies.

Benchmarking may be a one-off event, but is often treated as a continuous process in which organizations continually seek to challenge their practices. Benchmarking is a powerful management tool because it overcomes "the blindness paradigm" which is that "The way we do it is the best because this is the way we've always done it." Benchmarking opens organizations

---

*Quality Management in Intensive Care*, ed. Bertrand Guidet, Andreas Valentin and Hans Flaatten. Published by Cambridge University Press. © Cambridge University Press 2016.

to new methods, ideas, and tools to improve their effectiveness. It helps crack through resistance to change by demonstrating other methods of solving problems than the ones currently employed, and demonstrating that they work, because they are being used by others.

There are four types of benchmarking. Competitive benchmarking consists of making comparisons among competitors for a specific product. Internal benchmarking consists of making comparisons between yourself and similar operations within your own organization. Functional benchmarking consists of making comparisons to similar functions within the same industry. Generic benchmarking consists of making comparisons of processes independent of industry or overall functions. Competitive benchmarking stands for better understanding of the wants (expectations) of the customer because it is based on the reality of the market estimated in an objective way. It goes with a better economic planning of the purposes and the objectives of the company by centering on what takes place in a controlled and mastered fashion. Through the process of benchmarking, it is expected to obtain an increasing productivity, to implement better current practices, and to improve competitiveness.

## The benchmarking process

The process is very structured, with several steps:

- Identify your problem areas:
  - informal conversations with customers, employees, or suppliers;
  - exploratory research techniques such as focus group, quantitative research, surveys, questionnaires, quality control reports, financial analyses.
- Identify other industries that have similar processes.
- Identify organizations that are leaders in these areas.
- Survey companies for measures and practices.
- Visit the "best practice" companies to identify leading-edge practices.
- Implement new and improved business practices: take the leading edge practices, develop implementation plans.
- Fund the project and sell the ideas to the organization.

## Potential disadvantages and limitations

Benchmarking could be considered as spying on competitors or copying rather than promoting internal innovation. However, in Japan benchmarking is part of a manager's job description [3]. The major limitation is that benchmarking might help organizations measure efficiency of their operational metrics, but without any global measure of effectiveness. Another limitation is the ability of the managers to motivate the team and to engage in an action plan for change.

## Areas of benchmarking in critical care

### Structure and personnel

The minimal criteria defining an ICU vary across countries. A list of basic requirements is recommended by the ESICM [4]. According to French law, an ICU should have at least eight beds, a minimum of two nurses to every five patients, and a minimum of one helper to every four patients [5]. An on-site medical presence 24/7 is mandatory. The ICU director is fully dedicated to the ICU. There is at least one head nurse. Therefore, each ICU could compare its structure with other ICUs located in the same region or at the national level. In a recent survey of 215 medical French ICUs, the average number of beds was around 12 per unit; 32%, 58%, and 9% of ICUs reported, respectively, a patient:nurse ratio of 2–2.5, 2.5–3, and >3 [6]; 3%, 46%, 43%, and 8% of ICUs reported a patient:helper ratio of <3, 3–4, 4–5, >5.

Number and basic training of senior intensivists in each ICU is important to compare. Are physicians solely dedicated to the ICU or do they have other tasks or commitments in other departments? How is continuity of care organized? Is there a dedicated intensivist for night duties? Who is in charge of prescribing mechanical ventilation, renal replacement therapy, or antibiotics?

Number and qualification of nurses together with dedicated tasks are also important to consider. Is critical care nurses' training done within the ICU? Are they allowed tailored treatment according to pre-specified protocols such as glycemic control, sedation-analgesia, or vasopressor management? What is the availability of other allied healthcare professionals: helpers (or nurse-assistants), clinician pharmacist, physiotherapist, dieticians, and psychologists?

Besides quantitative assessment of the team, qualitative measures are also important to assess, such as burn-out level within a team (since burn-out might impact the quality of delivered care) [7,8] or team-satisfaction oriented culture. In a prospective study, we analyzed the answers to the COMIC questionnaire of ICU personnel from 26 ICUs located in the Paris area [9]. Organizational performance was assessed through a composite score related to five dimensions: coordination and adaptation to uncertainty; communication; conflict management; organizational change and organizational learning; and skills developed in relationship with patients and their families. Overall, there was a positive relationship between team-satisfaction oriented culture and good managerial practices and good job satisfaction. The multilevel analysis assessing the respective contribution of structural, contextual, and individual factors to the organizational score showed that only 9.5% of the variation was due to ICU-level factors. At an individual level, the significant variables were: lack of burn-out ($p < 0.001$), satisfaction at work ($p < 0.001$), and older mean age ($p = 0.02$), while at the ICU level a high physician and nurses/bed ratio ($p = 0.0001$) and a high workload per day ($p = 0.02$) were significant [9].

## Management

Several managerial aspects could be monitored, such as the presence of routine multidisciplinary clinical ward rounds, a standardized handover procedure, and a medical error reporting system. However, several factors hinder this approach, such as dictatorial behavior, lack of mutual respect, and fear of being stigmatized. New technology (e.g., a fancy ventilator or dialysis machine) has little chance of improving patients' outcome if a team-oriented culture is not promoted in ICUs and if human factors are not recognized as the main factors driving quality [10]. Based on data collected from 17,440 patients across 42 ICUs, Shortell *et al.* [11] were able to reveal that: technological availability is significantly associated with lower risk-adjusted mortality; diagnostic diversity is significantly associated with greater risk-adjusted mortality; and that caregiver interaction comprising the culture, leadership, coordination, communication, and conflict management abilities of the unit is significantly associated with lower risk-adjusted length of stay (LOS), lower nurse turnover, higher evaluated technical quality of care, and greater evaluated ability to meet family member needs.

## Processes

Several processes could be analyzed, such as the infection of central venous catheter (mortality is estimated at 10% and ICU LOS is increased by 5–8 days) and unplanned extubations (high rate of re-intubation and increased risk of nosocomial pneumonia and death). Some process indicators have been recommended by the ESICM [12]. The main concern is the lack of evidence that process improvement will translate into better outcomes.

## Outcomes

Clinical outcomes form the basis for performance appraisal of ICUs. Several outcome parameters have been proposed (re-admissions rate, unplanned night discharge rates, ICU LOS, or mortality) but most are highly dependent on external factors that cannot be modified, at least in the short-term. Indeed, all of them depend on the case-mix adjustments, on the number of ICU beds available in the structure, and the presence of an intermediate care, rehabilitation, or palliative care unit. At first sight, the standardized mortality ratio (SMR), which is the actual mortality divided by the predicted mortality, seems very attractive. Indeed, in a French study comparing outcome data across 25 ICUs, the authors found that the observed mortality varied by a factor of nearly three, whereas SMRs varied by a factor of about two [13]. Then, when additional information was included in the mortality prediction, reordering mainly occurred in the mid and upper range (Table 27.1). But in an

**Table 27.1** Ranking of ICU according to SMR: Model A with the customized SAPS2; Model B with the customized SAPS2 including diagnosis [13]

| Unit | n | H | SAPS II SMR | 95% CI | r | MODEL A SMR | 95% CI | r | MODEL B SMR | 95% CI | r |
|------|------|------|------|------|------|------|------|------|------|------|------|
| A | 368 | 0.12 | 0.58 | (0.42–0.77) | 1 | 0.74 | (0.54–0.99) | 1 | 0.67 | (0.48–0.90) | 1 |
| B | 523 | 0.19 | 0.64 | (0.52–0.78) | 2 | 0.82 | (0.67–1.00) | 2 | 0.73 | (0.59–0.88) | 2 |
| C | 747 | 0.19 | 0.66 | (0.56–0.78) | 3 | 0.84 | (0.71–1.00) | 3 | 0.84 | (0.71–0.99) | 4 |
| D | 454 | 0.21 | 0.67 | (0.55–0.82) | 4 | 0.85 | (0.69–1.04) | 4 | 0.82 | (0.67–1.01) | 3 |
| E | 434 | 0.20 | 0.68 | (0.54–0.84) | 5 | 0.88 | (0.70–1.08) | 6 | 0.85 | (0.68–1.05) | 5 |
| F | 542 | 0.24 | 0.68 | (0.57–0.81) | 6 | 0.85 | (0.71–1.01) | 5 | 0.88 | (0.74–1.05) | 6 |
| G | 850 | 0.17 | 0.69 | (0.58–0.81) | 7 | 0.89 | (0.75–1.05) | 7 | 1.04 | (0.88–1.23) | 15 |
| H | 607 | 0.23 | 0.77 | (0.64–0.91) | 8 | 0.96 | (0.81–1.14) | 8 | 1.01 | (0.85–1.20) | 11 |
| I | 470 | 0.28 | 0.77 | (0.65–0.91) | 9 | 0.97 | (0.81–1.15) | 9 | 1.01 | (0.85–1.20) | 10 |
| J | 1006 | 0.16 | 0.79 | (0.67–0.92) | 10 | 0.99 | (0.84–1.15) | 10 | 0.98 | (0.83–1.14) | 8 |
| K | 675 | 0.20 | 0.80 | (0.67–0.95) | 11 | 1.04 | (0.87–1.23) | 13 | 1.04 | (0.87–1.23) | 14 |
| L | 516 | 0.27 | 0.80 | (0.67–0.95) | 12 | 1.00 | (0.84–1.19) | 11 | 0.94 | (0.79–1.11) | 7 |
| M | 467 | 0.29 | 0.81 | (0.68–0.97) | 13 | 1.02 | (0.86–1.21) | 12 | 1.05 | (0.88–1.25) | 16 |
| N | 614 | 0.22 | 0.83 | (0.70–0.99) | 14 | 1.07 | (0.89–1.26) | 15 | 1.13 | (0.94–1.33) | 21 |
| O | 1059 | 0.20 | 0.84 | (0.73–0.96) | 15 | 1.06 | (0.92–1.21) | 14 | 1.03 | (0.89–1.17) | 12 |
| P | 665 | 0.28 | 0.84 | (0.73–0.97) | 16 | 1.07 | (0.92–1.23) | 16 | 1.11 | (0.96–1.28) | 18 |
| Q | 990 | 0.22 | 0.85 | (0.74–0.98) | 17 | 1.09 | (0.95–1.24) | 17 | 1.15 | (1.00–1.31) | 23 |
| R | 232 | 0.21 | 0.88 | (0.65–1.17) | 18 | 1.14 | (0.84–1.51) | 19 | 1.12 | (0.83–1.49) | 20 |
| S | 750 | 0.26 | 0.88 | (0.77–1.02) | 19 | 1.10 | (0.95–1.27) | 18 | 1.09 | (0.94–1.25) | 17 |
| T | 447 | 0.22 | 0.89 | (0.72–1.09) | 20 | 1.14 | (0.93–1.39) | 20 | 1.15 | (0.93–1.40) | 22 |
| U | 314 | 0.26 | 0.91 | (0.72–1.13) | 21 | 1.16 | (0.92–1.44) | 22 | 0.99 | (0.79–1.24) | 9 |
| V | 375 | 0.17 | 0.91 | (0.71–1.16) | 22 | 1.16 | (0.89–1.48) | 21 | 1.12 | (0.86–1.43) | 19 |
| W | 447 | 0.22 | 0.96 | (0.78–1.17) | 23 | 1.22 | (1.00–1.49) | 23 | 1.03 | (0.84–1.26) | 13 |
| X | 187 | 0.33 | 1.13 | (0.87–1.45) | 24 | 1.49 | (1.14–1.91) | 24 | 1.34 | (1.03–1.72) | 24 |

American study comparing the data of 47 ICUs, the authors found important discrepancies between the SMR computed with the different severity scores mainly due to differences in case-mix adjustment [14].

## Financial performance

The data collected vary according to the chosen perspective (at the ICU, hospital, or society level). There are two categories of costs: direct costs are attributable to a specific patient, whereas indirect costs (overhead costs) are shared by more than one patient. Each category can be divided into variable and fixed costs. Variable costs will be influenced by the activity (e.g., drugs, laboratory tests) while others are stable whatever the activity within the time period considered (e.g., wages for the head nurse and ICU director). Nurses' wages are usually classified as a direct variable costs but in fact in most countries, with public funding, there is no flexibility and no formal adaptation of the number of nurses according to beds, occupancy rate, and workload.

The structure of ICU cost has been studied in French ICUs (Figure 27.1). The cost-block method was tested for international comparison [15] (between France, Germany, Hungary, and the UK). Staff costs were found to be the major cost component in France, Germany, and the UK, where they can take up to 70% of total intensive care costs. Costs of clinical services include radiology, physiotherapy, blood gas analysis, and laboratory costs. Radiology costs were the highest in France and lowest in Hungary. Hospitals in the UK spent the most on blood products and drug costs. The total cost per patient day in the UK was nearly twice as expensive as in Germany and five times more expensive than in Hungary. Considering the ICU as an entity, the cost per patient-day is well suited to comparisons of expenditures between ICUs. There are large differences in resource use and costs among countries and also between national ICUs. The reasons for such differences are poorly understood. It is likely that differences in case-mix constitute the largest factor influencing these differences, but further studies will be necessary to ascertain this.

A modern directional distance function approach at the patient level enables a global appraisal of financial ICU performance [16]. The method estimates an efficient frontier that measures technical inefficiency of each patient by the use of relevant directional distance function. An ICU is technically inefficient in treating a patient if it does not minimize its

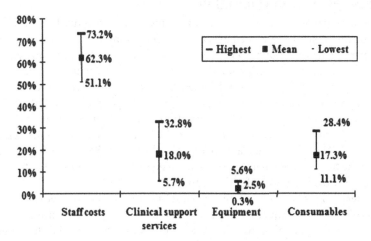

**Figure 27.1** Structure of ICU costs.

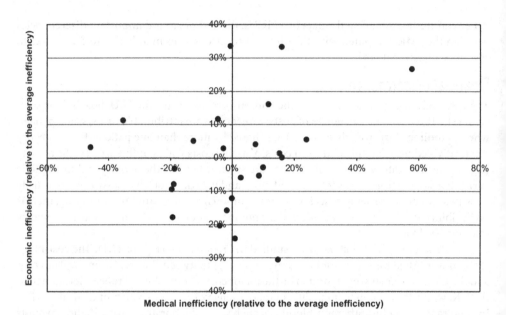

**Figure 27.2** Chart presenting both clinical performance assessed through SMR and economic performance assessed with econometric method. Study performed in French ICUs[16].

inputs given its outputs. The measure of an ICU's performance is the sum of its patients' inefficiencies. It is possible to produce a chart presenting econometric performance together with SMR. Well-performing ICUs are located in the lower left part – that is, low adjusted SMR and low technical inefficiency (Figure 27.2).

If costs are considered at the societal level, treatment after hospital discharge have to be considered.

To date, there is no parameter to measure costs associated with the burden of proxies of critical care patients.

## Academics: research and education

Several domains of research might be scrutinized, including: grant funding, number of publications, number of patients included in academic trials, number of collaborative studies, and being the primary investigator of trials. Several tools have been developed to assess the quantity and quality of scientific production. In France, scoring of scientific production as developed several years ago (Figure 27.3 and Table 27.1). Each journal is classified in its discipline (Category A gives 8 points, B = 6 points; C = 4 points; D = 3 points; E = 2 points; NC = 1 point). The points are multiplied according to the position of the author (first author ×4; second and last author ×3; third author ×2; others ×1). Only the best-ranked author is taken into account if several people from the same team coauthored the article. So an article published in the *Lancet* with the first author a member of the team gives $8 \times 4 = 32$ points. The total number of SIGAPS points provides funding for the hospital.

Faculty teaching is also quantitatively assessed, with number of medical students, residents, and fellows, but also qualitatively through satisfaction questionnaires. A list of criteria to be recognized as academic centers is usually applied, such as: journal club, multidisciplinary rounds, research meetings, inter-ICU meetings.

**Number of publications per year and category in our ICU in the last 5 years**

| Years | A | B | C | D | E | NC | Total | Score |
|-------|-----|-----|---|-----|---|-----|-------|-------|
| 2010 | 12 | 10 | 0 | 2 | 2 | 0 | 26 | 492 |
| 2011 | 18 | 2 | 2 | 1 | 0 | 2 | 25 | 442 |
| 2012 | 10 | 15 | 3 | 2 | 0 | 3 | 33 | 467 |
| 2013 | 13 | 8 | 1 | 2 | 2 | 4 | 30 | 398 |
| 2014 | 10 | 13 | 1 | 9 | 5 | 4 | 42 | 516 |
| Total | 63 | 48 | 7 | 16 | 9 | 13 | 156 | 2315 |

**Figure 27.3** Example of bibliometric assessment for a specific ICU since 2010.

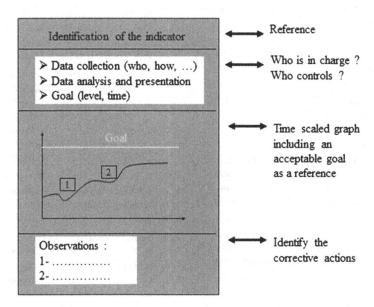

**Figure 27.4** How to improve an indicator?

# Driving changes using benchmarking

According to several indicators, some domains require changes. Most of the indicators do not provide obvious answers or plans for change. For example, excess LOS may be due to several reasons such as specific case-mix; discharge policy; absence of an intermediate care unit; presence of multi-resistant bacteria; homeless status; etc. The first step is to share the information with the team and think together in order to understand the root causes of this excess LOS. A schematic approach is depicted in Figure 27.4 and shows how to proceed to improve a specific indicator.

Recently, an ICU benchmarking program was conducted in the UK by Hutchings *et al.* [17]. This program gathered data for 96 ICUs between 1998 and 2006 and consisted of the adoption of key elements of modernization (creation of clinical networks sharing agreed protocols, the establishment of outreach services, and the adoption of care bundles) and increasing ICU capacities. This program resulted in enhanced ICU mortality adjusted to case-mix, reduction in transfers between units and in unplanned night discharges, and cost benefits.

## Conclusions

Critical care benchmarking is one method to enhance ICU performance. Benchmarking is feasible in many areas (structure and personnel, management, processes, outcomes, financial, and academic performance) and has few disadvantages and limitations. Adjustments to case-mix are essential to obtain accurate data.

## References

1. Camp R. 1989. *Benchmarking: The Search for Industry Best Practices that Leads to Superior Performance*, ASQC Quality Press, Milwaukee, WI.

2. Watson G. 1993. *Strategic Benchmarking: How to Rate Your Company's Performance Against the World's Best*, John Wiley & Sons, New York.

3. Boxwell RJ. Jr 1994. *Benchmarking for Competitive Advantage*. McGraw-Hill, New York.

4. Valentin A, Ferdinande P. ESICM Working Group on Quality Improvement: recommendations on basic requirements for intensive care units – structural and organizational aspects. *Intensive Care Med* 2011;37:1575–1587.

5. Décret n 2002-465 du 5 avril 2002 relatif aux établissements de santé publics et privés pratiquant la réanimation et modifiant le code de la santé publique (deuxième partie: Décrets en Conseil d'Etat).

6. Reignier J. Organisation de la réanimation française en 2013: état des lieux et référentiels. *Réanimation* 2013;22:1–23.9.

7. Embriaco N, Azoulay E, Barrau K, et al. High level of burnout in intensivists: prevalence and associated factors. *Am J Respir Crit Care Med* 2007;175:686–692.

8. Poncet MC, Toullic P, Papazian L, et al. Burnout syndrome in critical care nursing staff. *Am J Respir Crit Care Med* 2007;175:698–704.

9. Minvielle E, Aegerter P, Dervaux B, et al. Assessing organizational performance in ICU's: a French experience. *J Crit Care* 2008;23:236–244.

10. Festa MS. Clinical leadership in hospital care: leadership and teamwork skills are as important as clinical management skills. *BMJ*. 2005, 331:161–162.

11. Shortell SM, Zimmerman JE, Rousseau DM, et al. The performance of intensive care units: does good management make a difference?. *Med Car* 1994;32:508–525.

12. Rhodes A, Moreno RP, Azoulay E, et al., Prospectively defined indicators to improve the safety and quality of care for critically ill patients: a report from the Task Force on Safety and Quality of the European Society of Intensive Care Medicine (ESICM). *Intensive Care Med* 2012;38:598–605.

13. Aegerter Ph, Boumendil A, Retbi A, Minvielle E, Dervaux B, Guidet B. SAPS II revisited. *Intensive Care Med* 2005;31:416–423.

14. Kramer AA, Higgins TL, Zimmerman JE. Comparing observed and predicted mortality among ICUs using different prognostic systems: why do performance assessments differ? *Crit Care Med*. 2014. Epub ahead of print.

15. Negrini D, Sheppard L, Mills GH, et al. International programme for resource use in critical care (IPOC): a methodology and initial results of cost and provision in four European countries. *Acta Anaesthesiol Scandinavica* 2006;50:72–79.

16. Dervaux B, Leleu H, Minvielle E, Aegerter Ph, Guidet B. Performance of French intensive care units: a directional distance function approach at the patient level. *Int J Prod Econ*. 2009;120:585–594.

17. Hutchings A, Durand MA, Grieve R, Harrison D, Rowan K. Evaluation of modernisation of adult critical care services in England: time series and cost effectiveness analysis. *BMJ* 2009;339:b4353.

# Volume and outcome

Yên-Lan Nguyen and Bertrand Guidet

The volume of a structure is usually defined by the annual number of patients within the structure undergoing a procedure or with a medical condition. The systematic reviews by Halm *et al.* [1] and Gandjour *et al.* [2] suggest that, on average, patients requiring a high-risk medical or surgical procedure are more likely to survive in a high-volume centers. It means that there are also high-volume centers with poor outcomes and low-volume centers with good outcomes. These reviews highlight a large variation in the magnitude of the relationship between procedures, an inconsistent curve (linear or asymptote), and methodological quality discrepancies between studies (majority related to risk-adjustment methods). Both suffer from a publication bias (positive studies are more likely to be published).

Such observations lead to the creation of regionalized healthcare systems (e.g., trauma centers, high-risk surgeries, perinatal care) [3,4,5]. Regionalization of critical illness is particularly attractive in a period of increasing demand of critical care and in the setting of constrained resources [6]. Indeed, regionalization could both improve survival and reduce costs by concentrating high-risk critically ill patients at centers with concentrated resources and expertise to deliver high-quality care. Kahn *et al.* [7], using a Monte-Carlo simulation, suggested that the systematic transfer of invasive mechanically ventilated patient from low- to high-volume structures (with a median distance transfer of 8.5 miles) could save annually thousand of lives in the USA (representing a number needed to treat of 15.7). Implementing a regionalized critical care system is associated with potential risks (harm during transport, discontinuity of care, loss of medical skills in low-volume centers, overwhelming resources in high-volume centers) and barriers (lack of centralized authority, stakeholder resistance) [6]. Before implementing a critical care regionalized system, we need first to better characterize the volume–outcome relationship in critical illness.

## The potential mechanisms underlying the volume–outcome relationship

To date, besides the definition of volume and outcome used, the exact underlying mechanisms of the volume–outcome relationship remain unknown. Two potential mechanisms initially proposed by Luft were "practice makes perfect" and "selective referral" [8]. Two other mechanisms are the processes of care used and the structural factors. Understanding these different mechanisms will allow determination of whether we should expand the size of current

*Quality Management in Intensive Care*, ed. Bertrand Guidet, Andreas Valentin and Hans Flaatten. Published by Cambridge University Press. © Cambridge University Press 2016.

low-volume centers or whether we should implement within low-volume centers, specific characteristics from high-volume centers associated with enhanced outcomes.

## The definitions of volume and outcome used

The definitions of volume and outcome used influence the volume–outcome relationship. It is likely that current negative volume–outcome studies would have shown different results depending on the definitions of volume or outcome used.

For example, Macias *et al.* showed that in comparison to the volume of admissions of traumatic spinal cord injury, the volume of those patients requiring urgent spinal surgery was associated with enhanced outcome (reduced paralysis) [9]. Then, the curve of the relationship not being always linear, the narrower the selected ranges of volume studied, the greater the probability to obtain negative results.

The outcome most commonly used in critical care literature remains mortality. Recent data suggest the importance of studying other meaningful patient-centered outcomes, such as long-term quality of life or healthcare use [10]. To our knowledge, no study looking at the volume–outcome relationship in critical care has used such outcomes.

## "Practice makes perfect"

This first mechanism proposed by Luft [8] seems logical: the more you perform a complex task the better you will be at conducting this task in the future. It underlies that volume itself leads to better quality and improved outcomes. Unfortunately, longitudinal studies showing that volume change influences patient outcomes over time are lacking.

This mechanism seems particularly valid for complex, critically ill patients (e.g., hematology patients) [11], rare situations (e.g., acute respiratory distress syndrome with refractory hypoxemia) [12] or "exceptional" organ support (e.g., extra-corporeal membrane oxygenation) [13]. But thinking that expansion of the size of a small unit alone will enhance patient outcomes would be too simplistic. Indeed, taking care of complex patients, rare situations, or "exceptional" organ support requires long-term knowledge acquisition of all the medical and nursing staff and induces clinical practice (e.g., care bundles) and organizational changes. As shown in the medical literature, despite good access to technological tools and a large diffusion of international recommendations, the gap between evidence-based medicine and clinical practice remains large, even in high-volume academic centers [14].

## "Selective referral"

The second mechanism proposed by Luft [8] means that a center with good outcomes and reputation is more likely to recruit patients, to increase its annual volume, and to become a high-volume center. Such a mechanism may be true for scheduled surgery or medical conditions, but its application to critical care would be hazardous. Indeed, the admission to a critical care unit is most often a medical decision related to an acute situation (e.g., respiratory failure, shock, coma) requiring immediate therapeutics and not allowing long discussions on when or where treatments should be initiated.

## Processes of care

In critical care, bundles implementation (e.g., ventilator care, sepsis) is associated with improved outcomes [15,16]. Unfortunately, studies showing that volume change is associated with bundles implementation are lacking. Dres *et al.* found that patients with acute exacerbations of chronic obstructive pulmonary disease were more likely to receive non-invasive ventilation in high-volume ICUs, and with survival benefits [17]. In a case-vignettes study

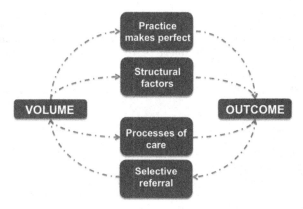

**Figure 28.1** Potential mechanisms of the volume–outcome relationship.

testing the clinical practice variability of French and Swiss intensivists on mechanical ventilation in 40 centers, we could not find any association between clinical practice and ICU annual volume (total of mechanically ventilated patients)[18]. The majority of participating centers had ventilator care bundles but we observed a gap between having them, knowing of their existence, and implementing them in daily practice.

## Structural factors

Several critical care structural factors are associated with improved outcomes (e.g., physician staffing, nurse:patient ratio, multidisciplinary rounds) [19]. Unfortunately, studies showing that volume change is associated with structural factors are lacking. Stub *et al.* [20] showed that volume itself did not influence the prognosis of patients suffering from out-of-hospital cardiac arrest. On the other hand, a survival benefit was observed among patients treated in hospitals with 24-hour cardiac interventional services. A proxy of structural factors might be the teaching status. Indeed, academic centers are more likely to be large structures and are supposed to have easier access to the most up-to-date knowledge.

## The volume–outcome relationship in critical illness: insights from the literature

Two systematic reviews on the volume–outcome relationship in critical illness have been published [21,22]. Both share the same conclusions: on average, high-volume structures are associated with improved outcomes but the relationship is not consistent across diagnostic groups, and when present may not always have a linear curve. High-risk critically ill patients (such as hematology patients), those requiring invasive mechanical ventilation, or those with severe sepsis seem to be more likely to benefit from high-volume structures.

Since these publications, several studies have been published. We will describe the results of the studies published after 2010 (not included in the systematic review of Kanhere *et al.* [22]), for two organ supports (invasive mechanical ventilation and renal replacement therapy) and for one common diagnosis (severe sepsis). The results of these studies are summarized in Table 28.1.

## Mechanical ventilation

Mechanical ventilation is the organ support most commonly used in critical care (concerns more than 40% of patients) and is associated with a high morbidity and mortality

**Table 28.1** Main characteristics of studies on the volume–outcome relationship published after 2010

| Population | Reference | Origin | Volume level | Structures | Patients | Clinical risk adjustment | Effect |
|---|---|---|---|---|---|---|---|
| Mechanical ventilation | Gopal, 2011 | UK | Hospital | 12 | 17,132 | Yes | No |
| | Cooke, 2012 | USA | Hospital | 119 | 5131 | Yes | No |
| | Moran, 2012 | Australia, New Zealand | ICU | 136 | 208,810 | Yes | No |
| | Fernandez, 2013 | Spain | ICU | 29 | 1923 | Yes | Yes |
| | Shahin, 2014 | UK | ICU | 193 | 104,844 | Yes | Yes |
| Renal replacement therapy | Nguyen, 2011 | France, USA | ICU | 108 | 12,947 | Yes | No |
| | Vaara, 2012 | Finland | ICU | 23 | 1558 | Yes | Yes |
| Sepsis | Powell, 2010 | USA | ED | 551 | 87,166 | Yes | Yes |
| | Banta, 2012 | USA | Hospital | ? | 1,213,219 | Yes | Yes |
| | Zuber, 2012 | France | ICU | 41 | 3437 | Yes | Yes |
| | Shahin, 2012 | UK | ICU | 170 | 30,727 | Yes | No |
| | Walkey, 2014 | USA | Hospital | 126 | 56,997 | Yes | Yes |

(around 30%) [23]. Several processes of care related to mechanical ventilation (sedation and analgesia, ventilator settings, weaning) are associated with improved outcomes and recommended by major critical care professional societies [24].

Since 2010, five studies looked at the volume–outcome relationship among patients requiring invasive mechanical ventilation and showed mixed results. These results should be interpreted with caution because they come from very different healthcare system organizations and consequently different case-mixes (e.g., universal single payer vs. fee for service payment system, high vs. low national density of ICU beds).

In comparison to the results of Shahin *et al.* [25], the negative results of the study by Gopal *et al.* [26] may be explained by a lack of power to detect any difference due to the much smaller sample size (regional vs. national perspective). The negative results of the study of Cooke *et al.* [27] may be explained either by a lack of power (median volume 40 [19;62]) (in comparison to the study of Kahn *et al.* with much larger volume ranges (median volume 274 [150;391]) [28]), either by the small variation across volume ranges or by the specific organization of the Veteran Affairs healthcare system. Moran *et al.* [29] found a relatively flat volume–outcome curve and their data even showed an association between higher volume and poorer outcomes (upper threshold of 353 patients per year). The lack of volume–outcome relationship observed in this very large database (15 years of data, more than 200,000 patients) may be related to the organization of critical care in these two countries (with only closed ICUs, a long-established training scheme, and routine transfers between structures). Overwhelming resources could be an explanation of the asymptote curve, regarding the very low median annual volume in this cohort (77 patients per year). The positive studies of Shahin *et al.* [25] and Fernandez *et al.* [30] did not look specifically at the bundles of care used or structural ICU factors.

## Renal replacement therapy

Renal replacement therapy concerns around 5% of patients with acute kidney injury and is associated with a very high morbidity and mortality (50%) [31]. To date, there are no recommendations in terms of type (continuous vs. intermittent), timing, or dose of renal replacement therapy.

Since 2010, two studies have looked specifically at the volume–outcome relationship among patients requiring renal replacement therapy; they showed mixed results. Nguyen *et al.* [32] studied the volume–outcome relationship in two different healthcare systems (France and the USA) and found no association between high-volume structures and patient outcomes. They adjusted their results to patient severity, ICU, and hospital characteristics. On the other hand, Vaara *et al.* [33] found a positive association among Finnish patients. The major differences between these two studies are the case-mix (Finnish patients were less severe), the volume ranges (RRT volume was much lower in Finland in comparison to France), and the lack of adjustments to ICU and hospital characteristics. Therefore, making comparisons or recommendations would be hazardous.

## Severe sepsis

The prevalence of sepsis is increasing and one in four critically ill patients with severe sepsis or septic shock will die [34]. Every four years, the Surviving Sepsis campaign, sponsored by major critical care professional societies, update guidelines for the management of septic patients [35]. The recommended bundles (six-hour resuscitation and 24-hour management bundles) are associated with improved outcomes.

Since 2010, five studies looked at the volume–outcome relationship of patients with sepsis. The majority of them (three studies from the USA [36,37,38] and one from France [39]) found a positive association. One from the UK [40], with a large database (from the Intensive Care National Audit and Research Center program (ICNARC), including more than 30,000 patients) found no relation between volume and outcome for all admissions of adult patients with sepsis in the UK. One of the underlying reasons may be the program ICNARC itself, which promotes bundle implementation, community outreach, and ICU benchmarking. Such a method is an incentive for ICUs to improve their clinical practice and subsequently patient outcomes.

To conclude, current data on the volume–outcome relationship in critical care suggest that, on average, higher volume leads to better outcome. A better understanding of the underlying mechanisms of this relationship and, particularly, the role of structural factors is essential before considering the possibility of the regionalization of critical illness.

## References

1. Halm EA, Lee C, Chassin MR. Is volume related to outcome in health care? A systematic review and methodologic critique of the literature. *Ann Intern Med.* 2002;137(6):511–520.

2. Gandjour A, Bannenberg A, Lauterbach KW. Threshold volumes associated with higher survival in health care: a systematic review. *Med Care.* 2003;41(10): 1129–1141.

3. Nathens AB, Jurkovich GJ, Maier RV, *et al.* Relationship between trauma center volume and outcomes. *JAMA.* 2001;285(9):1164–1171.

4. Studnicki J, Craver C, Blanchette CM, Fisher JW, Shahbazi S. A cross-sectional retrospective analysis of the regionalization of complex surgery. *BMC Surg.* 2014;14:55.

5. Lasswell SM, Barfield WD, Rochat RW, Blackmon L. Perinatal regionalization for very low-birth-weight and very preterm infants: a meta-analysis. *JAMA.* 2010;304(9):992–1000.

6. Nguyen Y-L, Kahn JM, Angus DC. Reorganizing adult critical care delivery: the role of regionalization, telemedicine, and community outreach. *Am J Respir Crit Care Med.* 2010;181(11):1164–1169.

7. Kahn JM, Linde-Zwirble WT, Wunsch H, *et al.* Potential value of regionalized intensive care for mechanically ventilated medical patients. *Am J Respir Crit Care Med.* 2008;177(3):285–291.

8. Luft HS, Bunker JP, Enthoven AC. Should operations be regionalized? The empirical relation between surgical volume and mortality. *N Engl J Med.* 1979;301(25):1364–1369.

9. Macias CA, Rosengart MR, Puyana J-C, *et al.* The effects of trauma center care, admission volume, and surgical volume on paralysis after traumatic spinal cord injury. *Ann Surg.* 2009;249(1):10–17.

10. Elliott D, Davidson JE, Harvey MA, *et al.* Exploring the scope of post-intensive care syndrome therapy and care: engagement of non-critical care providers and survivors in a second stakeholders meeting. *Crit Care Med.* 2014;42:2518–2526.

11. Lecuyer L, Chevret S, Guidet B, *et al.* Case volume and mortality in haematological patients with acute respiratory failure. *Eur Respir J.* 2008;32(3):748–754.

12. Darmon M, Azoulay E, Fulgencio J-P, *et al.* Procedure volume is one determinant of centre effect in mechanically ventilated patients. *Eur Respir J.* 2011;37(2):364–370.

13. Noah MA, Peek GJ, Finney SJ, *et al.* Referral to an extracorporeal membrane oxygenation center and mortality among patients with severe 2009 influenza A(H1N1). *JAMA.* 2011;306(15):1659–1668.

14. Tonelli MR, Curtis JR, Guntupalli KK, *et al.* An official multi-society statement: the role of clinical research results in the practice of critical care medicine. *Am J Respir Crit Care Med.* 2012;185(10):1117–1124.

15. Hutchings A, Durand MA, Grieve R, *et al.* Evaluation of modernisation of adult critical care services in England: time series and cost effectiveness analysis. *BMJ.* 2009;339:b4353.

16. van Zanten ARH, Brinkman S, Arbous MS, *et al.* Guideline bundles adherence and mortality in severe sepsis and septic shock. *Crit Care Med.* 2014;42(8):1890–1898.

17. Dres M, Tran T-C, Aegerter P, *et al.* Influence of ICU case-volume on the management and hospital outcomes of acute exacerbations of chronic obstructive pulmonary disease. *Crit Care Med.* 2013;41(8):1884–1892.

18. Nguyen Y-L, Perrodeau E, Guidet B, *et al.* Mechanical ventilation and clinical practice heterogeneity in intensive care units: a multicenter case-vignette study. *Ann Intensive Care.* 2014;4(1):2.

19. Nguyen Y-L, Wunsch H, Angus DC. Critical care: the impact of organization and management on outcomes. *Curr Opin Crit Care.* 2010;16(5):487–492.

20. Stub D, Smith K, Bray JE, Bernard S, Duffy SJ, Kaye DM. Hospital characteristics are associated with patient outcomes following out-of-hospital cardiac arrest. *Heart Br Card Soc.* 2011;97(18):1489–1494.

21. Abbenbroek B, Duffield CM, Elliott D. The intensive care unit volume–mortality relationship, is bigger better? An integrative literature review. *Aust Crit Care Off J Confed Aust Crit Care Nurses.* 2014;27:157–164.

22. Kanhere MH, Kanhere HA, Cameron A, Maddern GJ. Does patient volume affect clinical outcomes in adult intensive care units? *Intensive Care Med.* 2012;38(5):741–751.

23. Esteban A, Anzueto A, Frutos F, *et al.* Characteristics and outcomes in adult patients receiving mechanical ventilation: a 28-day international study. *JAMA.* 2002;287(3):345–355.

24. Tonelli MR, Curtis JR, Guntupalli KK, *et al.* An official multi-society statement: the role of clinical research results in the practice of critical care medicine. *Am J Respir Crit Care Med.* 2012;185(10):1117–1124.

25. Shahin J, Harrison DA, Rowan KM. Is the volume of mechanically ventilated admissions to UK critical care units associated with improved outcomes? *Intensive Care Med.* 2014;40(3):353–360.

26. Gopal S, O'Brien R, Pooni J. The relationship between hospital volume and mortality following mechanical ventilation in the Intensive Care Unit. *Minerva Anestesiol.* 2011;77(1):26–32.

27. Cooke CR, Kennedy EH, Wiitala WL, Almenoff PL, Sales AE, Iwashyna TJ. Despite variation in volume, Veterans

Affairs hospitals show consistent outcomes among patients with non-postoperative mechanical ventilation. *Crit Care Med.* 2012;40(9):2569–2575.

28. Kahn JM, Goss CH, Heagerty PJ, Kramer AA, O'Brien CR, Rubenfeld GD. Hospital volume and the outcomes of mechanical ventilation. *N Engl J Med.* 2006;355(1):41–50.

29. Moran JL, Bristow P, Solomon PJ, George C, Hart GK. Mortality and length-of-stay outcomes, 1993–2003, in the binational Australian and New Zealand intensive care adult patient database. *Crit Care Med.* 2008;36(1):46–61.

30. Fernández R, Altaba S, Cabre L, *et al.* Relationship between volume and survival in closed intensive care units is weak and apparent only in mechanically ventilated patients. *Anesthesiology.* 2013;119(4):871–879.

31. Uchino S, Kellum JA, Bellomo R, *et al.* Acute renal failure in critically ill patients: a multinational, multicenter study. *JAMA.* 2005;294(7):813–818.

32. Nguyen Y-L, Milbrandt EB, Weissfeld LA, *et al.* Intensive care unit renal support therapy volume is not associated with patient outcome. *Crit Care Med.* 2011;39(11):2470–2477.

33. Vaara ST, Reinikainen M, Kaukonen K-M, Pettilä V. Association of ICU size and annual case volume of renal replacement therapy patients with mortality. *Acta Anaesthesiol Scand.* 2012;56(9):1175–1182.

34. Angus DC, Linde-Zwirble WT, Lidicker J, Clermont G, Carcillo J, Pinsky MR. Epidemiology of severe sepsis in the United States: analysis of incidence, outcome, and associated costs of care. *Crit Care Med.* 2001;29(7):1303–1310.

35. Dellinger RP, Levy MM, Rhodes A, *et al.* Surviving Sepsis Campaign: international guidelines for management of severe sepsis and septic shock, 2012. *Intensive Care Med.* 2013;39(2):165–228.

36. Powell ES, Khare RK, Courtney DM, Feinglass J. Volume of emergency department admissions for sepsis is related to inpatient mortality: results of a nationwide cross-sectional analysis. *Crit Care Med.* 2010;38(11):2161–2168.

37. Banta JE, Joshi KP, Beeson L, Nguyen HB. Patient and hospital characteristics associated with inpatient severe sepsis mortality in California, 2005–2010. *Crit Care Med.* 2012;40(11):2960–2966.

38. Walkey AJ, Wiener RS. Hospital case volume and outcomes among patients hospitalized with severe sepsis. *Am J Respir Crit Care Med.* 2014;189(5):548–555.

39. Zuber B, Tran T-C, Aegerter P, *et al.* Impact of case volume on survival of septic shock in patients with malignancies. *Crit Care Med.* 2012;40(1):55–62.

40. Shahin J, Harrison DA, Rowan KM. Relation between volume and outcome for patients with severe sepsis in United Kingdom: retrospective cohort study. *BMJ.* 2012;344:e3394.

# Competence-based training and education

Francesca Rubulotta and Adrian Wong

## Definition of competence-based training and/or competence-based education

Competence-based training (CBT) supports individual learning and development by identifying the behaviour, knowledge, and skills that are necessary for a successful performance in a profession [1]. A 'competent' individual should have the ability to do something successfully or efficiently.

According to the Australian Medical Association a competency is a 'measurable ability'. It is an expertise that can be assessed with reliability and validity against a commonly agreed standard [2].

The concept of CBT does not originate from medical training but from the more complex world of vocational education. Vocational educational training provides practical experience in a particular occupational field, such as agriculture, home economics, or industry. Vocational education is linked to real life; traditional medical education instead has been criticized for its failure to ensure that all graduates are adequately prepared for clinical practice and independent work at the bedside [1].

The 2010 General Medical Council (GMC) training survey in the UK found that more than 10% of doctors coming towards the end of their training are not confident to take up a new role as a consultant or general practitioner [3]. The reason seemed to be that most medical training programmes around the world are still organized in terms of time spent on defined rotations rather than on the achievement of competencies. The GMC emphasized the need to ensure that medical training is fit for the purposes of delivering high-quality healthcare for the population served [3]. Medical education is therefore undergoing a paradigm shift, from the traditional time-based model (as a surrogate for experience) to a programme that requires documentation of proficiency [1,4].

Southgate defined CBT as being 'composed of cognitive, interpersonal skills, moral and personality attributes. It is in part the ability, in part the will, to consistently select and perform relevant clinical tasks in the context of the social environment, in order to resolve health problems of individuals in an efficient, effective economic and humane manner' [5].

Frank et al. published a more recent and elaborate definition of competency-based education (CBE) in medicine as a result of a systematic review of published definitions [6]. These

Quality Management in Intensive Care, ed. Bertrand Guidet, Andreas Valentin and Hans Flaatten. Published by Cambridge University Press. © Cambridge University Press 2016.

authors concluded that 'CBE is an approach to preparing physicians for practice that is fundamentally oriented to graduate outcome abilities and organized around competencies derived from an analysis of societal and patient needs. It de-emphasizes time-based training and promises greater accountability, flexibility, and learner-centeredness' [6]. CBE is clearly an emergent topic; however, Frank *et al.* showed that there 'is great heterogeneity in the medical CBE literature'. Several authors promoted the concept of 'progression of competence', meaning that learners advance along a series of defined milestones on their way to the explicit outcome goals of training [6]. Others presented the notion of 'outcome-based frameworks requiring a defined scheme of levels of progression towards the outcome' [6]. The structure of CBE is poorly defined and a new systematic review might be needed in the future to indicate keys elements. They have also identified ten recurring themes that form the fundamental concepts of the CBE but not the structure [6]. CBE curriculum and assessment methods need to be clarified at the beginning of the training and the competencies need to be the core of the process. Duration of training – i.e. time – is not crucial in CBE.

In 2004, competencies for intensive care medicine (ICM) were created by the Competency-Based Training in ICM (CoBaTrICE) collaborative, which was promoted by the European Society of Intensive Care Medicine (ESICM), supported by the Leonardo Da Vinci European Programme. The Leonardo programme was part of the European Union's Lifelong Learning Programme which supported vocational education and training (VET) organizations, staff, and learners as well as ICM to work together with European partners to improve training, skills, and employability. The CoBaTrICE collaboration was formed with the objective of developing an adequate CBT programme in ICM in Europe [7]. Members of the collaborative defined CBT as 'the ability to integrate generic professional attributes with specialist knowledge, skills and attitudes and apply them in the workplace' [7]. CoBaTrICE was designed to enhance life-long learning and to harmonize standards across national borders, thereby facilitating free movement of ICM professionals [7]. It was the first successful attempt in generating a curriculum and syllabus based on agreed minimum competencies required to become a specialist in ICM in Europe. There is no doubt that factors such as political, social, economic, health needs, and resources play some part in defining CBT at a national level [8].

## The challenge of using CBT in Europe

The process of CBT includes analysing the strains of a particular job before defining the final outcome and thus translating this into the basic essentials of the profession. A competency within medicine is rather challenging to define and to assess. The questions the trainer would ask are: What are we requiring this individual to do? Can this individual perform a specific task? How can we assess the ability of the individual to perform a certain task?

Adequate training is crucial to ensure doctors have the right attitudes, skills, knowledge, and qualities to practice. Training centres and training leaders are key to this process. However, a formal national system for quality assurance of training in ICM exists in only 18 (64%) of European countries according to a 2008 survey [9]. Consequently, there is considerable diversity in educational structures, processes, and quality assurance across Europe [9]. National training organizations (NTOs) or national accreditation bodies (NABs) should consider developing common standards for quality assurance based on CBT. More recently, the European Union of Medical Specialists (UEMS) Council named a similar path, 'common training framework' (CTF), applicable to several specialties with similar requirements for training and certification (directive 2005/36/EC for the free movement of professionals in Europe, amended 2013/55/EU) [10,11]. The ICM CTF has constructed the list of competencies needed and has described the characteristics of the trainers and the training centres. The CTF will enhance the use of CBT even further in the field of ICM. The current challenge is that all elements of medical training need to be planned so that trainees are able to achieve all competencies within the legal framework mandated by the European Working Time Directive (EWTD) [11,12]. The EWTD is a European Union (EU) initiative designed to prevent employers from forcing excessive hours on their employees. Prolonged working hours have implications for health and safety and these seem much greater than the ones anticipated by their original developers. The EWTD reduces the working time to an average of 48 hours per week. The EWTD (2003/88) and the directive describing the recognition of professional qualifications (2005/36/EU and 2013/55/EU) were not originally designed for healthcare delivery or healthcare professionals [12,13]. There are several concerns related to reduced training opportunities and training time [12,13]. Moreover, it is no longer acceptable, or appropriate, for trainees at any level of training to practice new skills on patients, even if they have a patient's explicit consent [1]. A primary aim is for trainees to practice skills in a safe environment, before performing them on the real patient. At present, simulation-based training is essential in high-reliability organizations (e.g. airline, nuclear, and oil industries) yet remains a niche player in medical education [1]. CBT ideally should use tools such as simulation and work-based assessment to face the challenge of achieving a long list of competence in an increasingly limited time frame.

## Training healthcare providers/professionals with a new method

The CoBaTrICE collaboration stated that CBT is 'a strategy which aims to standardize the outcome of training rather than the educational processes' [14]. Beyond the problem of training, competency is at the heart of the wider issues of accreditation, appraisals, and revalidations for all healthcare professionals.

CBT is increasingly used for delivering training at all levels of medical education, including undergraduate and postgraduate degrees [15]. Most of the time, CBT is combined with more traditional forms of training. However, when compared to the conventional approach, there is no fixed time period in CBT. The focus of CBE is on the learner and the achievement of required competencies. The demonstration of a competency at the time of assessment is the primary principle, and for those trainees who are able to demonstrate competence more rapidly, this will mean accelerated progression through the training. Nevertheless, it also means that training time could potentially be lengthened due to the amount of assessments required to complete each individual competency in the curriculum.

Development of CBT programmes can be summarized by the following steps [15,16,17]:
- Determine the appropriate competencies (knowledge, skills, attitude, behaviours).
- Devise the training programme.
- Promote reflective practices.
- Devise appropriate assessment and appraisal methods.
- Defining the pass standards.

In CBT the learner is given the responsibility for their own training and professional development. The programme defines the outcomes (competencies) required of physicians at different stages of training, and provides guidelines for the assessment of these outcomes and educational resources to support their acquisition within the workplace [17,18]. Outcomes, articulated as competency statements, are defined in a manner that facilitates integration of knowledge, skills and attitudes, and assessment of performance to a common standard during routine clinical work [7,9,18]. In CBT, teaching involves seminars, simulation, group discussions, active clinical learning experiences, reflective practice, and ongoing formative assessment, including peer review [18,19,20]. The workplace is part of the teaching, and therefore learning opportunities should be created [17,19]. The capability to reflect consciously upon one's professional practice is generally considered important for the development of expertise and, hence, education. Reflective practice and its application can be learned to gain a better understanding of its relation to competencies development in medicine.

## Assessments

The challenge is to measure the impact of training in terms of improved patient care and to assess the extent to which a physician is a self directed reflective thinker.

*MB Anderson, senior director of educational affairs, AAMC*

Assessment in CBT should include an appropriate balance of formative and summative assessment methods. It should provide insight into trainees' actual performance, as well as their capacity to adapt to changes. The CBT aims at generating new knowledge and improving overall performance. Each assessment is an objective decision that needs to be made based upon observations made by the trainer. Hence, it is crucial that as part of the training programme, there are tools and processes available to identify and support weaker candidates. Although various assessments tools have been developed, a common theme is that they need to be sufficiently robust and fit for purpose. Objective structured clinical examinations (OSCEs) were developed as the logical way of assessing candidates [17,18]. Standardization and the use of checklists are also advocated.

Training workplace-based assessment includes:

- Case-based discussion (CBD), which is a tool for assessing competencies related to a trainee's management of a patient. CBDs are used to judge clinical reasoning, decision-making, and use of knowledge in relation to a specific patient's care. This tool should include written records related to the patient's care (such as notes, discharge summary).
- Clinical evaluation (CEX) or mini CEX are learning tools used to evaluate a clinical skill such as history taking, clinical examination, and reasoning.
- Direct observation of procedural skills (DOPS) is an assessment tool designed to evaluate the functioning of a trainee undertaking a practical procedure. DOPS should ideally be performed using a structured checklist or following accepted clinical standards of practice. DOPS have been divided into routine and life-threatening procedures, with a clear differentiation of formative and summative sign off.
- The acute care assessment tool (ACAT) is designed for supervised learning in acute medical care. The ACAT looks at clinical appraisal, decision-making, team working, time management, prioritization, record keeping, communication, leadership skills, and handover for the whole time period and for multiple critically acutely ill patients.
- The audit assessment (AA) tool looks at a trainee's competence in completing an audit. The AA can be the review of audit documentation or a presentation of the audit at a department meeting.
- 360 degree evaluations and patient/family surveys are tools used to assess professionalism, including behaviour of the doctor and effectiveness of the consultation.
- Multisource feedback (MsF) is a method for assessing generic skills such as communication, leadership, team working, reliability, etc. This is based on the objective

systematic collection of feedback forms from a number of colleagues containing performance data on a trainee. The trainee will not see the individual responses. The summary of the MsF report is given by the educational supervisor.

- The multiple consultant report (MCR) is designed to capture consultants' views on a trainee's clinical performance.
- The quality improvement project assessment tool (QIPAT) is designed to assess a trainee's competence in completing a quality improvement project.
- Teaching observation (TO) is designed to provide structured, formative feedback to trainees on their competence in delivering teaching.

## Criticisms and limitations in CBT/CBE

Like most other professions, doctors are expected to perform a variety of complex tasks to a high level. Unfortunately, identifying the range of competencies required in medicine is challenging. Moreover, current patient care is complex due to the combination of the increase in patients' ages, expectations, and the increase of technologies. Doctors need to integrate new knowledge and skills and apply these appropriately in the treatment and care of their patients. ICM specialists need to rapidly assess benefit versus harm, uncertainty, and risks related to critical illness. These higher-order skills need to be developed progressively over time through significant patient contact, across a range of clinical settings, and through ongoing mentoring and feedback by senior clinicians. ICM doctors not only need to master individual competencies, but they must also learn how, when, and why to use them [1]. CBT has a particularly strong role in teaching and assessing the basics of procedural skills (e.g. suturing, urinary-catheter insertion, airway management skills). However, it has its limitations in assessing the candidate's professionalism and decision-making ability with regards to these skills and attitudes. Perhaps the greatest concern over CBT is that observing a trainee's proficiency in individual competencies alone does not ensure they are capable of integrating these skills into the comprehensive care of a wide range of patients and complex settings. Each 'competence' is context- and grade-specific. Competence (what a doctor can do) does not equate to performance (what a doctor does do) and certainly doesn't guarantee performance or safe practice. Proponents of CBT would argue that these limitations can be overcome by awareness that:

- competency is a broad objective and requires the integration of knowledge, skills, and behaviour;
- one needs to set the appropriate competencies for the appropriate level;
- achieving competency does not stop further learning and hence the pursuit of excellence.

## Why is CBT important for intensive care medicine?

CBT is important for the future of ICM because this discipline is not a recognized specialty in Europe. In November 2013, the directive 2005/36/EC for the free movement of professionals in Europe was amended by the Directive 2013/55/EU. This amendment has created the possibility of introducing new avenues for automatic recognition through the 'Common Training Principles' based on the harmonization of the minimum training requirements. In October 2014 a CTF for ICM was presented and accepted by UEMS, the oldest medical organization in Europe, with a current membership of 34 countries. It is the representative organization of the National Associations of Medical Specialists in the European Union and its associated countries. Its structure consists of a council responsible for 39 specialist sections and their European boards, addressing training in their respective specialty and incorporating representatives from academia (societies, colleges, and universities) with strong links to European institutions (European Commission and Parliament), other independent European medical organizations, and European medical/scientific societies. It sets high standards for healthcare practice throughout the EU. Competencies and the education related to the acquisition of listed competencies represent the main content of the CTF document. This will facilitate the safe movement of intensive care doctors even if ICM is not their primary specialty. This strategy is based on the call for tender CHAFEA/2014/Health/04 concerning the support for the definition of core competencies of healthcare assistants whose objective is to carry out a study that will explore the feasibility and prepare for a future suggestion for the establishment of a CTF for healthcare assistants (HCAs) in the EU. This is a new initiative and the European Board for ICM (EBICM) and the Multi Joint Commission for ICM (MJCICM) have achieved working together.

In conclusion, there are two main aspects related to CBT and CBE in ICM. The first is the model of teaching and adult education. The second is the need for an easily reproducible and adequate system to allow free movement of ICM specialists across Europe. The use of CBT could be the best way to achieve this. We are the first specialty to create and promote CTF in Europe. Other specialties will need to develop their own method of training that will maintain high standards within a reduced-hours environment. The pressure on ICM is higher compared to other specialties that can use automatic recognition of their training in Europe [10,11] As the total numbers of 'hands-on hours' in training has been reduced as a consequence of EWTD, CBT may become preferable if planned and structured adequately from the beginning. The new document describing the CTF suggests that ICM training in Europe should be a total of three years, with a maximum of two years in a core speciality. Implementation of the CTF will be done independently in each European member state and hopefully this will generate high-quality professionals able to work in the library as well as at the bedside.

# References

1. Aggarawl R, Darzi A. Technical skills training in the 21st century. *NEJM* 2006; 355: 2695–2696.
2. Australian Medical Association. Positional statement: Competency based training in medical education, 2010.
3. General Medical Council *National Training Surveys, Key Findings*. London: GMC, 2010.
4. Debas HT, Bass BL, Brennan MF, *et al.* American Surgical Association Blue Ribbon Committee Report on Surgical Education: 2004. *Ann Surg* 2005; 241: 1–8.
5. Southgate L. Professional competence in medicine. *Hospital Medicine* 1999; 60: 203–205.
6. Frank JR, Mungroo R, Ahmad Y, Wang M, De Rossi S, Horsley T. Toward a definition of competency-based education in medicine: a systematic review of published definitions. *Medical Teacher* 2010; 32 (8): 631–637.
7. Barrett H, Bion J. Development of core competencies for an international training programme in intensive care medicine. *Intensive Care Med* 2006; 32 (9): 1371–1383.
8. McGaghie WC, Miller GE, Sajid AW, Telder TV. *Competency-based Curriculum Development in Medical Education: An Introduction*. Geneva: World Health Organization, 1978.
9. CoBaTrICE Collaboration. The educational environment for training in intensive care medicine: structures, processes, outcomes and challenges in the European region. *Intensive Care Med* 2009; 35: 1575–1583.

10. Rhodes A, Chiche J-D, Moreno R. Improving the quality of training programs in intensive care: a view from the ESICM. *Intensive Care Med* 2011; 37: 377–379.

11. Directive 2005/36/EC of the European Parliament and of the Council of 7 September 2005 on the recognition of professional qualifications. http://eur-lex.europa.eu/legal-content/EN/TXT/PDF/?uri=CELEX:02005L0036-20140117&from=EN (accessed 20 March 2015).

12. Directive 2003/88/EC of the European Parliament and of the Council of 4 November 2003 concerning certain aspects of the organisation of working time. http://eur-lex.europa.eu/legal-content/EN/ALL/?uri=CELEX:32003L0088 (accessed 20 March 2015).

13. Rubulotta F, Moreno R, Rhodes A. Intensive care medicine: finding its way in the 'European labyrinth'. *Intensive Care Med* 2011; 37(2): 1907–1912.

14. Rubulotta F, Gullo A, Iapichino G, *et al.* (2009) The Competency-Based Training in Intensive Care Medicine in Europe (CoBaTrICE) Italian collaborative: national results from the Picker survey. *Minerva Anesthesiol* 75: 117–124.

15. Leung W-C. Competency based medical training: review. *BMJ* 2002;325:693–696.

16. Holmboe E, Snell L. Principles of competency-based education: better preparation for learners for practice. In *Educational Design: A CanMEDS Guide for Health Professionals*, edited by Sherbino J and Frank J. Ottawa: Royal College of Physicians and Surgeons of Canada, 2011.

17. Cook RJ, Pedley DK, Thakore S. A structured competency based training programme for junior trainees in emergency medicine: the 'Dundee Model'. *Emerg Med J* 2006; 23: 18–22.

18. Royal Colleges of Physicians Training Board. Recommendations for specialty trainee assessment and review incorporating lessons learnt from the workplace-based assessment pilot. 2014. www.jrcptb.org.uk/assessment (accessed 20 March 2015).

19. Mamede S, Schmidt HG. The structure of reflective practice in medicine. *Medical Education* 2004; 38: 1302–1308.

20. Frank, JR. *The CanMEDS 2005 Physician Competency Framework: Better Standards. Better Physicians. Better Care.* Ottawa: Royal College of Physicians and Surgeons of Canada, 2005.

# Applications of telemedicine in the intensive care unit

Rob Boots, Neil Widdicombe, and Jeffrey Lipman

## Introduction

Intensive care manages patients with complex and often life-threatening illnesses. Care is team based, provided by suitably trained staff around the clock, using appropriate equipment and work-practice guidelines. There is variable access to such resources. This review focuses on the clinical and economic utility of telemedicine in the intensive care unit (ICU). We searched the electronic databases of Medline-Ovid, PubMed, CINAHL, and EMBASE using the keywords critical care, intensive care, emergency medicine, and telemedicine, with no restriction on publication type, from the beginnings of their databases until September 2014. English-language abstracts and studies including their bibliographies were reviewed with no restrictions on publication type.

## Telemedicine and its application to the ICU

Although electronic communication can take many forms, telemedicine encompasses "real-time" clinical consultation using videoconferencing technology. Typically, clinical imaging and pathology are provided from "store and forward" technologies [1]. Applications have been described for emergency rooms, disaster management, patient visitors, remote, acute long-term, and academic medical centers for both adults and children using real-time continuous and intermittent interactions [2,3,4,5]. Development parallels advances in physiologic monitoring, telemetry, fast transmission communications, and computerized decision-support bringing current practice recommendations, alerts, pathology, and imaging to the bedside with the potential for clinical information system integration [6,7].

## Why the interest in telemedicine-ICU?

Health advisory authorities base recommendations for intensivist management of critically ill patients on reductions in hospital and ICU mortality [8]. There are specific guidelines for telemedicine use in the ICU [9,10,11]. Anticipated need for more critical care beds stems from an increasingly aged population with diverse medical problems. Although not necessarily a universal problem, North America faces shortages in both intensivists and nurses, with the former forming a 46% shortfall by 2030 in the setting of a workforce of young nurses and prolonged vacancies [12].

*Quality Management in Intensive Care*, ed. Bertrand Guidet, Andreas Valentin and Hans Flaatten. Published by Cambridge University Press. © Cambridge University Press 2016.

Although telemedicine would seem useful where access to specialist care is limited, enhanced contemporaneousness, quality, and consistency of care while providing collegial support and education occurs even in large tertiary centers [13]. Telemedicine has supplemented rather than replaced existing services [8]. Between 10% and 11% of critical care beds in the USA are now serviced by telemedicine-ICU [8,14], with several commercial vendors promoting both simple and complex systems (VISICU Corporation, Baltimore Maryland; CareAware, Cerner, Kansas City, Missouri; Metavision, IMDsoft, Needham, Massachusetts). Although the rate of adoption of telemedicine-ICU has slowed in the USA, early-adopting hospitals have been large teaching (>400 beds) or urban hospitals (>1 million residents), typically non-government, not-for-profit organizations where cardiothoracic and neurosurgical procedures are performed [15].

## Models of telemedicine care and management in the ICU

Many models of care for telemedicine-ICU are in use (Table 30.1). Clinical supervision may be time scheduled, continuous, or reactive to a problem with hybrid approaches spanning continuous multidisciplinary supervision to intermittent consultation liaison (Table 30.2) [5]. Data can be collected from monitoring systems, care devices including ventilators and pumps, camera and audio interactions, or from pathology and imaging systems and integrated into an electronic medical record, or can use existing systems and conventional clinical

**Table 30.1** Care organization using telemedicine in ICU

| Technical | Care team structure | Supervision |
|---|---|---|
| **Monitoring** | **Care model** | *Scheduled* |
| *Fixed* | *Consultation liaison* | *Continuous* |
| *Mobile/portable* | *Direct supervision* | *Reactive* |
| *Independently mobile* | *Robotic tele-presence* | |
| Vital signs monitoring | | |
| Visualization of patient | | |
| Data from devices | | |
| Decision support for alerts and alarms | | |
| **Communications architecture** | **Hub and spoke** | *Direct* |
| *Open* | *Collegial network* | *Indirect* |
| *Closed* | | |
| *Hybrid* | | |
| **Store and forward systems** | **Supervision team** | *Single* |
| | *Medical* | *Multiple sites* |
| | *Nursing* | |
| | *Allied health* | |
| | *Clinician assistants* | |
| | *Technicians* | |
| | **Direct patient care team** | |
| | *Trained clinicians* | |
| | *Clinician assistants* | |
| | *Technician-specific care teams* | |
| | **Service provision** | |
| | *Direct supervision of care* | |
| | *Direct prescription of care* | |
| | *Patient and practitioner education* | |
| | *Care plan protocol reinforcement* | |

**Table 30.2** Features of direct supervision and consultation liaison models for ICU-telemedicine (After [5])

| | |
|---|---|
| Direct supervision | Synchronous and often 24-hour supervision. |
| | Often central monitoring facility. |
| | Clinical progress including patient observations and pathology electronically available. |
| | Typically integrates an electronic medical record. |
| | Direct communication between supervising team and bedside care team or patient and family. |
| | Multiple-site supervision. |
| | Pre-emptive and reactive patient care. |
| | Robotic bedside attendance requires wireless networks. |
| Consultation liaison | Synchronous but generally not continuous. |
| | Video or telephone consultation. |
| | Uses available clinical and electronic infrastructures including pathology and imaging. |
| | Local direct care supervision and summary. |
| | Formats of routine rounds or response to problems. |
| | Generally reactive to patient problems. |

notes [5]. Communications can be "closed" using systems entirely contained within an organization or "open" using publicly accessed but encrypted communication systems, or hybrids. Clinicians communicating from a centralized hub or distributed sites can provide care to one or more patients. Technology at either the direct care unit or support end may be fixed, portable, or mobile (robotic tele-presence) [16]. Communication flow may follow a hub-and-spoke model between a principal center and distant units, a network of clinicians with service independent of any specific unit, or a combination approach.

Direct patient care staff can be specifically trained to function as individuals or care teams as needed. Typically, routine nursing rounds using continuous monitoring systems "house-keep" bedside care with evidence-based practice. An intensivist may routinely round, assist with new admissions, review patients with deteriorating trends, provide ad-hoc advice, write orders, supervise procedures, review and interpret investigations or provide consults, teaching, and support. A 1:2 nurse:patient ratio for direct care with one telemedicine nurse for 30–50 beds and one intensivist for 65–269 beds is common for continuous supervision models [17,18] but typically assesses only one patient in consultation-liaison systems [5].

A complex study from a single-site telemedicine-ICU project found 80% of telemedicine interactions were initiated by the telemedicine-ICU but contact initiated by the primary team increased over time [19]. There were significant favorable secular trends for timely responses to an event, including change detection, error detection, targeted monitoring, immediate patient risk detection with access to specialized expertise, and workload management including the coordination of tasks, adherence to best practice, and troubleshooting alarm and equipment problems. Patient safety interventions by the telemedicine-ICU nurses included patient rescue where immediate action was required (6%), prevention of adverse events such as falls, self-extubation, or recognizing inappropriately silenced alarms (19%), telemedicine-ICU initiated assistance in interventions (51%), and consultation, troubleshooting, and clinical coaching (24%) [20]. Consultations may directly supervise a patient, attend calls from home, or provide peer-review of therapy (98%), provide care plans (~30%) or bedside assessments (~40%), and direct supervision of procedures (~10%). Additionally, team teaching or communication and relative communication (~40%) are possible. Calls may involve any clinical team member in "one-to-one" or team interactions, occurring during daytime working hours or after-hours [20].

The quality of the communication is dependent upon secure telecommunication links of adequate bandwidth to allow 20–30 frames per second with clear audio. Using conventional telephone communications for remote direct assessment, team, and conference communication are either not possible or more complicated [21]. Team communications allow broader input, potentially avoiding miscommunications while achieving increased levels of clinician involvement.

# Evidence of utility and acceptability of telemedicine programs in the ICU

Telemedicine in the ICU represents more than a style of practice but rather a complex social, technical, and cultural change that adapts by incremental secular changes to transform a workflow. Service provision requirements are met by customizing the technology with changes to staff roles, responsibilities, and service performance targets. The impact of implementation depends upon the type of organization, the context of the telemedicine program and support by clinical staff. Without a commitment to change, outcome improvement does not occur. Time periods to demonstrate benefit need to be adequate. Interpersonal relationships, training, and understanding processes of care particularly in relation to comfort with peer review, unexpected disruptions of workflow and a disparity between the promises of the system and practical reality are key factors preventing acceptance [22].

Several systematic reviews have assessed the outcomes for telemedicine in the ICU [15,23–26]. Studies are generally a before–after design with varied descriptions of the telemedicine "dose" (e.g., frequency of rounds), the use of physiologic monitoring, laboratory or radiologic alerts, staffing models (closed or open units, high- or low-intensity staffing, academic or community care environments), the roles and responsibilities of the telemedicine practitioners (direct care supervision, orders authorities, or clinical consultation only), process of care adherence, outcome reporting, risk adjustment, secular trends, and intervention uptake. In addition, some studies measure processes of care as quality markers or use a case mix with an expected improved outcome with experienced input, such as the sickest patients or children cared for by non-specialist clinicians [27]. Such diverse issues limit the generalizability of findings.

Mortality rate improvements vary between 0.4% and 27% with 0.5–1 day reductions in ICU length of stay [14]. Based upon nearly 50,000 patients, both ICU and hospital mortality risk are improved (relative risk 0.79 and 0.83, respectively) and ICU and hospital lengths of stay reduced by 0.62 and 1.26 days, respectively [25]. Systems providing high-intensity supervision, such as continuous patient data monitoring with clinical alerts, appear to perform better than more passive consultation only systems (relative risk 0.78 for ICU mortality) but no differences were found when active interventions alone were considered. Significant reductions in risk adjusted mortality (23%), ICU (12%) and hospital lengths of stay (14%) may only be realized in well-established programs after 2–3 years, although dramatic effects within the first 12 months have been realized [28], or may not be realized at all [29,30,31]. In a very large study of nearly 120,000 patients without control for secular trends and self-selection of control and telemedicine-ICU hospitals, there were significant reductions in hospital mortality (hazard ratio 0.84) and ICU mortality (hazard ratio 0.74), ICU and hospital lengths of stay [13]. Important key factors for successful outcomes included improved physician review within an hour of admission, use of performance data, adherence to known ICU best practices, and reduced response times to alarms. A consultation liaison bedside review model using regular bedside ward rounds and faxed summaries to be included in the patient record with additional review by exception of nearly 1650 patients resulted in reductions of 30% in APACHE-III J standardized mortality ratio with comparable numbers of patients of similar disease severity, but at the expense of a prolonged length of stay in the remote hospital ICU [5].

Beneficial effects have not been confined to the introduction of telemedicine where ICU resources are limited [28]. Surgical and combined medical and surgical ICUs have also shown improved outcomes with a telemedicine program [32,33].

A recent multi-center study of a continuous monitoring telemedicine program to several large tertiary and regional Veteran Affairs hospitals with differing resource characteristics used matched control hospitals, risk adjustment, and sensitivity analysis for the type of unit; individual unit and regression modeling for secular trends found no outcome benefits for length of stay or mortality with a six-month pre- and post-implementation assessment [31]. Reductions in mortality were only seen in control hospitals. Thomas' study of more than 4000 patients found no mortality or length of stay benefits except in the sickest patients [30]. The meta-analysis of Young found that mortality and length of stay benefits in the ICU do not necessarily translate into hospital outcomes [26]. The effect of telemedicine as an adjunct to low-intensity staffing effects on mortality remains unclear [34]. The different findings of these studies possibly relates to processes of change management and implementation. Issues of adoption by bedside clinicians and integration of the program into a quality improvement program with clearly defined operating policies and patient care governance are important.

Where baseline ICU mortality and length of stay are considered optimal by objective benchmarking, the introduction of a telemedicine program may not be cost-effective. Even within telemedicine-ICU units, there are great practice disparities of local intensivist staffing, process, and performance review, governance structures, response rates to emergencies and who responds, use of interdisciplinary rounds, bedside documentation, handover and review frequency, case load, technical support, number of hours of telemedicine, case-mix, and teaching [35]. A multifaceted approach to knowledge exchange may enhance care despite no formal quality improvement interventions [36].

A large study of over 6000 patients in seven ICUs across two academic centers found significantly decreased practice variation and gaps in care for deep-venous thrombosis prophylaxis (OR 15.4), stress ulcer prophylaxis (OR 4.6), cardiovascular protection (OR 31), and ventilator-associated pneumonia bundles (OR 2.2), with an objective improvement in care quality for catheter blood stream infections (OR 0.5) and ventilator associated pneumonia (OR 0.15) [28]. Other studies have found significant improvements in sedation interruption [37], nursing satisfaction [38], ventilator bundle compliance reducing ventilation days [39,40], more appropriate prescribing [41], nosocomial sepsis rates [40], cardiopulmonary arrest rates [40], glycemic control [40], prevention of air embolism [40], organ donation referral [40], call-out for rapid response teams [40], and the need for transfers from local to major centers [42].

Perceptual studies are important in defining staff and patient acceptance and program success. Such studies generally use a before–after design and are small and lack objective measures of patient care and staff morale. In general, studies where objective assessment scales have been used, teamwork climate and clinical safety improve from access to physician support, increased supervision of patients, improved workflow [43], staff relations, communications, psychological working conditions, and education even in highly staffed units [13,44]. Even when programs already rate well in work performance, team and client communication, aspects of the working environment including autonomy of practice, work schedules, and worker clinical and psychological support may improve with the introduction of telemedicine [14]. However, telemedicine-ICU can also interrupt workflows [45]. The use of telemedicine in the ICU may be helpful in the management of burn-out and stress by providing support and the relieving of long hours of care [45].

Khunlertkit et al., using context analysis of semi-structured interviews, assessed general staff perceptions [17]. The principal advantages of the telemedicine-ICU program relate to peer review, more focused review from the limited distractions of telemedicine, emergency concentration of staff at the bedside, improved emergency response times, additional expertise to troubleshoot problems, review of care orders and medication plans, assessments for compliance with best practice providing quality improvement triggers, and the opportunity for real-time as well as scheduled education [17]. However, negative perceptions provide insights into areas which need to be managed which may compromise the success of the program, including: lack of acceptance of supervision; the inability of telemedicine staff to directly assist in patient care; telemedicine does not to prevent all errors; monitoring of large numbers of patients is not real-time; limitations of implementations preclude all information being available to the telemedicine clinicians; and patients can fall into care limbo where roles and responsibilities are not clearly defined [17].

Using the validated Schmidt Perception of Nursing Care Survey, 80% of patients believed they were monitored in privacy but there were no perceivable differences in individual patient review or time spent in explaining to, responding to, or watching over the patient [46].

The factors affecting nurse employment and satisfaction in the telemedicine-ICU are quite varied. In an environment of high stress and heavy workloads, the ICU has a high turnover of nursing staff and a young workforce. The quiet and flexible working environment of telemedicine-ICU can act as both a motivator and a detractor [47]. However, direct care is often missed, with telemedicine tasks described as monotonous and repetitive, especially at times of low activity, but stressful when simultaneous multiple patient care needs occur. Telemedicine-ICU staff often have senior experience as telemedicine provides a sustainable work practice for aging staff as most utilization occurs during day and evening working hours [48]. The novel team approach to patient care can be a workplace attractant, but limited acceptance and cooperation can jeopardize outcomes.

## Costs

There is great variability in telemedicine-ICU systems in terms of scope, complexity, start-up, and operational costs. Cost-effectiveness evaluations have not been performed with consistent rigor, often being derived from direct patient billing systems. Direct comparisons and complete cost estimates are difficult. Costs are incompletely apportioned for implementation, technology infrastructure, staffing, depreciation schedules, and differences in scope, such as the intensity of patient review and the need for information system integration. Cost benefits need to demonstrate improved care processes, outcomes, and reduced length of stay to allow economies of scale [49].

Returns on investment are difficult to ensure. Although the number of patients cared for may increase, reimbursement remains unclear in many jurisdictions. Incompatibility of legacy systems such as imaging, laboratory, admission, discharge and transfer systems are often expensive in terms of time and direct costs. Costs to be considered in the planning, implementation, and maintenance of a telemedicine-ICU system are detailed in Table 30.3.

The New England Healthcare Institute (NEHI) and the Massachusetts Technology Collaborative (MTC), working in collaboration with Price Waterhouse Coopers (PwC) reviewed the effectiveness of an academic university hospital and two community hospitals [50]. Mortality rates fell on average 13%, with a 20% fall in the academic center and an overall 30% reduction in length of stay and a 30–40% increase in admissions. Patient retention increased between 8% and 38%. In this environment, the central command set-up costs were $7 million, with operational costs of $3 million and some $400,000 capital investment and $40,000 per patient bed ongoing operational costs in the distant hospitals. With increased throughput and decreased length of stay, initial costs were recovered within the first year.

**Table 30.3** Cost considerations (After [23])

| | |
|---|---|
| Technology | Purchase, lease, support, and maintenance<br>Communications service fees (e.g., internet)<br>Licensing agreements<br>Hardware: bedside clinical equipment with appropriate data capture devices, monitors, audio-visual equipment, computers<br>Software: clinical information systems and communications<br>Communications: service agreements, servers and networking, telephony, facsimile, other office communication equipment |
| Staffing | Medical, nursing, administrative, and information technology support, salaries and wages – locally and remote<br>Training – locally and remote |
| Accommodation | Design, construction, outfit, and usage of central monitoring facility |
| Local infrastructure | Existing information, pharmacy, pathology, imaging and diagnostics, electronic medical record systems, and technology integration requirements. |
| Changes to direct care | Compliance with care models<br>Increase caseload<br>Altered case-mix<br>Procedural intervention and diagnostics<br>Allied health support – physiotherapy, rehabilitation, etc. |

A large multi-center installation run from an academic medical unit of 52 beds with an on-site intensivist and a worsening severity of illness reviewed some 35,000 days of critical care, finding a 20% crude mortality reduction and a halving of re-admission rates. Set-up costs were $22,000 and operating costs $23,000 per bed [51]. The break-even point was achieved when monitoring 100 beds.

Start-up costs have been reported as between $30,000 and $70,000 per bed for a comprehensive surveillance model and $45,000 (~30% of total costs) in operational costs in the first year [18,23]. In a systematic review, implementation and first-year operational costs ranged from $50,000 to $123,000 per ICU bed, with depreciation adjusting costs of $70,000–87,000 per bed [14]. Operational costs in Kumar's meta-analysis were $50,000–100,000 per bed [23]. There were potential costs savings between $2600 and $3000 per case, with overall hospital profits between $1000-$4000 per patient [14]. In the cost effectiveness study of Franzini *et al.*, the costs of installation for complex, continuous surveillance systems were estimated at $2–5 million, $50,000 per ICU bed, $0.5 million in direct operating costs, $1.2 million for clinician staffing per year [52] with annual operating costs in excess of $1.5 million [53]. Costs for maintenance [52], updating record systems, malfunction, downtime, and deployment of intensivists away from bedside have not been analyzed.

Cost savings were found with implementations in academic centers but may relate to case-mix and baseline work practices [32]. Between 50 and 60 ICU beds need to be serviced in the USA to achieve cost effectiveness [45,54]. Studies without vendor affiliation were not able to find such cost savings [23,55]. Only in the sickest patients with an APACHE II score of 50 or more were cost advantages shown, otherwise overall costs were increased 28% without outcome improvement [56]. Where the sickest patients represented 17% of the total admissions, there was no increase in costs but an improved mortality [56]. Breslow reported a 25% decrease in variable costs per patient, but this depends on the model of care, especially if patients are transferred to another institution resulting in reduced length of stay [53].

No data have been published on implementation or recurring costs of consultation only or hybrid systems. However, although a 4% reduction of retrievals representing a saving of AUS$7600 per patient can be accomplished (based upon quoted charges of Queensland Ambulance and Queensland Clinical Coordination 2012, Australia), keeping patients in the local center can result in a doubling of length of stay in the remote center, with the need for greater clinical care infrastructures in the local health facility [5].

## Issues to consider in the establishment of a telemedicine-ICU program

Developing an organizational vision for the introduction of telemedicine services needs to focus on process and outcome improvements, including patient flow, regional care delivery, integration of hospital information infrastructure, staff stress reduction from improved clinical support while containing staffing and cost challenges. Redundancy within the systems of patient care ensures timely review of patients, oversight, and feedback. Commercially, such systems may allow strengthening and greater healthcare market penetration [18]. However, the expectations of costs savings and a general approach to an IT strategy have not been found to be major project drivers [18].

Identified barriers to telemedicine-ICU implementation are similar to any large and complex organizational change. Major changes effect organizational culture with resistance to change increased by failure to get buy-in from clinicians, perceived threats to practice autonomy, the efficiency of distributed patient care, and inadequacy of training causing lack of confidence in the technology [14]. Perceptions of staffing adequacy, standards of direct clinical care, reimbursement, and cost benefits need to be recognized and managed. Accessibility, reliability, and simplicity, as keys to the utility of any system, require funding for a dedicated information system infrastructure. Unproductive user time rapidly erodes confidence in the system. However, what is promised is not always what is delivered. Expectations and realities must be clearly understood and aligned early in the project. Table 30.4 details the areas to consider in planning the introduction of a telemedicine-ICU system.

Implementation requires the establishment of stakeholder committees with clinical champions having both technical and operational expertise. There needs to be an understanding of impacts on workflows, agreed operational and best-practice policies, institutional and unit support, with recognition that there will invariably be problems with technologies and process applications, especially prescribing, therapy administration, and documentation systems, requiring patience and collaboration to resolve. Practical and supportive systems of communication and education need to be personalized and directly relevant for bedside staff and patients.

Assessment of the implementation should use time frames of several years and provide opportunities for refinement of work practice with objective assessment of outcomes including patient and staff experience [10]. Refinements need a rapid response to maintain enthusiasm for the program.

## Summary and conclusions

Telemedicine-ICU is adjunctive to bedside case management from a remote site by intensive care specialists, nursing, and allied staff using many models of audio-visual technology. Most information is available for complete remote 24-hour surveillance with less objective assessment of consultation liaison services. There has been a rapid adoption of such services especially in North America where ICU staff shortages exist. Improvements in processes of care, mortality, and length of stay can be demonstrated in many but not all implementations.

**Table 30.4** Planning considerations for the introduction of a telemedicine-ICU (After [57])

| | |
|---|---|
| Service gaps or enhancements | What are considered the needs in service delivery in the ICU?<br>– Enhanced trained staffing<br>– Care compliance<br>– Safety of patient care<br>– Quality of patient care<br>– Teaching and training opportunities<br>– Communication opportunities between clinicians and between clinical staff, patients, and relatives |
| Impacts of staffing | Identification of clinical groups presently providing the organization's intensive care and the potential impacts on job satisfaction, income and lifestyle of both participation and non-participation in telemedicine-ICU system of care.<br>Additional resource applied to patient care rather than a cost containment strategy.<br>Effects on existing care delivery structures within the ICU and the organization in general. |
| Care model | Extensive or limited supervision implementation.<br>Hours of operation. |
| System specification | Data communications bandwidth necessary for adequate quality.<br>Existing clinical data store and forward systems (radiology, laboratory).<br>Existing electronic medical records.<br>Interoperability with existing systems.<br>Need for real-time information from equipment such as pumps and ventilators, medication administration systems.<br>Security reliability and legislative compliance. |
| Credentialing [58] | Issues of jurisdictional accreditation and liability of telemedicine clinicians.<br>Defined roles, responsibilities, and scope of practice of telemedicine clinicians.<br>Defined local practice policy and procedures. |
| Reimbursement | Defined and approved processes for clinical practice billing by government authorities and insurers. |
| Hospital service impacts | Impacts on ICU and other hospital services either positively or negatively including effects on capital and operating costs.<br>Effects of transition periods.<br>Provision of redundancy, oversights, and impacts. |
| Performance measurements | Measures of effectiveness of telemedicine-ICU program<br>– Clinical incidents care standard compliance, standardized mortality, and length of stay, staff, patient, and relative satisfaction. |
| Training education | Training program for telemedicine-ICU system familiarization for clinicians.<br>Opportunities for staff and patient education. |

Little work formally reviews the impact and contribution of ICU-telemedicine to processes of care and staff, both organizationally and regionally. However, the technology is available with no evidence of worse patient outcomes. Telemedicine-ICU approaches to patient care are increasingly embraced but determining the most appropriate service for patient circumstances remains the challenge.

# Key point summary

1. Telemedicine care improves ICU mortality and length of stay with improved compliance with processes of care.
2. The clinical outcomes of telemedicine-ICU remain inconsistent across implementations, with baseline unit performance and clinical staff acceptance the major contributors to program success.

3. The introduction of a telemedicine-ICU program can range from complex 24-hour patient surveillance to an intermittent consultation liaison service.

4. Service provision requirements are met by customizing the technology with changes to staff roles and responsibilities and service performance criteria targets. The impact of implementation relates to the type of organization, the context for considering a telemedicine program, and the support by clinical staff.

# References

1. Wilson LS. Technologies for complex and critical care telemedicine. *Stud Health Technol Inform* 2008;131:117–130.

2. Mullen-Fortino M, Sites FD, Soisson M, Galen J. Innovative use of tele-ICU in long-term acute care hospitals. *AACN Adv Crit Care* 2012;23:330–336.

3. Nicholas B. Televisitation: virtual transportation of family to the bedside in an acute care setting. *Perm* 2013; 17:50–52.

4. Labarbera JM, Ellenby MS, Bouressa P, Burrell J, Flori HR, Marcin JP. The impact of telemedicine intensivist support and a pediatric hospitalist program on a community hospital. *Telemed J E Health* 2013;19:760–766.

5. Boots RJ, Singh S, Terblanche M, Widdicombe N, Lipman J. Remote care by telemedicine in the ICU: many models of care can be effective. *Curr Opin Crit Care* 2011;17:634–640.

6. Reynolds HN, Rogove H, Bander J, McCambridge M, Cowboy E, Niemeier M. A working lexicon for the tele-intensive care unit: we need to define tele-intensive care unit to grow and understand it. *Telemed J E Health* 2011;17:773–783.

7. Latifi R, Tilley EH. Telemedicine for disaster management: can it transform chaos into an organized, structured care from the distance? *Am J Disaster Med* 2014;9:25–37.

8. Lilly CM, Zubrow MT, Kempner KM, et al. Critical care telemedicine: evolution and state of the art. *Crit Care Med* 2014;42:2429–2436.

9. College of Intensive Care Medicine. Guidelines on the use of telemedicine in the intensive care unit. 2014. www.cicm. org.au/cms_files/Resources/Policy%20 Documents/IC-16-Guidelines on the Use of Telemedicine in Intensive Care.pdf (accessed September 2014).

10. Pronovost PJ, Berenholtz SM, Goeschel C, et al. Improving patient safety in intensive care units in Michigan. *J Crit Care* 2008;23:207–221.

11. The Leapfrog Group. Factsheet: ICU physician staffing (IPS). 2008. www. leapfroggroup.org/media/file/Leapfrog-ICU_Physician_Staffing_Fact_Sheet.pdf (accessed September 2014).

12. Nielsen M, Saracino J. Telemedicine in the intensive care unit. *Crit Care Nurs Clin North Am* 2012;24:491–500.

13. Lilly CM, McLaughlin JM, Zhao H, Baker SP, Cody S, Irwin RS. A multicenter study of ICU telemedicine reengineering of adult critical care. *Chest* 2014;145:500–507.

14. Deslich S, Coustasse A. Expanding technology in the ICU: the case for the utilization of telemedicine. *Telemed J E Health* 2014;20:485–492.

15. Kahn JM, Cicero BD, Wallace DJ, Iwashyna TJ. Adoption of ICU telemedicine in the United States. *Crit Care Med* 2014;42: 362–368.

16. Marttos A, Kelly E, Graygo J, et al. Usability of telepresence in a level 1 trauma center. *Telemed J E Health* 2013;19:248–251.

17. Khunlertkit A, Carayon P. Contributions of tele-intensive care unit (Tele-ICU) technology to quality of care and patient safety. *J Crit Care* 2013;28(315):e1–12.

18. Berenson RA, Grossman JM, November EA. Does telemonitoring of patients – the eICU – improve intensive care? *Health Aff (Millwood)* 2009;28:w937–947.

19. Anders SH, Woods DD, Schweikhart S, Ebright P, Patterson E. The effects of health information technology change over time: a study of tele-ICU functions. *Appl Clin Inform* 2012;3:239–247.

20. American Association of Critical Care Nurses. AACN tele-ICU nursing practice

guidelines. 2013. www.aacn.org/wd/
practice/docs/tele-icu-guidelines.pdf
(accessed September 2014).

21. Yager PH, Cummings BM, Whalen MJ,
Noviski N. Nighttime telecommunication
between remote staff intensivists and
bedside personnel in a pediatric intensive
care unit: a retrospective study. *Crit Care
Med* 2012;40:2700–2703.

22. Moeckli J, Cram P, Cunningham C,
Reisinger HS. Staff acceptance of a
telemedicine intensive care unit program:
a qualitative study. *J Crit Care* 2013;28:
890–901.

23. Kumar G, Falk DM, Bonello RS, Kahn JM,
Perencevich E, Cram P. The costs of critical
care telemedicine programs: a systematic
review and analysis. *Chest* 2013;143:19–29.

24. Ramnath VR, Ho L, Maggio LA, Khazeni
N. Centralized monitoring and virtual
consultant models of tele-ICU care: a
systematic review. *Telemed J E Health*
2014;20:936–961.

25. Wilcox ME, Adhikari NK. The effect
of telemedicine in critically ill patients:
systematic review and meta-analysis.
*Crit Care* 2012;16:R127.

26. Young LB, Chan PS, Lu X, Nallamothu
BK, Sasson C, Cram PM. Impact of
telemedicine intensive care unit coverage
on patient outcomes: a systematic review
and meta-analysis. *Arch Intern Med*
2011;171:498–506.

27. Dharmar M, Romano PS, Kuppermann N,
*et al.* Impact of critical care telemedicine
consultations on children in rural
emergency departments. *Crit Care Med*
2013;41:2388–2395.

28. Lilly CM, Cody S, Zhao H, *et al.* Hospital
mortality, length of stay, and preventable
complications among critically ill patients
before and after tele-ICU reengineering
of critical care processes. *JAMA*
2011;305:2175–2183.

29. Willmitch B, Golembeski S, Kim SS,
Nelson LD, Gidel L. Clinical outcomes
after telemedicine intensive care
unit implementation. *Crit Care Med*
2012;40:450–454.

30. Thomas EJ, Lucke JF, Wueste L, Weavind L,
Patel B. Association of telemedicine for
remote monitoring of intensive care

patients with mortality, complications, and
length of stay. *JAMA* 2009;302:2671–2678.

31. Nassar BS, Vaughan-Sarrazin MS, Jiang L,
Reisinger HS, Bonello R, Cram P. Impact
of an intensive care unit telemedicine
program on patient outcomes in an
integrated health care system. *JAMA Intern
Med* 2014;174:1160–1167.

32. Kohl BA, Fortino-Mullen M, Praestgaard
A, Hanson CW, Dimartino J, Ochroch
EA. The effect of ICU telemedicine on
mortality and length of stay. *J Telemed
Telecare* 2012;18:282–286.

33. Wilcox ME, Chong CA, Niven DJ, *et al.*
Do intensivist staffing patterns influence
hospital mortality following ICU
admission? A systematic review and
meta-analyses. *Crit Care Med* 2013;41:
2253–2274.

34. Wallace DJ, Angus DC, Barnato AE,
Kramer AA, Kahn JM. Nighttime
intensivist staffing and mortality among
critically ill patients. *N Engl J Med*
2012;366:2093–2101.

35. Lilly CM, Fisher KA, Ries M, *et al.*
A national ICU telemedicine survey:
validation and results. *Chest* 2012;142:
40–47.

36. Scales DC, Dainty K, Hales B, *et al.*
A multifaceted intervention for quality
improvement in a network of intensive care
units: a cluster randomized trial. *JAMA*
2011;305:363–372.

37. Forni A, Skehan N, Hartman CA, *et al.*
Evaluation of the impact of a tele-ICU
pharmacist on the management of sedation
in critically ill mechanically ventilated
patients. *Ann Pharmacother* 2010;44:
432–438.

38. Rincon F, Vibbert M, Childs V, *et al.*
Implementation of a model of robotic tele-
presence (RTP) in the neuro-ICU: effect
on critical care nursing team satisfaction.
*Neurocrit Care* 2012;17:97–101.

39. Kalb T, Raikhelkar J, Meyer S, *et al.*
A multicenter population-based
effectiveness study of teleintensive care unit-
directed ventilator rounds demonstrating
improved adherence to a protective lung
strategy, decreased ventilator duration, and
decreased intensive care unit mortality.
*J Crit Care* 2014;29:691 e7–14.

40. Goran SF. Measuring tele-ICU impact: does it optimize quality outcomes for the critically ill patient? *J Nurs Manag* 2012;20:414–428.

41. Dharmar M, Kuppermann N, Romano PS, *et al.* Telemedicine consultations and medication errors in rural emergency departments. *Pediatrics* 2013;132:1090–1097.

42. Webb CL, Waugh CL, Grigsby J, *et al.* Impact of telemedicine on hospital transport, length of stay, and medical outcomes in infants with suspected heart disease: a multicenter study. *J Am Soc Echocardiogr* 2013;26:1090–1098.

43. Chu-Weininger MY, Wueste L, Lucke JF, Weavind L, Mazabob J, Thomas EJ. The impact of a tele-ICU on provider attitudes about teamwork and safety climate. *Qual Saf Health Care* 2010;19:e39.

44. Romig MC, Latif A, Gill RS, Pronovost PJ, Sapirstein A. Perceived benefit of a telemedicine consultative service in a highly staffed intensive care unit. *J Crit Care* 2012;27(426): e9–16.

45. Ries M. Tele-ICU: a new paradigm in critical care. *Int Anesthesiol Clin* 2009;47:153–170.

46. Golembeski S, Willmitch B, Kim SS. Perceptions of the care experience in critical care units enhanced by a tele-ICU. *AACN Adv Crit Care* 2012;23:323–329.

47. Hoonakker PLT, Carayon P, McGuire K, *et al.* Motivation and job satisfaction of tele-ICU nurses. *J Crit Care* 2013;28(315): e13–21.

48. Reynolds EM, Grujovski A, Wright T, Foster M, Reynolds HN. Utilization of robotic "remote presence" technology within North American intensive care units. *Telemed J E Health* 2012;18:507–515.

49. Cummings J, Krsek C, Vermoch K, Matuszewski K. Intensive care unit telemedicine: review and consensus recommendations. *Am J Med Qual* 2007;22:239–250.

50. New England Health Care Institute and Massachusetts Technology Collaborative. Critical care, critical choices: the case for tele-ICUs in intensive care. 2010. www.masstech.org/sites/mtc/files/documents/2010 TeleICU Report.pdf (accessed September 2014).

51. Fortis S, Weinert C, Bushinski R, Koehler AG, Beilman G. A health system-based critical care program with a novel tele-ICU: implementation, cost, and structure details. *J Am Coll Surg* 2014;19:676–683.

52. Franzini L, Thomas E. Costs and effectiveness of tele-ICUs in reducing morbidity and mortality in intensive care units. *J Med Econ* 2008;11:165–169.

53. Breslow MJ, Rosenfeld BA, Doerfler M, *et al.* Effect of a multiple-site intensive care unit telemedicine program on clinical and economic outcomes: an alternative paradigm for intensivist staffing. *Crit Care Med* 2004;32:31–38.

54. Breslow MJ. Remote ICU care programs: current status. *J Crit Care* 2007;22:66–76.

55. Morrison JL, Cai Q, Davis N, *et al.* Clinical and economic outcomes of the electronic intensive care unit: results from two community hospitals. *Crit Care Med* 2010;38:2–8.

56. Franzini L, Sail KR, Thomas EJ, Wueste L. Costs and cost-effectiveness of a telemedicine intensive care unit program in 6 intensive care units in a large health care system. *J Crit Care* 2011;26(329):e1–6.

57. Rogove HJ, McArthur D, Demaerschalk BM, Vespa PM. Barriers to telemedicine: survey of current users in acute care units. *Telemed J E Health* 2012;18:48–53.

58. Davis TM, Barden C, Olff C, *et al.* Professional accountability in the tele-ICU: the CCRN-E. *Crit Care Nurs Q* 2012;35:353–356.

# Epilogue

## Bertrand Guidet, Andreas Valentin, and Hans Flatten

The goal of all hospitals is to provide optimal care for their patients. The patients and their families trust us and expect the best care, which today includes delivery with high quality. They are often in search of information and are in a difficult situation related to illness, stress, anxiety, and possible financial difficulties. We, the intensive care community, are responsible for fulfilling their expectations, and all of us must contribute to achieve this high level of quality. Thus, the perspective in intensive care has clearly changed and should be patient-centered, and every step of the hospital pathway should be scrutinized.

The ICU differs from most other wards in the hospital. Contrary to other specialties, most of the patients do not choose to be admitted to a specific ICU. They are "captive" in the unit, and hence we have a great responsibility to give them the highest quality of care.

There are numerous questions that a patient and his or her relatives might go through when considering our ICUs.

*How organized was the ICU admission? Is there a shared policy between ICU physicians and other physicians within the same hospital in the need of intensive care and hence the refusal rate and the cause of refusal? What is a triage process, and how is it discussed and decided? Was the physician in charge of the admission listening to patients' and relatives' wishes and were we asked for any advanced directives?*

*While in the ICU is there a systemic evaluation of the daily goal for the patient in order to decide whether full-code treatment should be applied? If necessary, how are end-of-life decisions taken, and who participates in the discussion, and in what way are patient and/or family members involved?*

*How is the ICU organized to avoid iatrogenic events? Do they use protocols, abide to quality indicators, and do they use checklists when appropriate? When there is an adverse event how is it reported and analyzed to avoid similar mishaps in the future? Do the team analyze their practice and compare the practice to the state of the art? Are handover procedure formalized in a way to avoid missing information or lack of continuity of care?*

*In this unit, where I am treated or where my family member is treated, do the people really work together? How do they exchange information and do they share the same values?*

*During the ICU stay I would like to rest so I would like to sleep but all those alarms are constantly ringing! They alarm much too often and when it does nobody is checking what is going on. I felt pain but it looks like there is no regular pain protocol in this unit. Recently, they decided to order a CT scan; it was a nightmare since I had to wait 30 minutes in a cold corridor and we were out of oxygen. For sure, there is no checklist for patient transport and no shared procedures between the radiology department and the ICU.*

*All along my ICU stay, I want to know why the different procedures are performed in order to understand what is going on. I want to be part of the process. If I am comatose or unable to*

Quality Management in Intensive Care, ed. Bertrand Guidet, Andreas Valentin and Hans Flaatten. Published by Cambridge University Press. © Cambridge University Press 2016.

*respond then I want my relatives to be informed. This implies that ICU nurses and physicians must improve their communication skills. Multidisciplinary rounds should be performed, along with interviews in order to have several points of view (nurses, junior doctor, senior doctors, family members).*

The tasks are enormous and the answer lies in the ICU team. There must be a leader setting the goal. The ICU director is a manager, in charge of choosing priority, the right people in the right place. The team must share the same values and goals. The culture should be people-oriented rather than task- or procedure-oriented. This is not always easy because we are working in a complex environment with urgent and stressful situations. We are dealing with issues concerning life and death and with the suffering of patients and families. Certainly, we face conflict within the team or with other hospital teams. We might disagree but we need to find ways to exchange opinions, feelings, and grief. In the end, the conflict process could be beneficial if it is handled correctly and openly.

What are the tools that a manager may use to improve quality? We need objective data to documents the managerial diagnosis; from that perspective a database with activity data, severity scores, and performance indicators are helpful. We must also be open about our data and share them on regional or national levels. Here, intensive care registries can be most helpful, and may foster friendly "competition" and learning from each other.

There is a constant need to educate all members of the team. For this purpose we can use mortality–morbidity conferences, simulation, group works, and educational lectures. Promoting research is certainly also important since good research translates into good clinical practice. People actively involved in research programs feel part of the team. This is also important for the nurses and may contribute to the decrease of turnover and burn-out.

In order to improve the global process of care, we need to get feedback from our customers. Hence we should promote and rely on patient/family satisfaction questionnaires. In the future new technology will help us recruit more respondents and offer automatic analysis.

Intensive care plays a central role in the hospital, with round-the-clock coverage for critically ill patients. Therefore, we need to direct messages to the health authorities to make them aware of our vital role in a modern hospital. In addition, we need to recognize the changing role of intensivists as protectors and managers of the critically ill during the desired continuum of care in their journey through the hospital. We should also contribute to the discussion about structure of ICUs within a region or even at country level. Today we know that for some procedures there is a volume–outcome relationship, with small units providing suboptimal care. Benchmarking techniques are able to identify outliers with below average performance. Those units should be either closed, merged with larger units, integrated into a network, or upgraded. To set such standards is a responsibility for national as well as European scientific societies, and we as intensivists also must work through such channels.

To conclude, quality is mainly human driven. As a consequence, the organization should schedule time for communication and multidisciplinary discussion. Usually such time is not included in workload indexes and in funding of ICUs. Quality cannot be seen as parallel to our work in the ICU; it is an integrated part of our practice. And remember: The customer is always right, so let's listen to what our patients and their relatives tell us!

# Index

*Note: Italic* page numbers indicate figures and tables.

Printed in the United States
By Bookmasters